Microbiology

PreTest™ Self-Assessment and Review

Notice

Medicine is an ever-changing science. As new research and clinical experience broaden our knowledge, changes in treatment and drug therapy are required. The authors and the publisher of this work have checked with sources believed to be reliable in their efforts to provide information that is complete and generally in accord with the standards accepted at the time of publication. However, in view of the possibility of human error or changes in medical sciences, neither the authors nor the publisher nor any other party who has been involved in the preparation or publication of this work warrants that the information contained herein is in every respect accurate or complete, and they disclaim all responsibility for any errors or omissions or for the results obtained from use of the information contained in this work. Readers are encouraged to confirm the information contained herein with other sources. For example and in particular, readers are advised to check the product information sheet included in the package of each drug they plan to administer to be certain that the information contained in this work is accurate and that changes have not been made in the recommended dose or in the contraindications for administration. This recommendation is of particular importance in connection with new or infrequently used drugs.

Microbiology

PreTest™ Self-Assessment and Review

Thirteenth Edition

James D. Kettering, PhD
Emeritus Professor of Microbiology
Loma Linda University
Loma Linda, California

Craig A. Seheult, MD, MS
Contributor—Immunology
Loma Linda University
School of Medicine
Loma Linda, California
Class of 2009

New York Chicago San Francisco Lisbon London Madrid Mexico City
Milan New Delhi San Juan Seoul Singapore Sydney Toronto

The **McGraw·Hill** Companies

Microbiology: PreTest™ Self-Assessment and Review, Thirteenth Edition

1 2 3 4 5 6 7 8 9 0   DOC/DOC   14 13 12 11 10

ISBN-13 978-0-07-162335-3
ISBN-10 0-07-162335-3

This book was set in Berkeley by Glyph International.
The editors were Kirsten Funk and Cindy Yoo.
The production supervisor was Sherri Souffrance.
Project management was provided by Somya Rustagi, Glyph International.
The cover designer was Maria Scharf.
RR Donnelley was printer and binder.

This book is printed on acid-free paper.

Library of Congress Cataloging-in-Publication Data

    Microbiology : PreTest self-assessment and review.—13th ed. / [edited by] James D. Kettering.
       p. ; cm.
    Includes bibliographical references and index.
    ISBN-13: 978-0-07-162335-3 (pbk. : alk. paper)
    ISBN-10: 0-07-162335-3 (pbk. : alk. paper)
    1. Medicalmicrobiology—Examinations, questions, etc.   I. Kettering, James D.
    [DNLM: 1. Microbiological Phenomena—Examination Questions.   QW 18.2
    M626   2010]
    QR46.M544   2010
    616.9'041—dc22   2009047491

Student Reviewers

Jodie Bachman
UMDNJ School of Osteopathic Medicine
Class of 2011

Anne Doughtie
Texas Tech University Health Science Center
Class of 2009

Russel Kamkhe
SUNY Upstate Medical University
Class of 2010

Contents

Immunology

Introduction

Microbiology: PreTest™ Self-Assessment and Review, Thirteenth Edition, allows medical students to comprehensively and conveniently assess and review their knowledge of microbiology and immunology. The 500 questions provided here have been written with the goal to parallel the topics, format, and degree of difficulty of the questions found in the United States Medical Licensing Examination (USMLE) Step 1.

The High-Yield Facts in the beginning of the book are provided to facilitate a rapid review of microbiology. It is anticipated that the reader will use these High-Yield Facts as a "memory jog" before proceeding through the questions.

Each question in the book is followed by four or more answer options to choose from. In each case, select the one best response to the question. Each answer is accompanied by a specific page reference to a text that provides background to the answer, and a short discussion of issues raised by the question and answer. A bibliography listing all the sources can be found following the last chapter.

To simulate the time constraints imposed by the licensing exam, an effective way to use this book is to allow yourself one minute to answer each question in a given chapter. After you finish going through the questions in the section, spend as much time as you need verifying your answers and carefully reading the explanations provided. Special attention should be given to the explanations for the questions you answered incorrectly; however, you should read every explanation even if you've answered correctly. The explanations are designed to reinforce and supplement the information tested by the questions. For those seeking further information about the material covered, consult the references listed in the bibliography or other standard medical texts.

Acknowledgments

The author wishes to thank Betty J. Kettering, MSPH, and David E. Kettering, Esq., for expert assistance in the production of the manuscript for this revision.

High-Yield Facts

PHYSIOLOGY AND MOLECULAR BIOLOGY

- Koch postulates: (1) specific organism must be in diseased animal; (2) organism must be isolated in pure culture; (3) organism should produce exact disease in healthy, susceptible animal; (4) organism re-isolated from infected animal.
- Gram stain: (1) fixation; (2) crystal violet; (3) iodine treatment; (4) decolorization (alcohol/acetone); (5) counterstain (safranin). Gram-positive when the color is purple; gram-negative when the color turns red.
- Gram stain poor for: *Chlamydia* (intracellular location), *Mycoplasma* (no cell wall), *Rickettsia* (small size), *Treponema* (too thin, spirochete, use darkfield microscope), *Mycobacterium* (use acid-fast stain), *Legionella* (use silver stain).
- Bacterial shapes: bacilli (rod), cocci (spherical), spirilla (spiral).
- Bacterial aggregates: diplococci (eg, *Neisseriae*), streptococci (chains), tetrads (fours), staphylococci (clusters), sarccinae (cubes).
- Flagella: monotrichous—single polar flagellum; lophotrichous—cluster of flagella at pole; amphitrichous—flagella at both poles; peritrichous—flagella encircling the cell.
- Type VII pili = F (sex) pili; important in bacterial conjugation.
- Conjugation—DNA transferred from one bacterium to another; transduction—viral transfer of DNA from one cell to another; transformation—cellular uptake of purified DNA or naked DNA from the environment.
- Peptidoglycan (murein or mucopeptide) layer: unique to prokaryotes (glycan polymers of sugar N-acetylglucosamine [NAG] and N-acetylmuramic acid [NAM] cross-linked by a short peptide). Cross-linking enzymes are transpeptidases (targets for β-lactam antibiotics).
- Bacterial structures: peptidoglycan (support); cell wall/membrane (antigenic); outer membrane (lipopolysaccharide [LPS]/endotoxin); plasma membrane (oxidative/transport enzymes); ribosome (protein synthesis); periplasmic space (hydrolytic enzymes and β-lactamases); capsule (antiphagocytic polysaccharide except *Bacillus anthracis,* which is D-glutamate); pilus/fimbria (adherence, conjugation); flagellum (motility); spore (heat, chemical, dehydration resistance, consists of dipicolinic acid); plasmid (genes for

toxins, enzymes, antibiotic resistance); glycocalyx (adherence, made of polysaccharide); inclusion bodies (no membrane; store glycogen, polyphosphate, poly-β-hydroxybutyric acid).

- Gram-positive: teichoic acid unique.
- Gram-negative: LPS/endotoxin unique.
- LPS/endotoxin: lipid A covalently linked to polysaccharide core outer membrane and then unique "O antigen" polysaccharide repeat; LPS/endotoxin causes an acute-phase protein response in vivo (release of TNF-α, IL-1, IL-6), causing fever, and the like.
- Lysozyme: breaks down glycan backbone bonds of peptidoglycan. Spheroplast: partial cell wall lysozyme digestion.
- Protoplast: complete cell wall lysozyme digestion, causing a spherical shape of bacteria.
- Exponential or geometric growth: cell number = a (2^n), where a is number of starting cells, n equals number of generations.
- Bacterial growth curves (four phases): (1) lag (no cellular division, cell size increases); (2) exponential (regular doubling time, essential nutrients decrease, toxins increase); (3) stationary (cell division rate = cell death rate) stage at which spores are formed; (4) death (cell energy stores deplete, exponential death due to low population equilibrium).
- Bacteriostatic: agent **inhibits** multiplication; growth resumes upon removal of agent.
- Bactericidal: agent **kills** bacteria; irreversible.
- Sterile: free from all forms of life.
- Disinfectant: chemical kills bacteria but is toxic to tissue.
- Septic: pathogenic organism is present in living tissue.
- Aseptic: pathogenic organism is not present in living tissue. (Virology— no bacterial agents are present.)
- Passive transport: no energy required, movement down the concentration gradient, no carrier molecule (protein molecule that attaches to metabolic molecule needed inside the bacterium) that can cross the cell wall and cell membrane. The food goes in and the waste goes out.
- Active transport: requires energy, movement against the concentration gradient.
- Fluoride ion (water, toothpaste, and the like): inhibits several cellular bacterial enzymes, especially enolase.
- Bacterial pathogenesis: (1) antiphagocytic (cell wall proteins—protein A in *Staphylococcus aureus* and protein M in *Streptococcus pyogenes*, capsules,

pili/fimbriae *Neisseria gonorrhoea*); (2) adherence factors (pili/fimbriae, lipoteichoic acid, glycocalyx, adhesion); (3) enzymes (coagulase, collagenase, fibrinolysin, hyaluronidase, lecithinase, mucinase); (4) toxins (exotoxins, endotoxins/LPS).

• Exotoxins: polypeptide, highly fatal even in low doses, toxoids as vaccines, mostly heat labile, secreted, both gram-negative and gram-positive.
• Endotoxins: LPS, low toxicity, no toxoids, no vaccines, heat stable, released on lysis, only gram-negative.
• Free radicals of oxygen (superoxides) kill anaerobic bacteria exposed to air. Superoxide dismutase is a potent bacterial antioxidant. The peroxidases in bacteria are protective.
• Obligate anaerobes: lack catalase and/or superoxide dismutase and are susceptible to oxidative damage, foul smelling, produce gas in tissue (eg, *Actinomyces*, *Bacteroides*, and *Clostridium*).
• Superoxide dismutase catalyzes: $2O_2^- + 2H^+ \rightarrow H_2O_2 + O_2$
• Catalase catalyzes: $2H_2O_2 \rightarrow 2H_2O + O_2$
• Myeloperoxidase catalyzes: $Cl^- + H_2O_2 \rightarrow ClO^- + H_2O$
• NADPH oxidase catalyzes: $NADPH + 2O_2 \rightarrow 2O_2^- + H^+NADP^+$
• Sites of action of antimicrobial agents include cell wall synthesis, cell-membrane integrity, DNA replication, protein synthesis, DNA-dependent RNA polymerase, folic acid metabolism.

VIROLOGY

Virology basics: commonly used terms are virion, capsid, capsomere, nucleocapsid.
• All DNA viruses are double-stranded (ds), except Parvovirus.
• All DNA viruses have linear DNA, except papovaviruses (ds, circular) and hepadnaviruses (ds, circular, segmented).
• All RNA viruses have single-stranded RNA (ssRNA), except reoviruses (ds, circular).
• Segmented RNA viruses include orthomyxoviruses, reoviruses, and bunyaviruses (hantavirus).
• Positive-sense RNA (same as mRNA) includes picornaviruses, caliciviruses, flaviviruses, retroviruses, and coronaviruses. All other RNA viruses are negative sense (need viral RNA polymerase within the virion).
• Obligate intracellular parasites, using viral receptors to attach to host cell receptors.

- Growth cycle: attachment, entry, eclipse (production of viral components), maturation, release.
- Viral disease patterns: acute, chronic, latent (persistent).
- DNA viruses replicate in the host nucleus (except poxviruses).
- RNA viruses replicate in the host cytoplasm (except influenza and retroviruses).

Hepatitis Viruses

- Hepatitis A virus (HAV)—RNA picornavirus, fecal-oral transmission, no chronic carriers
- Hepatitis B virus (HBV)—DNA hepadnavirus; parental or sexual transmission; transplacental, acute, and chronic disease; HBV possesses a reverse transcriptase polymerase
- Hepatitis C virus (HCV)—Flavivirus; +ssRNA; parental or sexual transmission, acute and chronic disease
- Hepatitis D virus (HDV)—"delta" hepatitis—defective RNA virus, requires HBV coinfection, acute and chronic infections
- Hepatitis E virus (HEV)—Calicivirus, +ssRNA, fecal-oral transmission, no chronic carriers
- HAV and HBV have approved vaccines.

DNA Viruses

- Parvovirus B19—ssDNA—causes fifth disease/erythema infectiosum (slapped cheek appearance).
- Papovavirus.
  - Papillomavirus—ds circular DNA—causes warts (human papillomavirus [HPV] type 1 and 4—benign; type 6 and 11—anogenital; type 16 and 18—cervical carcinoma)
  - Polyoma virus—BK—causes kidney disease; JC (progressive multifocal leukoencepalopathy)
- Adenovirus (ds linear DNA)—causes conjunctivitis and respiratory diseases in kids. Strains 10, 41 cause gastroenteritis.
- Herpesviruses.
  - Herpes simplex—latent infections are common.
- HSV-1—affects trigeminal ganglia; causes cold sores, conjunctivitis, and encephalitis (treat with acyclovir).
- HSV-2—affects sacral nerve ganglia—sexually transmitted.

- Varicella-zoster—chicken pox-shingles—lesions are asynchronous (all forms present). "Shingles"—dermatomal distribution. Vaccine is attenuated.
- Cytomegalovirus (CMV)—common; ubiquitous; direct and sexual contact for transmission; causes retinitis and pneumonitis in immunocompromised; neonates suffer from CMV inclusion disease.
- Epstein-Barr virus (EBV)—infects B lymphocytes; causes infectious mononucleosis; positive for heterophile antibodies (monospot test)— EBV—early antigen (EA), viral capsid antigen (VCA), epstein barr nuclear antigen (EBNA)—diagnostic value.
- Poxvirus—largest, most complex viruses, dsDNA—grow in cytoplasm, complex envelope.
- Variola—smallpox, extinct since 1977; bioterrorism agent; Vaccinia virus—vaccine strain
- Molluscum contagiosum—benign tumors

Positive ssRNA Viruses

- Picornavirus (+ssRNA).
  - Poliovirus, coxsackie A and B viruses, echovirus, HAV—polio—Salk (inactivated)/Sabin (live, attenuated) vaccines; the United States now uses killed vaccine, especially pediatric.
  - All strains cause upper respiratory infections (URIs), rashes, limited central nervous system (CNS) infections (glucose is normal, protein is slightly elevated), gastrointestinal infections (GI), hemorrhagic conjunctivitis, and myocarditis.
- Rhinoviruses—causes common cold.
- Flaviviruses—HCV, yellow fever, dengue, Saint Louis encephalitis.
- Togaviruses—arboviruses; Western Equine encephalitis, Eastern Equine encephalitis, Venezuelan Equine encephalitis, West Nile virus (birds and horses are normal hosts).
- Rubella virus—causes German measles; no insect vector; causes severe birth defects.
- Coronaviruses—mostly causes common cold; also severe acute respiratory syndrome (SARS).
- Retroviruses—the genome is diploid—*gag* genes—p 24, p 7, p 9, and p 17; env—gp 120 and gp 41; *pol* gene which encodes for reverse transcriptase/integrase; *pro* gene which encodes for protease; AIDS (CD4)

< 200 lymphocytes/mm³. Opportunistic infections include *Candida*, *Mycobacterium* species, multiple viruses, and protozoan.

Negative ssRNA Viruses

Require virion-associated RNA-dependent RNA polymerase.

- Paramyxoviruses
  - Measles—fever, conjunctivitis, Koplik spots—rash
  - Complications—pneumonia, encephalitis; good vaccine
  - Mumps—salivary, parotid glands; orchitis; good liver vaccine
  - Respiratory syncytial virus—major cause of URI; treat infants with ribovirin
- Rhabdovirus (rabies)—bullet-shaped appearance; skunks, raccoons, foxes, coyotes/dogs, and bats are main reservoirs in United States; animal bite transmission through saliva; control animal vectors; Negri body— eosinophilic intracytoplasmic inclusion body in neural tissues
- Orthomyxoviruses.
  - Influenza A and B, segmented genomes
  - Genetic drift—minor antigen changes; genetic shift—major new hemagglutinin (H) and/or neuraminidase (N) changes
- Bunyaviruses—California encephalitis virus; hantavirus
- Arenavirus—causes lymphocytic choriomenigitis virus, causes Lassa fever

dsRNA Viruses—Double-Shelled Capsids

- Rotaviruses—causes infantile diarrhea
- Reoviruses—common in humans, causes febrile diseases

BACTERIOLOGY

- Gram-positive cocci: staphylococci catalase +, streptococci catalase –.
- *Staphylococcus aureus*: Mannitol-salt agar (selective and differential), yellow colonies, **coagulase** +, mannitol +, catalase +; some are methicillin resistant (MRSA), some have vancomycin resistance emerging (VISA); protein A binds IgG Fc inhibiting phagocytosis, causes rapid-onset food poisoning (preformed enterotoxin), toxic shock syndrome, scalded skin syndrome, osteomyelitis, acute bacterial endocarditis (IV drug users), abscesses, recurrent infection in chronic granulomatous disease (CGD).
- *Staphylococcus saprophyticus*: second leading cause of urinary tract infection (UTI) in young sexually active females.

- Streptococci: β-hemolytic divided into groups (13 groups: A-O) based on cell wall carbohydrate antigens. Group A divided into > 50 types based on M proteins (virulence, specific immunity), catalase negative.
- *Streptococcus pyogenes* (group A): Hyaluronic acid capsule, carbohydrate antigen, M protein, bacitracin sensitive, cellulitis, rheumatic fever, glomerulonephritis, necrotizing fasciitis, erysipelas, scarlet fever.
- Viridans: include *S viridans, S mitis, and so on.* Normal oral flora, α-hemolytic, subacute bacterial endocarditis after dental/oral surgery.
- *Enterococcus* (Streptococcus) *faecalis* (group D): normal intestinal flora, subacute bacterial endocarditis after pelvic/abdominal surgery, UTIs, growth in 6.5% NaCl.
- *Streptococcus agalactiae* (group B): normal vaginal flora; in dairy products (cattle pathogen); neonatal sepsis; Christie, Atkins, Munch-Peterson (CAMP) test +.
- Peptostreptococci: normal oral/vaginal flora, endocarditis, lung abscess.
- *Streptococcus pneumoniae:* pneumonia, meningitis, otitis media (children), optochin sensitive, bile soluble, use quellung reaction (capsule Ags, host Abs), pneumococcal polyvalent vaccine.
- Dick test: test susceptibility to scarlet fever.
- Shultz-Charlton test: Determine if rash is due to erythrogenic toxin of scarlet fever.
- Gram-negative cocci (*Neisseria*): oxidase +, diplococci, polysaccharide capsule, associated with C5, C6, V7, C8 complement deficiency; pathogenic forms: Thayer-Martin agar −, chocolate agar +, nutrient agar −, 37°C growth +, room temperature −; nonpathogenic forms: Thayer-Martin agar −, chocolate agar +, nutrient agar +, 37°C growth +, room temperature +.
- *Neisseria meningitidis:* capsule, endotoxin, toxemia, petechiae, hemorrhage, disseminated intravascular coagulation (DIC), Waterhouse-Friderichsen syndrome.
- Bacterial meningitis: in < 40-year-old = *S pneumoniae;* > 40-year-old = *S pneumoniae;* 2 to 6 months + neonates = Group B streptococci, *Escherichia coli;* neonates to 5-year-old children = *N meningitidis.*
- *Neisseria gonorrhoeae:* pili, IgA protease, pharyngitis, proctitis, pelvic inflammatory disease (PID), urethritis, cervicitis.
- Gram-positive bacilli: aerobic (*Bacillus*); anaerobic (*Clostridium*), killed by autoclave.
- *Bacillus anthracis:* polypeptide capsule, exotoxin, anthrax (woolsorters' disease).

- *Bacillus cereus:* food poisoning (food reheated once), enterotoxin.
- *Clostridium:* no cytochrome enzymes, no catalase, no superoxide dismutase.
- *Clostridium tetani:* noninvasive, neurotoxins (prevents release of neural inhibitory transmitters such as γ-aminobutyric acid [GABA] and glycine), lockjaw, spastic paralysis; give toxoid/antitoxin.
- *Clostridium botulinum:* noninvasive, exotoxins (prevents acetylcholine release), flaccid paralysis, antitoxin (honey ingestion in infancy).
- *Clostridium perfringens:* invasive, enterotoxin, food poisoning, myonecrosis, collagenase, lecithinase, gas gangrene.
- *Clostridium difficile:* Pseudomembranous colitis can occur after broad-spectrum antibiotic usage.
- *Corynebacterium diphtheria:* gram-positive rod, metachromatic granules, exotoxin (inhibits EF-2 and protein synthesis).
- *Listeria monocytogenes:* gram-positive rod in cerebrospinal fluid (CSF), compromised host, neonate, diarrhea after eating raw cheeses, tumbling motility.
- *Salmonella:* motile gram-negative rod, enteric fever, food poisoning; *Salmonella typhi* = human pathogen; other species = animal pathogens; motile; nonlactose fermenter.
- *Shigella:* nonmotile gram-negative rod, more virulent than *Salmonella,* bloody diarrhea, shigellosis is human disease, oral-anal route (fingers, flies, food, and feces), toxin inhibits protein synthesis.
- *Escherichia coli:* gram-negative rod, most common UTI, sepsis (serious); enterohemorrhagic *E coli* (EHEC) (colitis, hemolytic uremic syndrome-verotoxin, hamburger, beef); enteroinvasive *E coli* (EIEC) (fever, bloody stool, diarrhea); enterotoxigenic *E coli* (ETEC) (traveler's diarrhea); enteropathogenic *E coli* (EPEC) (infant fever and diarrhea, nonbloody stool).

E	E	E	E
Hamburger	Invasive	Traveler's Diarrhea	Pediatric
E	E	E	E
C	C	C	C

- *Pseudomonas aeruginosa:* gram-negative rod, antibiotic resistance, blue-green pigments; causes UTI, wounds, burns, greenish-yellow sputum.
- *Klebsiella:* large capsule; causes UTI, pneumonia, especially in alcoholics (currant jelly sputum).

- *Haemophilus influenzae:* gram-negative rod; causes meningitis, otitis, sinusitis, epiglottitis.
- *Proteus:* gram-negative rod, result in swarming growth; produce urease (urea → NH_3); also produced by *Helicobacter pylori* and *Ureaplasma urealyticum;* causes UTI, wounds, renal stones, large staghorn caliculi.
- *Gardnerella vaginalis:* "clue cells"; vaginitis with discharge (fishy smell, conduct whiff test).
- *Bordetella pertussis:* capsule form, pili, killed vaccine, causes whooping cough.
- *Yersinia pestis:* "safety pin" (bipolar staining), causes plague (bubonic/ pneumonic), spread by rat flea.
- *Francisella tularensis:* spread by skinning rabbits (jackrabbits), causes tularemia.
- *Pasteurella multocida:* spread by cat/dog bites; causes cellulitis, "shipping fever."
- *Brucella:* detected by dye sensitivity test; causes undulant fever.
- *Mycobacterium tuberculosis:* causes tuberculosis, detected by acid-fast stain, Lowenstein-Jensen medium, purified protein derivative (PPD) testing.
- *Mycobacterium leprae:* causes leprosy, cannot be cultured.
- *Haemophilus ducreyi:* causes painful lesion, chancroid (syphilis: painless chancre).
- *Treponema pallidum:* detected by Venereal Disease Research Laboratories (VDRL) tests, fluorescent treponemal antibody absorption (FTA-ABS), and IgM antibody; use penicillin G for treatment; has three stages, spirochetes, dark-field microscopy.
- *Borrelia:* aniline dyes (Wright/Giemsa), *Ixodes* tick, relapsing fever, Lyme disease, acute necrotizing ulcerative gingivitis, spirochete.
- *Legionella pneumophila:* Legionnaires' disease, fulminating pneumonia, gram-negative rod, airborne through contaminated water (air-conditioner cooling system).
  - Exotoxin: heat labile
  - Endotoxin (LPS): heat stable
- Diphtheria/Pseudomonas exotoxin: act via ADP-ribosylation of EF-2, thus protein synthesis inhibited.
- *Escherichia coli, Vibrio cholerae, B cereus* heat-labile enterotoxin: ADP-ribosylation of G_s protein turns G_s protein on, thus activating adenylate cyclase, leading to ↑cAMP and diarrhea.

- *Bordetella pertussis* heat-labile enterotoxin: ADP-ribosylation of G_i protein turns off G_i protein, thereby activating adenylate cyclase, leading to ↑cAMP and diarrhea.
- *Vibrio:* oxidase positive; one flagellum; curved, "comma-shaped" gram-negative rod; halophilic (except *V cholerae*).
- *Vibrio parahaemolyticus:* spread by contaminated seafood, causes diarrhea.
- *Vibrio vulnificus:* spread by contaminated marine animals (oyster ingestion), causes diarrhea, skin lesions (handling).
- Resistant nosocomial infections: vancomycin-resistant enterococci (VRE), treat with quinupristin-dalfopristin, methicillin-resistant *S aureus* (MRSA) treat with vancomycin, and vancomycin-indeterminate *S aureus* (VISA) consider new treatment options such as linezolid or quinupristin-dalfopristin.
- *Mycobacterium tuberculosis* causes initial primary pulmonary infection which may enter chronic latent granulomatosis stage; or result in reactivation of disease characterized by hemoptysis, loss of weight, and fever.
- Penicillin-resistant pneumococci (*S pneumoniae*) may account for up to 40% of isolates of *S pneumoniae*. Third- or fourth-generation cephalosporins may be used as alternative treatment as well as vancomycin and rifampin.
- *Campylobacter* (GE) and *Helicobacter* (PUD) are both helical-shaped bacteria. *Campylobacter* causes a food-borne GI illness, most commonly from undercooked meat. Both bacteria are susceptible to antibiotics such as tetracycline. *Helicobacter* may be treated with Pepto-Bismol, metronidazole, and amoxicillin.

Media-Selective Examples
- Bile esculin agar—used to identify Enterococcus from non-Group D cocci
- Bordet-Gengou agar—used for isolating *B pertussis*
- Chocolate agar—used to identify fastidious organisms (*Neisseria and Haemophilus*)
- Thayer-Martin agar—used to identify *Neisseria*
- Meuller-Hinton agar—used for susceptibility testing
- EMB agar and MacConkey agar—used to identify enterobacteriaceae (enterics)
- Fletcher medium—used to identify *Listeria*
- Loeffler medium—used to identify *C diphtheriae*

- Lowenstein-Jensen medium—used to identify mycobacteria
- Middlebrook 7H10—used to identify mycobacteria
- Mannitol salt agar—used to identify staphylococci, specific for *S aureus*
- Selenite broth—used to identify enrichment for *Salmonella/Shigella*

RICKETTSIAE, CHLAMYDIAE, MYCOPLASMAS

Rickettsiae

- *Rickettsia, Coxiella, Bartonella (Rochalimaea)*, and *Ehrlichia*—main genera. All are obligate intracellular parasites due to limited adenosine triphosphate (ATP) production. Insect vectors include ticks, mites, and body lice.
- Rocky Mountain spotted fever—*caused by Rickettsia rickettsii*, spread by ticks, invades capillaries, causing vasculitis. Rash commonly progresses from extremities to trunk. Diagnosis is usually serologic, using cross-reacting antibodies to *Proteus vulgaris* OX strains.
- Treat with tetracyclines, doxycycline
- *Coxiella burnetii*—reservoir is livestock; inhalation transmission. Causes Q fever, an atypical pneumonia.
- *Bartonella*—pericellular, not intracellular infection (*B quintana, B henselae*). Causes trench fever, septicemia, cat scratch disease.
- *Ehrlichia*—infects monocytes, granulocytes; tick transmission.

Chlamydiae

- Obligate intracellular parasites that require host ATP. Possess a modified gram-negative cell wall, a true bacterium.
- Unusual life cycle—infectious elementary bodies bind to receptors, enter cells, forming an intracellular reticulate body. Dividing reticulate bodies form new elementary bodies. Reticulate bodies form inclusion bodies in the host cell.
- *Chlamydia trachomatis* is sensitive to sulfa drugs, stains with iodine (glycogen staining). Serotypes A, B, and C cause trachoma, a chronic follicular keratoconjunctivitis, often resulting in blindness (leading cause worldwide).
- Serotypes D to K cause reproductive tract infections, pneumonia, and inclusion conjunctivitis. Chlamydial genital infections are widespread and common. Neonatal infections often result in inclusion conjunctivitis. Treat with erythromycins or tetracyclines.
- Serotypes L1, L2, and L3 cause lymphogranuloma venereum.

- Identify genital infections with molecular probes, fluorescent antibody (FA) staining for tissues, grow in McCoy cell cultures.
- *Chlamydia psittaci* uses birds as primary hosts. Humans develop an atypical pneumonia from inhaling the organism. Diagnosis is usually serology, not iodine staining.
- *Chlamydia pneumoniae* (TWAR) causes human bronchitis, pneumonia, and sinusitis. Treat with azithromycin.

Mycoplasma

Bacteria with no cell wall.
- Grown on laboratory media; do not Gram stain
- *Mycoplasma pneumoniae*—causes sore throat through atypical pneumonia (walking pneumonia); treat with tetracyclines or erythromycins
- *Ureaplasma urealyticum*—urethritis, prostatitis; forms tiny colonies

MYCOLOGY

- Fungi (molds and yeasts) are eukaryotic—cell membranes have ergosterol (not cholesterol); target for imidazole, amphoteracin B, and nystatin antifungal.
- Fungal structures—hyphae (molds) or yeast. ("Mold in the cold, yeast in the beast.")
  - Dimorphism—change from hyphae to yeast forms.
  - Hyphae grow into a mycelium; septate hyphae have cross-walls; nonseptate hyphae have no cross-walls.
  - Yeasts—oval cells that replicate by budding.
  - Spores—reproductive devices—blastoconidia—yeast buds, conidia—hyphae (macro- and microforms); endospores—*Coccidioides immitis*; arthroconidia—hyphae fragmentation.
- Laboratory test—Sabouraud agar is standard fungal medium.
  - Identity—based on morphology, biochemical test, immunologic tests, or genetic probes
- Dermatophytes.
  - *Malassezia furfur*—hypopigmentation of skin, spaghetti and meatballs appearance
  - *Trichophyton*—affects skin, hair, nails; *Microsporum* affects hair and skin; *Epidermophyton* affects nail and skin
  - *Tineas*—ringworm (*T capitis* affects hair, *T corporis* affects skin, *T cruris* affects groin, causes jock itch, *T pedis* causes athlete's foot)

- *Candida*—shows up in pseudohyphae and yeast forms; affects normal flora; causes opportunist infection, such as thrush, in immunocompromised patients
- *Sporothrix schenckii*—dimorphic fungus found in plants; transmitted while handling thorny plants and the like; lymphatics involved (rose gardener's disease)
- Thermally dimorphic fungi—systemic infections, rose gardener's disease.
  - *Histoplasma capsulatum*—caused by fungus in the environment with tuberculate macroconidia; small, oval budding yeast in cells of the reticuloendothelial system (RES)
  - Central United States—river valleys, especially important—birds and caves
  - Primary disease—asymptomatic to pneumonia
  - Systematic—especially in AIDS patients with mucocutaneous lesions common
  - Laboratory tests—history plus blood smears and culture
- *Coccidioides immitis*—found in sandy environment, especially deserts (southwest United States); hyphae develop into arthroconidia; inhaled arthroconidia develop into spherules (endospores).
  - Primary disease—valley fever—asymptomatic to self-limited pneumonia; disseminated form certain HLA types; pregnant women and immunocompromised patients are at a greater risk; affects skin, bone, joints, and meninges.
  - Laboratory—culture is hazardous and proper technique is necessary if done; sputum, urine, bronchial washes may show spherules.
- *Blastomyces dermatitidis*—environment includes hyphae with conidia on stalks; tissue—large yeast with broad-based bud.
- Same geographical area (Ohio and Mississippi River valley) as *Histoplasma* conidia are inhaled.
- Primary disease—pneumonia.
- Laboratory tests show large yeast, broad-based buds.

Opportunistic Fungi

- *Aspergillus fumigatus*—hyphae with branches at acute angles and small conidia; ubiquitous in environment; fungus balls in lung cavities; invasive disease possible; opportunist infection
- *Candida albicans*—yeast and pseudohyphae normal mucocutaneous flora; causes oral thrush in infants and antibiotic users

- Endocarditis (right side of heart)—patients are mainly IV drug abusers or those who have indwelling catheters
- *Cryptococcus neoformans*—yeast with large capsule
  - Environment—soil with bird droppings
  - Disease—pulmonary (often asymptomatic) in pigeon breeders; fungal meningitis in AIDS patients and cancer patients
  - Laboratory test—latex agglutination—CSF (capsular antigen); India ink wet mount, capsule stains
- *Mucor, Rhizopus, Absidia*—nonseptate hyphae
  - Environment—common organisms
  - Opportunist infections—rhinocerebral infections; diabetics
  - Laboratory test—broad, nonseptate hyphae with 90° angles on branching
- *Pneumocystis jiroveci*—exposure common—seldom causes disease except in immunocompromised (AIDS patients and the like); causes interstitial pneumonia (old name: *P carinii*, isolated from rats)
  - Laboratory tests—H and E tissue stains, silver stains, cup-shaped cysts, Tx-TMP-SMX, pentamidine

PARASITOLOGY

- Protozoa are single-celled animals. Trophozoites are motile, while cysts are involved in transmission.
- Amoebas.
  - *Entamoeba histolytica*—disease of the large intestine; amebic dysentery—trophozoites feed on red blood cells (RBCs), causing flask-shaped ulcers. Also liver and lung abscesses possible.
  - *Naegleria*—free-living amoeba in hot water sources; causes primary amebic meningoencephalitis (PAM); rapid onset of symptoms, with death possible in days.
  - Acanthamoeba—free-living amoebas; cause granulomatous amoebic encephalitis (GAE); found in tap water, freshwater, seawater, and other such sources.
- Flagellates.
  - *Giardia lamblia*—worldwide distribution, animal reservoirs; cysts in water sources. Trophozoites attach to intestine, causing watery diarrhea and malabsorption. Cramping, light-colored, fatty stools; also acquired from day-care centers or while camping.

- *Trichomonas vaginalis*—trophozoite with undulating membrane and polar flagella; presents with yellow discharge which has a fishy odor; males usually asymptomatic; sexually transmitted.
- *Trypanosoma*—flagellates transmitted by tsetse fly; cause African sleeping sickness.
- *Trypanosoma cruzi*—Chagas disease transmitted by kissing bug; prevalent mostly in South and Central America; causes cardiomegaly, megacolon.
- *Leishmania*—sandfly vectors; cause visceral, cutaneous, and mucocutaneous lesions.
- Sporozoans—sexual and asexual life cycle forms; worse in HIV, immunocompromised patients.
- *Cryptosporidium parvum*—found in US waters; causes a self-limited diarrhea.
- *Plasmodium* species cause malaria. *Anopheles* mosquito vectors; complicated life cycles; *P vivax, P ovale, P malariae, P falciparum.*
- *Toxoplasma gondii*—reservoir is cats. Humans ingest cysts from cat feces or undercooked meats. Specially dangerous to human fetus as it affects congenital development.
- Flukes.
  - *Fasciolopsis buski*—affects intestines; cysts on water plants ingested; causes diarrhea.
  - *Clonorchis sinensis*—affects liver; transmitted from raw or undercooked fish; biliary tree localization and liver location.
  - *Fasciola hepatica*—sheep liver fluke; humans can become infected by ingestion of metacercariae on aquatic plants.
  - *Schistosoma*—also called blood flukes; species include *S hematobium* cystitis; causes bladder cancer, squamous cell carcinoma.
- Cestodes—segmented flatworms with complicated life cycles.
  - *Taenia solium* (pork) and *T saginata* (beef)—larval forms (cysticercosis) found in undercooked meat. Adult tapeworms develop in the intestine.
  - *Diphyllobothrium latum*—fish tapeworm; fish in freshwater lakes, undercooked fish ingested; depletes host of vitamin B_{12}.
  - *Echinococcus granulosis*—tissue cestode. Humans are intermediate hosts and ingest eggs from sheepdog feces, hydatid cysts of liver, anaphylaxis if burst.

- Nematodes—roundworms.
- *Ascaris lumbricoides*—may cause intestinal blockage.
- *Enterobius vermicularis* (pinworm)—eggs in bedclothes, detected in scotch tape test, etc; autoinoculation common; widespread in the United States.
- *Necator americanus*—New World hookworm.
- *Ancylostoma duodenale*—Old World hookworm; eggs found in soil; penetrate bare feet.
- *Strongyloides stercoralis* (threadworm)—found in tropics, southwest United States; is similar to hookworms; no eggs, only larval forms.
- *Trichuris trichiura* (whipworm)—found in tropics; spreads when eggs are ingested, or due to poor sanitation; causes mucoid or bloody diarrhea, anal prolapse.
- *Trichinella spiralis* (pork roundworm)—larvae ingested in pork or wild game meat. Larvae may calcify in muscle of intermediate host.
- Tissue nematodes—filarial worms. None are significant in the United States.
- *Onchocerca volvulus*—also called river blindness. Blackfly is the vector of disease. The preferred treatment is ivermectin.
- *Loa loa*—biting fly is the vector.
- *Wuchereria bancrofti*—mosquito vectors; may cause elephantiasis by blocking lymphatics.

IMMUNOLOGY

- Two types of immune response: (1) adaptive or acquired (specific, but slow), (2) innate (native or nonadaptive, rapid).
- Innate immunity: nonspecific, no immunological memory, first line of defense (epithelial), biochemical defenses (stomach $\downarrow$pH, GI proteolytic enzymes, and bile), phagocytes (polymorphonuclear neutrophils [PMNs] and monocytes, macrophages), soluble mediators (complement, acute-phase proteins such as C-reactive protein, cytokines such as ILs, IFNs, CSFs), inflammation (C5a: chemotaxis, C3b: opsonization, neutrophils).
- Adaptive immunity: specific, antigen-driven, possesses discrimination and memory, divided into (1) humoral immunity (B cells, plasma cells) and (2) cell-mediated immunity (T helper, T cytotoxic).
- Antibodies (B lymphocytes/plasma cells): main functions are (1) *neutralize* toxins/viruses, (2) *opsonize* bacteria, and (3) *complement activation*.

- Antibodies (five isotypes): IgG, IgA, IgM, IgD, IgE (based on Fc heavy-chain differences), two light chains and two heavy chains held together by S-H bridges, hinge region is polyproline, paratope binds antigen and is composed of heavy and light chains. Pepsin yields $F(ab)_2$, papain yields two "useless arms."
- Antibody concentrations (serum): IgG > IgA > IgM > IgD > IgE.
- IgG: crosses the placenta (Rh incompatibility, hemolytic disease of newborn), 80% of serum antibody, binds (activates) complement, four subclasses, main antibody in secondary response.
- IgA: secretory antibody, serum (monomer), secretions (dimers), two subclasses, dimer (J chain), does not bind complement.
- IgM: pentamer; binds complement, first to appear after infection, elevated in congenital/perinatal infections.
- IgD: susceptible to proteolytic degradation, found with surface IgM on mature B lymphocytes.
- IgE: cytotropic/reaginic antibody, allergy antibody, type I hypersensitivity (mast cells/basophils protective in worm infections), lowest concentration in serum.
- Bence Jones proteins: multiple myeloma—large amounts of κ/γ light chains in urine excretion.
- Natural killer cells: marker is CD16 (IgG Fc receptor).
- B cells: antibody producers contributing to allergy (IgE), autoimmunity, host defense (opsonize, neutralize, complement activate).
- B-cell markers: Fc receptor, C3 receptor, CD21 (receptor for EB virus), CD10 (common acute lymphoblastic leukemia antigen [CALLA]).
- T cells: host defense (fungi, viruses, *M tuberculosis*), allergy (type IV—delayed hypersensitivity), antibody regulation, graft/tumor rejection.
- T-cell markers: CD2, TCRαβ-CD3, CD4 (HIV) or CD8, CD44 (migration).
- Complement deficiencies: (1) C1 esterase inhibitor: angioedema; (2) decay-accelerating factor (DAF): paroxysmal nocturnal hemoglubinuria; (3) C3 deficiency: severe, recurrent infections (sinus and respiratory)—pneumonococci; (4) C5 to C9 deficiency: disseminated gonococcemia.
- Major histocompatibility complex (MHC) Class I: exists on all nucleated cells—MHC I > CD8.
- MHC Class II: exists on antigen-presenting cells (macrophages/dendritic cells), important to organ rejection—MHC II > CD4.
- Cytokines: IFN (antiviral), TNF (inflammation, fever, acute-phase reactants, cachexia), IL-1 (fever/pyrogen, acute-phase proteins), IL-2 (T-cell

stimulator), IL-3 (bone marrow stimulator), IL-4 (IgE production), IL-5 (proeosinophil, antihelminths), IL-6 (acute-phase proteins, B-cell differentiation), IL-8 (inflammation, chemotaxis), IL-12 (NK cell stimulator, T_H1 stimulator, active cytotoxic lymphocyte stimulator, promotes cell-mediated immunity).

- Acute-phase cytokines: IL-1, IL-6, TNF-α.
- Mitogens: B lymphocytes (LPS), T lymphocytes (phytohemagglutinin [PHA] and Con A), both B and T cells (pokeweed mitogen [PWM]).
- Enzyme-linked immunosorbent assay (ELISA)-sensitive presumptive diagnosis of HIV infection, Western blot specific, definitive diagnosis of HIV infection → both detecting anti-HIV antibodies in patient sera; detection of HIV RNA by nucleic acid amplification of viral load is best predictor of "progression to AIDS."
- Immunodeficiencies: (1) primary—rare and *cause* disease; (2) secondary—common and the *result* of disease.
- Primary immunodeficiencies: Bruton agammaglobulinemia—no B cells, low antibodies, small tonsils, only males; DiGeorge syndrome (congenital thymic aplasia)—third and fourth pharyngeal pouches development failure, no thymus, no T cells, no parathyroid (hypocalcemia), and recurrent viral, fungal, protozoal infections; severe combined immunodeficiency disease (SCID)—no T or B cells, defective IL-2 receptor, deficiency adenosine enzyme, recurrent infections (viral, bacterial, fungal, protozoal); Wiskott Aldrich syndrome—B and T cell deficiency, low IgM, high IgA, normal IgE; ataxia telangiectasia—defective DNA repair; Chèdiak-Higashi disease—autosomal-recessive defect in phagocytosis; CGD—NADPH oxidase deficiency, increased opportunistic pathogens, phagocytic deficiency; chronic mucocutaneous candidiasis—*C albicans* T-cell dysfunction.
- Immunodeficiency characterized by unusual and recurrent infections.
  - B-cell (antibody) deficiency—bacterial infections
  - T-cell deficiency—viral, fungal, and protozoal infections
  - Phagocytic cells deficiency—pyogenic infections (bacterial), skin infections, systemic bacterial opportunistic infections
  - Complement deficiencies—pyogenic infections (bacterial)
- Hypersensitivity: (1) type I (anaphylaxis, immediate-type hypersensitivity, IgE); (2) type II (cytotoxic hypersensitivity); (3) type III (immune complex hypersensitivity); (4) type IV (cell-mediated, delayed-type hypersensitivity).

- Type I: mast cell/basophil, IgE, vasoactive amines, asthma, anaphylaxis, local wheal, and flare.
- Type II: IgM, IgG bind antigen and lyse cell, autoimmune hemolytic anemia, Goodpasture syndrome, erythroblastosis fetalis.
- Type III: immune complex, serum sickness, Arthus reaction → antibody-antigen complexes.
- Type IV: lymphokines released from activated T lymphocytes, TB skin test, contact dermatitis, transplant rejection, lupus (SLE).
- Autoantibodies: systemic lupus erythematosus (antinuclear antibodies, anti-dsDNA, anti-Smith); drug-induced lupus (antihistone); rheumatoid arthritis (anti-IgG); celiac disease (antigliadin), Goodpasture syndrome (antibasement membrane); Hashimoto thyroiditis (antimicrosomal); scleroderma Calcinosis Raynaud Esophagus Sclerosis Teleangiectasiae (CREST) (anticentromere); scleroderma diffuse (anti-scl-70).
- Active immunity: induced after exposure to foreign antigens, memory established, slow onset.
- Vaccines: (1) capsular polysaccharide vaccines (*Streptococcus, N meningitidis, H influenzae*); (2) toxoid vaccines (*C diphtheriae, C tetani, B pertussis*); (3) purified protein vaccines (*B pertussis, Borrelia burgdorferi, B anthracis*); (4) live, attenuated bacterial vaccines (*M bovis* for tuberculosis/BCG, *F tularensis*); (5) killed bacterial vaccines (*V cholerae, Y pestis, R rickettsiae*/typhus, *C burnetii*/Q fever); (6) killed, live, attenuated, and polysaccharide vaccines (*S typhi*).
- Adjuvants (human vaccines): aluminum hydroxide or lipid.
- Passive immunity: administration of preformed antibody in immune globulin preparations, no memory established, rapid onset (eg, tetanus antitoxin, botulinum antitoxin, diphtheria antitoxin), antitoxin = immune globulins.

Physiology and Molecular Microbiology

Questions

1. A 28-year-old female with folliculitis who is not responsive to a 10-day treatment course with penicillin. Which of the following numbered bonds of the 6-amino-penicillanic acid (structure shown below) would be broken by the penicillinase isolated from the etiologic agent?

a. 1
b. 2
c. 3
d. 4
e. 5

2. Following an ineffective antibiotic therapy using glycopeptides, a gram-negative rod was isolated from a 35-year-old male who presented with symptoms of a urinary tract infection. Which of the following bacterial transport methods is energy independent and is most likely not involved in transport of the antibiotics into the cell?

a. ATP-dependent active transport
b. Facilitated diffusion
c. Group translocation
d. Proton gradient energized active transport
e. Simple diffusion

3. A 36-year-old male developed a painful purulent urethral discharge following a 2-week vacation to Thailand. A Gram stain reveals gram-negative diplococci. Iron is essential for the expression of its virulence factors. Which of the following macromolecules is important in iron metabolism?

a. Ferric oxide
b. Lactoferrin
c. Lipopolysaccharide (LPS)
d. Siderophores
e. Transferrin

4. A medical student is admitted to the emergency department with symptoms of hemorrhagic colitis. An aliquot of *Escherichia coli*, which is considered the etiologic agent of the infection, is treated with ethylenediaminetetraacetic acid (EDTA). The first wash is analyzed and found to contain alkaline phosphatase, DNase, and penicillinase. Which of the following is the anatomic area of the cell most likely affected by the EDTA?

a. Chromosome
b. Mesosomal space
c. Periplasmic space
d. Plasma membrane
e. Slime layer

Questions 5 and 6

A 52-year-old male develops abscesses following surgery to repair an abdominal gunshot wound. Gram stain of the exudates from his foul-smelling abscess reveals numerous polymorphonuclear neutrophils (PMNs) and several gram-negative rods that did not grow on blood plates in the presence of O_2. Metabolism of O_2 results in toxic reactive oxygen species.

5. Which of the following enzymes is most likely involved in the following reaction?

$$2O^{2-} + 2H^+ \rightarrow H_2O_2 + O_2$$

a. ATPase
b. Catalase
c. Oxygen permease
d. Peroxidase
e. Superoxide dismutase

6. Which of the following enzymes is most likely involved in the following reaction?

$$H_2O_2 + H_2A^* \rightarrow 2H_2O + A \text{ ("A" may be a number of chemical groups).}$$

a. ATPase
b. Flavoprotein oxidase
c. Oxygen permease
d. Peroxidase
e. Superoxide dismutase

7. A teenaged boy suffered a foot laceration while swimming in a polluted water area in a river. He did not seek medical treatment, and the wound developed a foul-smelling exudate. One of the bacteria isolated from the abscess exudate was missing superoxide dismutase, catalase, and a peroxidase. Which of the following statements best describes this microorganism?

a. Aminoglycoside antibiotics will be effective against this bacterium.
b. This bacterium is a facultative aerobe.
c. This bacterium is an anaerobe.
d. This bacterium is more virulent than one containing the three enzymes.
e. This bacterium will survive in an O_2 environment.

Questions 8 and 9

A 20-year-old pregnant female patient presents to the emergency room with a 4-day history of fever, chills, and myalgia. Two days prior to this, she had noted painful genital lesions. Pelvic examination revealed extensive vesicular and ulcerative lesions on the left labia minora and majora with marked edema. The cervix had exophytic (outward-growing) necrotic ulcerations. Specimens were taken to test for *Neisseria gonorrhoeae, Treponema pallidum, Haemophilus ducreyi, Chlamydia trachomatis*, and herpes simplex virus type 2 (HSV-2).

8. You decide to use newly purchased cutting-edge technology to rapidly identify the infecting pathogen. Real-time polymerase chain reaction (PCR) requires which of the following reaction ingredient sets?

a. Specimen (template DNA), forward primer, reverse primer, polymerase (Taq), dNTPs, $MgCl_2$ hepes buffer, H_2O, and fluorescent reporter (ie, SYBR-green I)
b. Specimen (template DNA), forward primer, reverse primer, polymerase (Taq), dNTPs, $MgCl_2$, hepes buffer, and H_2O
c. Specimen (template DNA), forward primer only, polymerase (Taq), dNTPs, $MgCl_2$, hepes buffer, and H_2O
d. Specimen (template DNA), reverse primer only, polymerase (Taq), dNTPs, $MgCl_2$, hepes buffer, and H_2O
e. Specimen (template DNA), forward primer, reverse primer, dNTPs, $MgCl_2$, hepes buffer, H_2O, and fluorescent reporter (ie, SYBR-green I)

9. Real-time SYBR-green PCR reveals the following results:

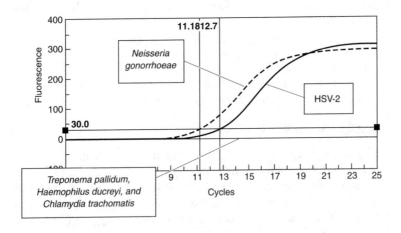

Which of the following is she infected with?

a. The woman is infected with N gonorrhoeae, T pallidum, H ducreyi, C trachomatis, and HSV-2.
b. The woman is infected with only HSV-2.
c. The woman is infected with only N gonorrhoeae.
d. The woman is infected with both N gonorrhoeae and HSV-2.
e. The woman is not infected with any of the above-mentioned pathogens.

10. A gram-negative diplococci identified as *N gonorrhoeae* is isolated from an 18-year-old male, who presented with symptoms of urethritis. Continuous passage of this strain on laboratory medium results in the reversion of a fimbriated to a nonfimbriated strain. Which of the following is the most likely implication of this phenomenon?

a. A negative capsule strain
b. Death of the organism
c. Inability of *N gonorrhoeae* to colonize the mucosal epithelium
d. Loss of serologic specificity
e. Reversion to a gram-positive stain

11. Eighteen hours after eating undercooked chicken, a 50-year-old farmer presents to the emergency room with abdominal pain, cramping, bloody diarrhea, and nausea. An isolate from the stool is serologically recognized as *Salmonella enteritidis* serovar *newport*. A mutant of this organism has lost region 1 (O-specific polysaccharide) of its LPS. This mutant would be identified as which of the following?

a. *Arizona*
b. *Salmonella typhi*
c. *Salmonella newport*
d. *Salmonella enteritidis*
e. *Salmonella enteritidis* serovar *newport*

12. A 10-week-old infant is diagnosed with meningitis. A lumbar puncture reveals numerous neutrophils and gram-positive rods. She is admitted to the hospital and started on IV β-lactams. Which of the following targets would most likely play a role in the development of resistance to the antibiotics?

a. Bactoprenol
b. DNA gyrase
c. Penicillin-binding proteins (PBPs)
d. Reverse transcriptase
e. RNA polymerase

13. A cattle farmer develops necrotic lesions on his hands following a traumatic encounter with a bull. Selective inhibition of synthesis of dipicolinic acid (structure shown below) from the etiologic agent of the infection would most likely inhibit the formation of which of the following structures?

a. Bacterial flagella
b. Bacterial spores
c. Eukaryotic cilia
d. Eukaryotic flagella
e. Fimbriae

Questions 14 and 15

A 30-year-old male presents to the emergency room with high fever and malaise which he reports began 4 days ago and got progressively worse each day. He appears underweight and very ill. Physical examination reveals needle marks in both antecubital fossae. Listening for heart sounds, you hear a distinctive systolic heart murmur. You order blood cultures and make a presumptive diagnosis of acute bacterial endocarditis. Following is the growth curve of the organism growing in a nutrient medium at 35°C with both O_2 and added CO_2 present.

Growth curve—*Escherichia coli*

14. Which of the following phases would most likely be missing detectable growth and hence would be resistant to β-lactam antibiotics?

a. Lag phase
b. Log phase
c. Stationary phase
d. Death phase

15. On which of the following growth phases would treatment with gentamicin have a maximal effect?

a. Lag phase
b. Log phase
c. Stationary phase
d. Death phase

16. An outbreak of diarrhea is thought to be related to a group of vendors who were selling hotdogs at the county fair. Stool cultures are positive for *Salmonella* in almost all the patients. Growth of the isolated colonies in nutrient liquid medium without the transfer to fresh medium will eventually induce the death phase of the organism. Which of the following is a limiting factor in microbial growth under laboratory conditions?

a. Accumulation of oxygen-free radicals
b. Accumulation of peroxide
c. Accumulation of toxic products in the growth medium
d. Loss of superoxide dismutase
e. Oxygen

17. A 62-year-old woman with diagnosed type 2 diabetes lived alone and did essentially nothing to manage her illness, including disregarding her physician's instructions. She was taken to her local emergency room (ER) with severe, multiple infected foot lesions, which yielded a variety of opportunistic microbes with a mixture of antibiotic sensitivities. The successful treatment of infectious diseases is based on the principle of selective toxicity. Which of the following antimicrobial agents is the most toxic to humans?

a. Bacitracin
b. Cephalosporin
c. Mitomycin
d. Penicillin
e. Vancomycin

18. A 42-year-old alcoholic man presents with fever, chills, cough, and chest x-ray suggestive of pneumonia. The Gram-stained smear of sputum shows many PMNs and gram-positive cocci in pairs and chains. Which of the following is the correct order of the procedural steps when performing the Gram stain?

a. Fixation, crystal violet, alcohol/acetone decolorization, safranin
b. Fixation, crystal violet, iodine treatment, alcohol/acetone decolorization, safranin
c. Fixation, crystal violet, iodine treatment, safranin
d. Fixation, crystal violet, safranin
e. Fixation, safranin, iodine treatment, alcohol/acetone decolorization, crystal violet

19. A 78-year-old man presents to the local emergency department with a severe headache and stiff neck. The cerebrospinal fluid (CSF) specimen is cloudy. Analysis reveals 400 white blood cells per cubic millimeter (95% PMNs), a protein concentration of 75 mg/dL, and a glucose concentration of 20 mg/dL. While in the ER, a resident does a Gram stain of the CSF but mistakenly forgets the iodine treatment step. If the meningitis is caused by *Streptococcus pneumoniae*, how will the bacteria seen on the resident's slide appear?

a. All the cells will be blue.
b. All the cells will be decolorized.
c. All the cells will be purple.
d. All the cells will be red.
e. All the cells will lyse, thus no Gram stain results will be obtained.
f. Half of the cells will be red and the other half will be blue.

20. A 28-year-old female just returned from a 1-week cruise with stops along the coast of Mexico. Forty-eight hours after her return she is reported to have headache, fever, abdominal cramps, and constipation. Over the next 5 days, her fever increases with continued complaints of myalgias, malaise, and anorexia. A blood culture is positive for *S typhi*. Her condition improves with a treatment course of a cephalosporin. Which of the following is the function of porins that would prevent the effective use of other antimicrobials?

a. Hydrolysis of hydrophilic antimicrobials
b. Metabolism of phosphorylated intermediates
c. Serologic stabilization of the O antigen
d. Inactivation of hydrophobic antimicrobials
e. Transfer of small molecules through the outer membrane

21. A 21-year-old man was bitten by a tick in Oregon. Two years later, during the course of routine screening for an unknown ailment, a screening for Lyme disease test was performed, which was negative. A Western blot strip (IgG) showed the following pattern:

Which of the following is an accurate interpretation of the test?
a. The patient has acute Lyme disease.
b. The patient has chronic Lyme disease.
c. The patient should be tested for HIV on the basis of the Western blot.
d. The pattern may represent nonspecific reactivity.
e. The screening test should be repeated.

22. Over 30 individuals attending a home improvement conference are hospitalized with bloody diarrhea and severe hematological abnormalities. An investigation establishes that all of these individuals developed symptoms following consumption of hamburgers from the same fast-food restaurant chain. Although other individuals ate the same hamburgers, they did not report any symptoms. An analysis is initiated using PCR to evaluate the *E coli* strains from all the individuals, looking for the major virulence factor associated with *E coli* 0157/H7, the etiologic bacterium responsible for the outbreak. Early attempts at the PCR used *E coli* DNA polymerase. This was replaced with DNA polymerase from *Thermus aquaticus* ("Taq" polymerase). Which of the following is the primary advantage in using this enzyme?

a. It is cheaper than *E coli* polymerase.
b. Specificity is increased because nonspecific hybridization of primers does not occur.
c. Use of Taq polymerase enables lower temperatures to be used.
d. Use of Taq polymerase results in fewer PCR cycles.
e. Upon repeated cycling, Taq polymerase becomes denatured, which causes less interference with the hybridization process.

Questions 23 to 25

A healthy 45-year-old female had root canal treatment about 3 weeks ago. She now presents with a new heart murmur, fever, painful skin nodules, and abdominal pain with an abnormal liver function test. In addition, there are other systemic complications that cannot be attributed to α-hemolytic streptococci, the major suspected organism. Because several patients from the same county had a similar clinical presentation, an exploration for defining all the microorganisms in the oral cavity is initiated.

You have been asked to design a nucleic acid amplification test for a rarely isolated bacterium. There are several questions that you must ask in order to develop a test that can be used to diagnose disease.

23. Assume, initially, that the PCR will amplify any DNA, human or microbial. Which of the following is the best way to prevent contamination of the PCR process?

a. Do all of the work under a hood.
b. Incorporate self-sterilizing agents into the PCR mixture.
c. Use universal precautions.
d. Wash benches with bleach.
e. Wear gloves.

24. You must choose primers for this PCR. *Primers* are small pieces of nucleic acid that recognize a pair of unique sites on the bacterial chromosome. For an optimum test to be developed, which of the following characteristics is the least desirable?

a. Ability to be constructed by a synthesizer
b. Ability to serve as a template for replication
c. Complementary to sequences on the bacterial chromosome
d. That the sequences are widely recognized by many bacterial species
e. Uniqueness to the organism that you wish to detect

25. You have chosen the primers for the PCR that you designed. You have also developed a reaction mixture that contains, among other substances, a polymerase enzyme. After the primer pairs have been amplified, they must be detected. Which of the following detection methods is most sensitive (ie, will detect the highest number of amplicons)?

a. Capture of the amplicons on a solid phase followed by an enzyme immunoassay
b. Ethidium staining of the amplified products (amplicons)
c. Labeling of the amplicons with fluorescent dyes
d. Microscopy
e. Southern blot

26. A high school-aged young woman presented to her family physician with what appeared to be an acute uncomplicated urinary tract infection. She was treated with a β-lactam antimicrobial, but her symptoms persisted. *Escherichia coli* was isolated from the infection but many of the organisms appeared Gram-stain variable and rounded. The rounded forms were identified as spheroplasts. Which of the following statements about the *E coli* cells shown in the microphotograph below is most characteristic of the organism observed in this infection?

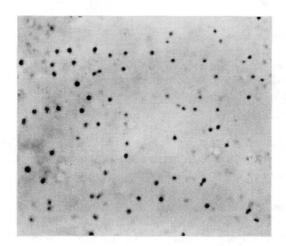

a. The rounded forms are commonly referred to as endospores.
b. The rounded forms are osmotically stable.
c. The rounded forms can result from treatment with penicillin.
d. The rounded forms have formed cell walls but have become coccoid.
e. Treatment of the parent *E coli* with lysozyme has no effect.

27. A 3-year-old girl from a family that does not believe in immunization presents to the emergency room with a sore throat, fever, malaise, and difficulty breathing. A gray membrane covering the pharynx is observed on physical examination. *Corynebacterium diphtheriae* is confirmed as the etiologic agent of this infection.

Analysis of the gene for the major virulence factor is needed by a graduate student for further study. The sequence of the cloning process is critical to the production of clones which will facilitate amplification of the cloned fragment. Which of the following steps initializes the cloning process?

a. Amplification of source DNA
b. Detection and purification of clones
c. Incorporation of a cloning vector into the host cell
d. Isolation and fragmentation/amplication of source DNA
e. Joining of host DNA to a cloning vector

28. A 3-year-old girl from a day care center is brought to the local public health clinic because of a severe, intractable cough. During the previous 10 days, she had a persistent cold that had worsened. The cough developed the previous day and was so severe that vomiting frequently followed it. The child appears exhausted from the coughing episodes. A blood cell count shows a marked leukocytosis with a predominance of lymphocytes. To rule out the infection of other children and staff at the day care, samples taken from them are evaluated with a *Bordetella*-specific DNA probe. Which of the following is usually true of nucleic acid probes?

a. Nucleic acid probes are not as sensitive as traditional culture methods for detection of pathogenic microorganisms.
b. Only DNA can be used as a probe.
c. Primers are labeled to allow detection, but probes are unlabeled.
d. Probes can be designed so that they can detect very specific pieces of a nucleic acid, for example, a penicillin-resistant gene.

29. A 55-year-old male presents with severe bilateral pulmonary infiltrate, elevated temperature, leucocytosis, elevated enzymes, and elevated creatine kinase. He and six of his friends had recently visited their favorite restaurant, which had a large water fountain that was misty on the day of his visit. He is diagnosed with Legionnaires' disease; however, his friends do not yet have similar symptoms. To evaluate their infectious state, specimens are taken from these individuals and analysed by PCR. Which of the following is usually required for PCR?

a. A heat-sensitive DNA polymerase enzyme
b. A single nucleotide primer
c. An ultracentrifuge
d. A universal probe to detect the amplified product
e. Knowledge of the genetic sequence to be amplified

Questions 30 to 33

The following five growth curves are lettered (A-E) corresponding to an expected growth curve if certain antibiotics were added to an exponentially growing culture of *E coli*. The arrow indicates when antibiotics were added to the growing culture.

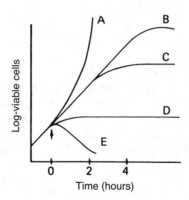

30. Chloramphenicol treatment would be expected to produce which one of the following growth curves?

a. A
b. B
c. C
d. D
e. E

31. Penicillin would be expected to produce which one of the following growth curves?

a. A
b. B
c. C
d. D
e. E

32. Sulfonamide would be expected to produce which one of the following growth curves?

a. A
b. B
c. C
d. D
e. E

33. If no antibiotics were added to the exponentially growing culture, which one of the following growth curves would result?

a. A
b. B
c. C
d. D
e. E

34. Several strains of S pneumoniae are isolated from various patients. Some demonstrate high virulence while others appear to be nonvirulent. Mixing these cultures in the laboratory causes the nonvirulent strains to become pathogenic in laboratory animal experiments. Uptake by a recipient cell of soluble DNA released from a donor cell is defined as which of the following?

a. Competence
b. Conjugation
c. Recombination
d. Transduction
e. Transformation

35. A non-spore-forming, gram-positive bacillus was isolated from a throat specimen from a primary school-aged child who had not been vaccinated with the DTaP vaccine. A diphtheroid gram-positive rod may develop into a pathogenic *C diphtheriae* by means of a bacteriophage infection. Transfer of a donor chromosome fragment by a temperate bacterial virus is defined as which one of the following?

a. Competence
b. Conjugation
c. Recombination
d. Transduction
e. Transformation

36. An increase in antibiotic resistance has been observed in microbial *Staphylococcus, Pseudomonas, and E coli* strains isolated from patients in medical centers. Direct transfer of a plasmid between two bacteria is defined as which of the following?

a. Competence
b. Conjugation
c. Recombination
d. Transduction
e. Transformation

37. After incubating a culture of five *E coli* bacteria for 2 hours, the following graph was constructed. Which of the following represents the number of *E coli* now present in this culture?

a. 32
b. 64
c. 160
d. 320
e. 640

38. Which of the following is an accurate description of Koch postulates?

a. The causal organism must be isolated, grown in pure culture, cause disease in a healthy susceptible animal, and ultimately be recovered from the inoculated animal.
b. The causal organism must be isolated, grown in pure culture, cause disease in a previously immunized (to the causal organism) animal, and ultimately be recovered from the inoculated animal.
c. The causal organism need only be isolated and grown in pure culture.
d. The causal organism may be inferred through an extensive history and physical of the diseased animal.
e. The causal organism must cause repeated symptoms (illness) in the same (original) animal.

39. A young child suffered from skin lesions that resulted from a bicycle accident. A mixed culture (gram-negative and gram-positive bacteria) was isolated by the clinical laboratory, complicating antibiotic sensitivity testing. The treating physician needed to make a decision about which antibiotic to use immediately, but also needed to consider whether there might be natural resistance to any medications used. The following diagram illustrates the cell walls of gram-positive and gram-negative bacteria. Which of the following statements is indicative of the contents of the indicated (arrow) portion in the diagram?

a. Genetic material such as DNA or RNA
b. Hydrolytic enzymes such as β-lactamases
c. Lipid A
d. LPS
e. Teichoic acid

40. A 55-year-old British teacher presents with weight loss, weakness, muscle atrophy, and declining cognitive function. Her history reveals that her favorite meal is soup made with cow brain, which she has eaten almost every week since she was 10 years old. She is suspected to suffer from bovine spongiform encephalopathy (BSE). In comparing viruses with prions, which of the following is most likely?

a. Both prions and viruses contain some form and quantity of nucleic acid, either DNA, RNA, or both.

b. Both viruses and prions upon infection induce an antibody response in the host.

c. Both viruses and prions upon infection induce an inflammatory response in the host.

d. Conventional viruses are rapidly inactivated by ultraviolet light or heat, whereas prions are not.

e. Both viral and prion proteins are encoded by viral genes.

41. Over 200 isoniazid-resistant strains of *Mycobacterium tuberculosis* isolated from different patients in the northwestern region of Russia are screened by a PCR-restriction fragment length polymorphism assay. This analysis reveals a 93.6% prevalence of a specific G to C mutation in the *katG* in strains from patients with both newly and previously diagnosed cases of tuberculosis. Which of the following best describes the type of mutation that resulted in isoniazid resistance in these strains?

a. Inversion

b. Missense

c. Nonsense

d. Transition

e. Transversion

42. Posaconazole (SCH56592) is a potent, novel, broad-spectrum triazole in Phase III trials. Both in vitro and in vivo testing have demonstrated that posaconazole is more effective than fluconazole against *Candida* spp and *Aspergillus* spp. Seven closely related isolates of *Candida albicans* exhibited progressive decreases in susceptibility to both posaconazole and itraconazole. Four of the isolates had amino acid changes, which were previously associated with azole resistance. Which of the following best describes the type of mutation that has resulted in decreased sensitivity to posaconazole resistance in these strains?

a. Inversion
b. Missense
c. Nonsense
d. Transition
e. Transversion

43. A patient presents to the emergency room with vomiting, diarrhea, high fever, and delirium. Upon physical examination, you notice large, painful buboes, and disseminated intravascular coagulation. Laboratory diagnosis of aspirate taken from the bubo reveals a gram-negative rod with bipolar staining resembling a safety pin. Which of the following antibiotics is most appropriate as part of your immediate treatment?

a. Ceftazidime
b. Ceftriaxone
c. Penicillin
d. Streptomycin
e. Vancomycin

44. A 3-year-old girl who has missed several scheduled immunizations presents to the emergency room with a high fever. She is irritable and has a stiff neck. Fluid from a spinal tap reveals 20,000 white blood cells per milliliter with 85% polymorphonuclear cells. Which of the following is the preferred third-generation cephalosporin with good activity against organisms of childhood meningitis?

a. Ceftazidime
b. Ceftriaxone
c. Penicillin
d. Streptomycin
e. Vancomycin

45. A patient presents to the emergency room with a progressive fever, cough, and general malaise. History determines that he works with sheep on a farm and had just been involved in wool harvesting. Which of the following antibiotics is most appropriate as part of your immediate treatment?
a. Ceftazidime
b. Ceftriaxone
c. Penicillin
d. Streptomycin
e. Vancomycin

46. During the course of his hospital stay, a severely burned 60-year-old male develops a rapidly disseminating bacterial infection. Small gram-negative rods that are oxidase positive are cultured from green pus taken from the burn tissue. Which one of the following third-generation cephalosporins will most likely have the best primary activity against this etiologic agent?
a. Ceftazidime
b. Ceftriaxone
c. Penicillin
d. Streptomycin
e. Vancomycin

47. Laboratory results of a clinical specimen from a patient with hospital-acquired pneumonia reveal the presence of *Staphylococcus aureus* with a methicillin-resistant plasmid. Which of the following drugs is the best immediate treatment?
a. Ceftazidime
b. Ceftriaxone
c. Penicillin
d. Streptomycin
e. Vancomycin

48. A young, essentially healthy woman was concerned about her loss of job time due to recurrent urinary tract infections. Her physician prescribed an antibiotic, which would control microbial nucleotide synthesis by inhibiting dihydrofolic acid reductase in bacteria up to 50,000 times more than in mammalian cells. Which of the following agents work by this mechanism?

a. Amdinocillin
b. Amphotericin
c. Chloramphenicol
d. Penicillin
e. Trimethoprim

49. An 18-year-old college freshman presents with fever of 103°F, headache, right flank pain, nausea and vomiting, and urinary frequency with hematuria and dysuria. Renal ultrasound demonstrates a right urinary stone with right hydronephrosis. Which of the following antibiotics binds to PBP-2 and is the most appropriate treatment option?

a. Amdinocillin
b. Amphotericin
c. Chloramphenicol
d. Penicillin
e. Trimethoprim

50. A 75-year-old African American male with neurogenic bladder presents to the emergency room with hypertension, fever up to 104.6°F, and nausea and vomiting. The urine from his foley catheter gives a positive culture for *Enterococcus faecalis*. Which of the following antibiotics inhibits the final peptide bond between D-alanine and glycine and is the most appropriate treatment for this patient?

a. Amdinocillin
b. Amphotericin
c. Chloramphenicol
d. Penicillin
e. Trimethoprim

51. A patient with leukemia has a chest CT finding that suggests aspergillosis. Which of the following antimicrobial binds sterols and alters membrane permeability, and would most likely be used in this patient's treatment?

a. Amdinocillin
b. Amphotericin
c. Chloramphenicol
d. Penicillin
e. Trimethoprim

52. A 10-week-old infant is diagnosed with meningitis. A lumbar puncture reveals numerous neutrophils and gram-positive rods. She is admitted to the hospital and is thought to be allergic to β-lactams. Which of the following antibiotics attaches to the 50S ribosome, inhibits peptidyl transferase, and would most likely be used to treat this patient?

a. Amdinocillin
b. Amphotericin
c. Chloramphenicol
d. Penicillin
e. Trimethoprim

Questions 53 to 57

An outbreak of diarrhea is thought to be related to a group of vendors who were selling snow cones at a local carnival. Stool cultures are positive for *Salmonella* in almost all the patients. To determine the relatedness of the strains and the source of the infection, DNA is isolated from all the strains. The following diagram illustrates the amplification of a conserved region of the DNA by PCR. There are at least four points in the PCR process (A-D) that are critical to the reaction.

53. The Southern blot detection system for amplified PCR products fails to function. Which of the following would most likely be affected?

a. A
b. B
c. C
d. D

54. DNA does not hybridize with the primers. Which of the following would most likely be affected?

a. A
b. B
c. C
d. D

55. The laboratory observes a series of false-positive results. Which of the following processes is most likely faulty?

a. A
b. B
c. C
d. D

56. The DNA strands fail to re-anneal. Which of the following processes is most likely faulty?

a. A
b. B
c. C
d. D

57. The laboratory observes a series of false-negative results. Which of the following processes is most likely faulty?

a. A
b. B
c. C
d. D

58. *Neisseria meningitidis*, group B, is identified as the cause of a local meningitis outbreak in a military training camp. This organism is characterized by which one of the following?

a. γ-Glutamyl polypeptide
b. Hyaluronic acid
c. Outer-membrane proteins
d. Por A and Por B proteins
e. Repeating polysaccharide capsule of glucose and glucuronic acid

59. A child attended classes, and the teacher noted several skin lesions on his arms that looked like vesicular areas broken down and denuded areas that contained pus and crusted over areas. The school nurse recognized that such lesions probably contained highly communicable bacteria and sent him home. Group A streptococci (GAS) produce beta (clear zone) hemolysis and are frequently the cause of pharyngitis, impetigo, rheumatic fever, and toxic shock syndrome. Which chemical component listed below is routinely characteristic of GAS?

a. γ-Glutamyl polypeptide
b. Hyaluronic acid
c. Outer-membrane proteins
d. Repeating polysaccharide capsule of glucose and glucuronic acid
e. Sialic acid polymers

60. In an area where severe weather damaged water purification facilities, numerous cases of intestinal infections occurred due to the ingestion of water contaminated with fecal bacteria. The cases, in general, responded to appropriate antimicrobial treatments. Bacterial endotoxins are integral parts of the cell wall LPS of gram-negative bacteria that appear to be capable of inducing inflammation by activating complement, resulting in hypotension. Bacterial LPS is characterized by which of the following?

a. Glycolipids (waxes)
b. Ketodeoxyoctulonate (KDO)
c. Phospholipid
d. Repeating polysaccharide capsule of glucose and glucuronic acid
e. Ribitol teichoic acid

61. A 64-year old female with a history of COPD visited her physician because of recent poor health symptoms. Examination of her 20-year-old pulmonary x-rays demonstrated possible old TB lesions. Laboratory specimen staining revealed acid-fast organisms, which were later identified as *M avium* complex. Mycobacteria are stained by the acid-fast technique because their cell walls are characterized by which of the following?

a. Glycolipids (waxes)
b. Ketodeoxyoctulonate
c. Phospholipid
d. Repeating polysaccharide capsule of glucose and glucuronic acid
e. Ribitol teichoic acid

62. Several governmental offices received mailed envelopes that contained an unknown white powder. Several employees were contaminated and isolated for diagnosis and any necessary treatment. *Bacillus anthracis* is frequently described as a bioterrorism agent. Among its virulence factors can be found toxins (PA, EF, LF) as well as capsules, which consist of which of the following materials?

a. Poly-D-glutamic acid
b. Hyaluronic acid
c. Outer-membrane proteins
d. Repeating polysaccharide capsule of glucose and glucuronic acid
e. Sialic acid polymers

63. A number of elderly residents living in an assisted care facility suffered from sinusitis, otitis media, and mild pneumonias during midwinter. Several strains of *S pneumoniae* were isolated from a number of the patients. Most were treated with amoxicillin and responded well to the therapy. *Streptococcus pneumoniae* can cause significant morbidity and mortality due to capsular virulence factors. These capsules (55 antigenic types) are characterized by which of the following?

a. γ-Glutamyl polypeptide
b. Hyaluronic acid
c. Outer-membrane proteins
d. Repeating polysaccharide capsule of glucose and glucuronic acid
e. Sialic acid polymers

Physiology and Molecular Microbiology

Answers

1. The answer is d. (*Brooks, pp 174-181. Levinson, pp 69-73. Ryan, p 197.*) The structural integrity of the β-lactam ring in penicillins is essential for their antimicrobial activity. Many resistant strains of staphylococci produce an enzyme, penicillinase (β-lactamase), that cleaves the β-lactam ring at the carbon-nitrogen bond. Other organisms, including certain coliform bacteria, produce an amidase enzyme that inactivates penicillin by disrupting the bond between the radical and nitrogen in the free amino group (1 in the diagram). Bonds 2, 3, and 5 are not commonly broken by bacterial enzymes.

2. The answer is e. (*Brooks, pp 15-19. Levinson, p 10. Ryan, pp 28-29.*) Almost no important nutrients enter the bacterial cell through simple diffusion, exceptions being carbon dioxide and oxygen. Some diffusion, however, is facilitated by specific protein carriers. Most transport (ATP-dependent transport, facilitated diffusion, group translocation, and proton gradient active transport), except simple diffusion, is energy dependent, particularly in gram-negative bacteria. Group translocation occurs in the absence of oxygen. For example, a simple carbohydrate such as glucose is phosphorylated enzymatically and is then transported into the cell.

3. The answer is d. (*Brooks, pp 19, 65, 168. Ryan, p 29.*) Siderophores such as aerobactin and enterobactin are compounds that chelate iron (Fe^{3+}) and promote its transport as a soluble compound. The iron-chelator complex is actively transported into the cell by the cooperative action of a group of proteins that span the outer membrane, periplasm, and inner membrane. Transferrin and lactoferrin are iron-binding proteins found in blood and milk and use a fundamentally different mechanism involving specific receptors that bind these molecules. Ferric or iron oxide is rust, and LPS is a microbial cell-wall constituent.

4. The answer is c. *(Brooks, p 29. Levinson, pp 6-7, 13. Ryan, p 19.)* The periplasm is the space between the outer membrane and the plasma membrane of bacteria. The periplasmic space in *E coli* has been shown to contain a number of proteins, sugars, amino acids, and inorganic ions. Ethylenediaminetetraacetic acid is a chelating agent that disrupts the cell walls of gram-negative bacteria. The chromosome contains the genetic information of the organism and is found within the cytoplasmic contents, which would make it difficult to be affected by EDTA as described. Mesosomes are large, irregular, convoluted invaginations of the cytoplasmic membrane. The plasma (cytoplasmic) membrane surrounds the cytoplasmic contents, while the slime layer (along with the term "capsule") describe external polysaccharide layers which are often protective of the organism by inhibiting phagocytosis by WBCs.

5 and 6. The answers are 5-e, 6-d. *(Brooks, pp 67-68. Levinson, pp 15-16, 102-104. Ryan, p 31.)* Oxygen, when it is metabolized, gives rise to hydrogen peroxide (H_2O_2) and superoxide-anion (O_2^-). Both of these by-products are extremely toxic to cells. Peroxide is produced by many bacteria, particularly facultative anaerobes that use flavoprotein intermediates. H_2O_2 is degraded by peroxidases, as illustrated in equation 2. Superoxide is detoxified by a critical enzyme known as *superoxide dismutase*. Such metabolism also results in H_2O_2 production (equation 1). *Peroxidase* and *catalase* are often used interchangeably to describe H_2O_2 reactions. However, in equation 2 when the H_2A reactant is another H_2O_2 molecule, the enzyme is known as *catalase*. If H_2A is another intermediate, then the enzyme is known as *peroxidase*. ATPase breaks down adenosine triphosphate to phosphate and energy. Oxygen-permease enzymes facilitate the transfer of oxygen across membranes. An oxidase enzyme is present in animals and plants that catalyzes an oxidation reaction (the process of a substance [eg, flavoprotein]) combining with oxygen.

7. The answer is c. *(Brooks, pp 67-68. Levinson, pp 15-16, 102-104. Ryan, p 31.)* Superoxide dismutase is an enzyme found in both prokaryotic and eukaryotic cells that can survive in an environment of O_2. Lack of this enzyme, as well as peroxidase and catalase, ensures that a bacterium will not grow in the presence of O_2.

Absence of these enzymes is not related to virulence, although ability to survive in an O_2-rich atmosphere may impart certain benefits to the proliferation of bacteria in the human host. Aminoglycosides and trimethoprim-sulfa drugs are never active against anaerobes.

8 and 9. The answers are 8-a, 9-d. (*Brooks, pp 377, 380, 710. Levinson, pp 67, 255. Murray-2009, pp 165-168. Ryan, pp 251-254.*) Although traditional PCR had many advantages in speeding up the process of detecting the presence/absence of DNA/RNA in a sample, it had many limitations, with end-point detection being its largest problem. End-point detection involves the need for running agarose gel electrophoresis of the PCR product to visualize the presence/absence of DNA/RNA in a sample. This is time consuming, messy, and, overall, not ideal in the clinical setting. This led to the development of an enhanced modality known as *real-time PCR*.

With the advent of real-time PCR, many of the limitations of traditional PCR have been overcome. Real-time PCR allows for the detection of PCR amplification during the early phases of the PCR reaction and therefore avoids the need for gel electrophoresis, thus minimizing time to detection. The same stage cycling (denaturation, annealing, extension) used in traditional PCR is also utilized in the real-time PCR system. The difference, however, exists in the dependence of real-time PCR on a fluorescent reporter for the detection and quantitation of target DNA. This reporter signal increases in direct proportion to the amount of PCR product (amplicon) in a reaction. By recording the amount of fluorescence emission at each cycle, it is possible to monitor the PCR during the exponential phase where the first significant increase in the amount of PCR product correlates to the initial amount of target template. There are two general methods for the quantitative detection of the amplicon: (1) fluorescent probes (FAM, TAMRA, TET, ROX, and the like) or (2) DNA-binding agents (SYBR-green I, ethidium bromide, and the like).

SYBR-green is a dye that binds the minor groove of double-stranded DNA (dsDNA). When SYBR-green binds to dsDNA, the intensity of the fluorescent emissions increases. As more dsDNA amplicons are produced, the SYBR-green signal will increase, allowing for real-time analysis while the PCR is running.

Real-time PCR is a powerful improvement over the traditional PCR system and can be applied to such investigations as (1) viral quantitation, (2) quantitation of gene expression, (3) array verification, (4) drug therapy efficacy, (5) DNA damage measurement, (6) quality control and assay validation, (7) pathogen detection (rapid and accurate), and (8) genotyping. A real-time PCR, in addition to requiring the same ingredients as a regular PCR (ie, specimen/template DNA, forward primer, reverse primer, polymerase [Taq], dNTPs, $MgCl_2$, hepes buffer, H_2O), also requires the presence of a fluorescent reporter such as SYBR-green I. The diagram represented in Question 9 was obtained using a Smart Cycler II real-time PCR machine purchased from Cepheid. Sigmoidal-shaped curves indicate amplification in vitro and, hence, presence of *N gonorrhoeae* and HSV-2 in the collected clinical sample. Horizontal lines represent no amplification and the absence of *T pallidum*, *H ducreyi*, and *C trachomatis* in the obtained clinical sample. Real-time PCR is becoming increasingly important in the clinical setting for rapid and sensitive identification of pathogens from clinically obtained samples, and thus should be a familiar process to every health care professional.

10. The answer is c. (*Brooks, pp 296-301. Levinson, pp 11-12, 33, 39. Ryan, p 22.*) Bacteria may shift rapidly between the fimbriated (fim +) and the nonfimbriated (fim −) states. Fimbriae function as adhesions to specific surfaces and, consequently, play a major role in pathogenesis. Lack of fimbriae prevents colonization of the mucosal surface by the bacterium. Pili (fimbriae) are hairlike appendages that extend several millimeters from the gonococcal surface. Fim changes would have no effect on capsule presence or loss of serologic specificity. Such changes would not cause the death of the organism, and *Neisseria* organisms never revert to a gram-positive staining result due to the major differences found in the structures of gram-positive and gram-negative cell walls.

11. The answer is d. (*Brooks, pp 257-260. Levinson, pp 140-142, 475s. Ryan, pp 354, 362-363.*) Region 1 (the O antigenic side chain of LPS) is responsible for the many serotypes of *Salmonella*. A mutant of *Salmonella* deficient in region 1 is not identified as a "newport," at least by virtue of its somatic antigen; biochemical identification of this mutant would be *S enteritidis* (*enterica*). Loss of region 1 does not affect genus and species classification of *Salmonella*. Loss of O groups is associated with a change from smooth to rough colony form. H antigens are related to motility (flagella presence or absence) while Vi antigens relate to virulence. There are more than 2500 serotypes of *Salmonella*, and DNA-DNA studies demonstrated seven evolutionary groups. Nearly all *Salmonella* human infections are in

DNA hybridization group I. Laboratory reports may use antigenic formulas following the species name because they impart more precise information about the isolates.

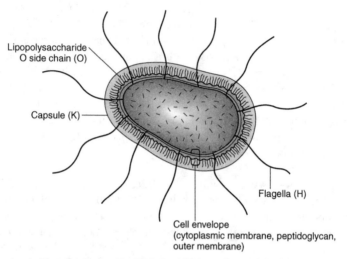

Lipopolysaccharide
O side chain (O)

Capsule (K)

Flagella (H)

Cell envelope
(cytoplasmic membrane, peptidoglycan,
outer membrane)

(Reproduced with permission from Toy EC, DeBord C, Wanger A, et al. Case Files: Microbiology. 2nd ed. New York, NY: McGraw-Hill; 2008:78.)

12. The answer is c. *(Brooks, pp 174-182. Levinson, pp 9, 69-72. Ryan, pp 36, 196.)* Transpeptidases or PBPs combine with penicillin to keep the final cross-linking step in the synthesis of peptidoglycan in the cell wall. All of the other choices are involved in polymerization processes. Examples of polymerization include the cell membrane (bactoprenol) and synthesis of DNA and RNA.

13. The answer is b. *(Brooks, pp 85-86. Levinson, pp 12-13. Ryan, pp 24-25.)* Dipicolinic acid, formed in the synthesis of diaminopimelate (DAP), is a prominent component of bacterial spores but is not found in vegetative cells or eukaryotic appendages or fimbrial structures. The calcium salt of dipicolinic acid apparently plays an important role in stabilizing spore proteins, but its mechanism of action is unknown. Dipicolinic acid synthetase is an enzyme unique to bacterial spores. Bacterial flagella and fimbriae (pili) and eukaryotic flagella and cilia have never been found to contain dipicolinic acid molecules.

14 and 15. The answers are 14-a, 15-b. *(Brooks, pp 52-54. Levinson, p 15. Ryan, pp 40-42.)* Bacterial growth curves are multiphasic. The lag phase is characterized by lack of growth but not necessarily metabolic activity. The bacteria are "adjusting" to their new environment. Depending on the bacteria, the temperature, nutrients, and pH, the microorganisms start dividing after a few hours and grow logarithmically for 12 to 18 hours. Toxins accumulate in the medium and nutrients become limiting. Oxygen and carbon dioxide are usually not limiting, as the gases freely diffuse into the growing culture. When death and growth of cells are equal, the stationary phase occurs. The death phase is characterized by a death rate that is more rapid than the growth rate. An antibiotic that inhibits protein synthesis would be optimally active in a rapidly dividing culture, where proteins are being rapidly synthesized, that is, the logarithmic phase. Bacteria introduced into the human host may undergo similar phases of growth. However, other factors such as host defenses play a major role in limiting logarithmic growth, as do accumulation of toxic by-products as might occur in a closed-space infection such as an abscess.

16. The answer is c. *(Brooks, pp 52-54. Levinson, pp 15-16. Ryan, pp 40-42.)* As described in the explanations for Questions 14 and 15, if fresh medium is not added during the logarithmic growth phase, toxic metabolic end products will accumulate in the growth medium. Bacteria may be maintained in the log growth phase by removing small amounts of growth medium and replacing it with that of fresh, new medium. No toxin accumulation sufficient to inhibit bacterial growth will occur. Without such treatment, however, bacterial growth will be inhibited by toxic metabolic products. The remaining options (accumulation of oxygen-free radicals, peroxidase, oxygen, or loss of SOD) may occur but would most likely not be as effective individually in limiting microbial growth.

17. The answer is c. *(Brooks, p 164. Levinson, pp 77-79. Ryan, pp 215-216.)* Ideally, antibiotics should attack a microbial structure or function not found in human cells. Except for mitomycin, all the antibiotics listed in the question interfere with cell wall synthesis in bacteria. Mitomycin inhibits DNA synthesis in both mammalian and microbial systems; viral DNA synthesis, however, is relatively resistant to mitomycin.

18 and 19. The answers are 18-b, 19-d. (*Brooks, p 39. Levinson, pp 7-8. Ryan, pp 16, 232-233.*) First described in 1884 by a Danish physician, Hans Christian Gram, the Gram stain has proved to be one of the most useful diagnostic laboratory procedures in microbiology and medicine. The Gram stain procedure is characterized by the following steps: (1) *fixation* of the bacteria to the slide, (2) crystal violet (acridine dye) treatment, (3) iodine treatment, (4) *decolorization* using alcohol/acetone wash, and (4) *counterstaining* using safranin. Gram-positive bacteria have thick outer walls with no lipids, whereas gram-negative bacteria have a thin wall and an outer membrane. The difference between gram-positive and gram-negative organisms is in the cell-wall permeability to these complexes on treatment with mixtures of acetone and alcohol solvents. Thus, gram-positive bacteria retain purple iodine-dye complexes, whereas gram-negative bacteria do not retain these complexes when decolorized using an alcohol/acetone wash. If the iodine treatment step is omitted during the Gram stain process, the purple iodine-dye complexes will not form. The crystal violet will wash away during the alcohol/acetone decolorization washing step and all cells will appear *red*. Gram staining of pus or fluids along with clinical findings can guide the management of an infection before culture results are available in the clinical setting.

20. The answer is e. (*Brooks, pp 25-27. Levinson, p 6. Ryan, pp 19, 21.*) A porin is a protein trimer with each subunit containing a pore with a diameter of 1 nm. Porins function in outer-membrane (OM) permeability. While porins are known to permit the transfer of small molecules (sugars, amino acids, and certain ions) across the OM, specific porins may also influence the diffusion of larger molecules. Also, porins can regulate the passage of many antimicrobial drugs such as ampicillin. Depending on charge, porins may also repel certain molecules, such as bile salts, found in the intestinal environment. Since porins are related only to the passive diffusion of low molecular weight hydrophilic compounds, they would play no role in the metabolism required for hydrolysis of antimicrobials, metabolism of metabolic intermediates, serologic stabilization of the O antigen, or inactivation of hydrophobic antimicrobials.

21. The answer is d. (*Brooks, pp 337-339. Levinson, pp 24, 176-177. Ryan, pp 434-437.*) The serologic diagnosis of Lyme disease is fraught with difficulty. Enzyme immunoassay (EIA) may be insensitive in the early stages of disease and may lack specificity in advanced stages. Western blot analysis of the antibody is the confirmatory test for Lyme disease, but it, too, is not 100% sensitive and specific. The Western blot test detects antibodies to proteins and glycoproteins of *Borrelia burgdorferi*. Not all of these proteins are specific for the organism. For example, antibodies to Gp66 may reflect a cross-reaction, as many gram-negative bacteria have similar glycoproteins. For this reason, a Western blot showing only antibodies to Gp66 is thought to be a nonspecific immune response.

In some symptomatic patients, the diagnosis of early Lyme disease can be established by observing the unique skin lesion (erythema migrans). If the lesion is absent or at a later stage of disease, specific Lyme disease must be differentiated from many other diseases. No one test is sensitive and specific. Blood is collected for serology, but culture is not usually performed. IFA, EIA, and Western Blot assays may not accurately identify Lyme disease specifically. PCR has been applied to the detection of *B burgdorferi* DNA in many body fluids and has been found to be rapid, sensitive, and specific, but it does not differentiate between live from dead (antibiotic treated) organisms. A screening test does not need to be repeated and differentiation between acute and chronic disease may depend upon the physician's interpretation of laboratory results. The specificity of a PCR test would be sufficient to rule out HIV testing while the significant Western Blot results for HIV correspond to p24, gp41, and gp120/160 (not Gp66).

22. The answer is b. (*Ryan, pp 251-253.*) DNA polymerase isolated from the hot springs thermophilic bacterium named *T aquaticus* is essential for the PCR process because of its stability at high temperatures (95°C). While the *E coli* enzyme can be used, the enzyme itself becomes denatured, fewer cycles are possible, and nonspecific reactions occur because of hybridization of primers to nontarget DNA. The use of Taq polymerase allows DNA copying at 72°C rather than 37°C, which further reduces nonspecific hybridization.

23 to 25. The answers are 23-b, 24-d, 25-e. (*Murray-2009, pp 165-168. Ryan, pp 251-255.*) The PCR has revolutionized the detection of infectious microorganisms, particularly those that are difficult to grow. During their normal practice, physicians will usually not be required to design a PCR test, but they should know some of the design elements of PCR so that they might better understand the results from these widely used tests.

One of the major problems of PCR in the past was contamination from extraneous nucleic acid. There are several ways to prevent contamination and the resulting falsely positive results. They include the use of separate laboratories, hoods, gloves, and surface disinfectants. The most effective method, however, is the use of internal sterilizing agents such as uracil N-glycosyls (UNG). These agents cross-link extraneous DNA so that the product cannot be amplified. Primers can now be purchased from a catalog and their sequence obtained online. Primers are easily synthesized, must be complementary to sequences on the bacterial chromosome, and when coupled to such sequences must promote replication. The specificity of PCR is a function of choosing a primer pair that is unique to the organism that you wish to detect. The PCR process is best explained by the "needle in the haystack" analogy. One needle in a haystack is difficult to find. However, if one needle becomes a million needles, then detection is easy. The same is true for nucleic acids. The amplicons (amplified nucleic acids) can be detected by a number of methods because they are so plentiful. These methods include specific staining with ethidium bromide of a gel containing these amplicons, and Southern blotting of the amplicons "tags" them so that they can be seen on photographic film. Amplicons are also bound to solid phases and detected with labeled enzymes or an instrument that reads a fluorescent tag. Microscopy is not used.

26. The answer is c. (*Brooks, pp 30, 161, 348. Levinson, pp 8-9, 89. Ryan, p 19.*) The organisms illustrated in the question are spheroplasts of *E coli*. Lysozyme cleaves the β-1-4-glycosidic bond between N-acetylmuramic acid and N-acetylglucosamine. Spheroplasts are bacteria with cell walls that have been partially removed by the action of lysozyme or penicillin. Ordinarily, with disintegration of the walls, the cells undergo lysis; however, in a hypertonic medium, the cells persist and assume a spherical configuration. Endospores are formed by gram-positive bacteria in the genera *Bacillus* and *Clostridium*. It has also been shown that for *E coli* and other gram-negative rods, exposure to minimal concentrations of antibiotics does not rupture the cell wall but promotes elongation of the cell by inhibiting the division cycle.

27. The answer is d. (*Brooks, pp 112-119. Ryan, pp 252-253.*) Gene cloning is a basic step in virtually every genetic engineering process. First, the source DNA is isolated and cut into small pieces and then attached to a cloning vector with DNA ligase. The cloning vectors are inserted into the host organism (usually a bacterium), and then the cloned DNA is isolated, identified, and purified. Amplification of source DNA is not a necessary step.

28. The answer is d. *(Brooks, pp 117-119. Ryan, pp 251-255.)* Nucleic acid probes, either DNA or RNA, are commonly used in clinical and research microbiology laboratories. These complementary pieces of nucleic acid bind to genes or gene parts of interest and are detected by their label, which may be either radioactive or nonradioactive. Probes, in general, are more sensitive than traditional growth-dependent methods, particularly for those microorganisms that either cannot be cultured or grow very slowly.

29. The answer is e. *(Brooks, pp 118-119. Murray-2009, pp 165-168. Ryan, pp 251-255.)* PCR is a widely used tool for amplification of small pieces of nucleic acid present in minute quantities. Once the sequence to be amplified is known, a specific forward and reverse primer is added. The temperature is alternately raised and lowered up to 45 to 50 times in the presence of a heat-resistant DNA polymerase from *T aquaticus*. The amplified gene product is then detected by one of a number of techniques such as cloning, direct hybridization, agarose gel electrophoresis, and southern hybridization. A heat-sensitive DNA polymerase would be destroyed by the PCR heating-cooling steps. Two primers are necessary to get both strands replicated. A small bench-top centrifuge is used in DNA preparation, not an ultra-centrifuge. A probe used to detect an amplified products needs to be extremely specific, not "universal."

30 to 33. The answers are 30-d, 31-e, 32-c, 33-b. *(Brooks, pp 52-60. Levinson, pp 15-16, 69-82. Ryan, pp 35, 41-42, 194-204.)* Penicillin causes lysis of growing bacterial cells. Its antimicrobial effect stems from impairment of cell-wall synthesis. Because penicillin is bactericidal, the number of viable cells should fall immediately after introduction of the drug into the medium.

Both chloramphenicol and sulfonamides are bacteriostatic—that is, they retard cell growth without causing cell death. Chloramphenicol causes an immediate, reversible, bacteriostatic inhibition of protein synthesis. Sulfonamides, on the other hand, compete with para-aminobenzoic acid in the synthesis of folate; intracellular stores of folate are depleted gradually as the cells continue to grow.

The number of viable cells in a culture eventually will level off, even if no antibiotic is added to the environment. A key factor in this phenomenon is the limited availability of substrate.

34 to 36.   The answers are 34-e, 35-d, 36-b. (Brooks, pp 103-107. Levinson, pp 17-22. Ryan, pp 57-64.) Transformation, transduction, and conjugation are critical processes in which DNA is transferred from one bacterium to another. Transformation, the passage of high-molecular-weight DNA from one bacterium to another, was first observed in pneumococci. Later studies have shown that, at least in S pneumoniae, double-stranded DNA is "nicked" by a membrane-bound endonuclease, initiating DNA entry into the host cell. One of the nicked DNA strands is digested, and the other is integrated into the host genome. Transduction, which can affect many bacteria, is a process in which a fragment of donor chromosome is carried to a recipient cell by a temperate virus (bacteriophage). In generalized transduction, the phage virus can carry any segment of the donor chromosome; in restricted transduction, the phage carries only those chromosomal segments immediately adjacent to the site of prophage attachment. In conjugation, too, DNA is passed from one bacterium to another. However, instead of the transfer of soluble DNA, a small loop of DNA, called a *plasmid*, is passed between cells. Examples of plasmids are the sex factors and the resistance (R) factors.

37.   The answer is d. (Brooks, pp 40-42, 52-55. Levinson, pp 15-16.) Bacteria reproduce by binary fission and thus undergo exponential (logarithmic) growth. In this question, the chart indicates a doubling time for E coli as 20 minutes. Therefore, after 2 hours there will be six doubling times. Using the equation 2^n, where n equals the number of generations, and remembering that we started with five E coli cells in the start culture, we rewrite this equation after 2 hours as "5×2^n"; thus, the number of E coli cells in the culture after 2 hours is $5 \times 2^6 = 320$.

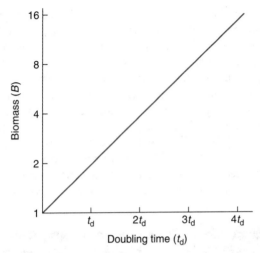

(Reproduced, with permission, from Brooks GF, et al. Jawetz's Medical Microbiology. 24th ed. New York, NY: McGraw-Hill; 2007:53.)

38. The answer is a. *(Brooks, pp 148-149. Levinson, pp 48-49. Ryan, pp 305-306.)* Koch postulates, formulated by Robert Koch in 1877, were an attempt to determine the cause of infectious disease. Simply stated, they consist of four statements: (1) a specific organism must be isolated from every diseased patient; (2) the organism must be isolated in vitro in pure culture; (3) when inoculated, the pure organism must cause the disease in a healthy, susceptible animal; and (4) the organism must be reisolated from the infected animal.

39. The answer is b. *(Brooks, p 29. Levinson, pp 6-7. Ryan, pp 15-31.)* The area indicated by the arrow in the diagram is known as the *periplasmic space*, which is the space between the plasma membrane and the outer membrane. This space contains many hydrolytic enzymes such as alkaline phosphatase, antibiotic-inactivating enzymes such as β-lactamases, and various binding proteins involved in chemotaxis and the active transport of solutes into the cell. RNA and DNA are in the cellular cytoplasm. Lipid A and LPS are part of the gram-negative cell wall, while techoic acid residues are found in some gram-positive cell walls.

40. The answer is d. (*Brooks, pp 2-3, 581-582. Levinson, pp 196-197, 317-321. Ryan, pp 80, 624-628.*) Prions are infectious particles that are composed solely of protein (ie, they contain no detectable nucleic acid). On the other hand, viruses contain both protein and nucleic acid. Prions give rise to a number of "slow" diseases known as transmissible spongiform encephalopathies such as Creutzfeldt-Jakob disease in humans, bovine spongiform encephalopathy in cows, and scrapie in sheep. Prions are unusually resistant to ultraviolet irradiation, alcohol, formalin, boiling, proteases, and nucleases. They can be inactivated by prolonged exposure to steam autoclaving or 1N or 2N NaOH. This has strong implications in the sterilization procedure used for certain medical instruments. The following table is an excellent comparison between conventional viruses and prions.

COMPARISON OF PRIONS AND CONVENTIONAL VIRUSES

Feature	Prions	Conventional Viruses
Particle contains nucleic acid	No	Yes
Particle contains protein	Yes, encoded by cellular genes	Yes, encoded by viral genes
Inactivated rapidly by UV light or heat	No	Yes
Appearance in electron microscope	Filamentous rods (amyloid-like)	Icosahedral or helical symmetry
Infection induces antibody	No	Yes
Infection induces inflammation	No	Yes

(*Reprinted, with permission, from Levinson W, Jawetz E. Medical Microbiology and Immunology. 7th ed. New York, NY: McGraw-Hill; 2002.*)

41 and 42. The answers are 41-e, 42-b. (*Brooks, pp 107-110. Levinson, pp 17-22. Ryan, pp 54-57. Mokrousov, pp 1417-142. Li, pp 74-80.*) Mutations result from three types of molecular changes, namely, base substitution mutation, frame shift mutation, and transposon or insertion sequences causing mutations. Inversion mutations are caused by insertion sequences (ISs) or IS-like elements. Missense mutation refers to base substitution resulting in a codon that causes a different amino acid to be inserted. Nonsense mutation refers to base substitution generating a termination codon that prematurely stops protein synthesis. Transition mutations are the replacement of a pyrimidine (C, T) by a pyrimidine or a purine (A, G) by a purine. Transversion mutations are the replacement of a purine by a pyrimidine or pyrimidine by a purine.

43 to 47. The answers are 43-d, 44-b, 45-c, 46-a, 47-e. *(Brooks, pp 182-184, 291-292. Levinson, pp 69-84. Murray-2009, pp 199-209. Ryan, pp 198, 220-221, 269-270, 305-307, 484-488.)* The patient in Question 43 is infected with *Yersinia pestis* and has bubonic plague. Ceftriaxone or cefotaxime are preferred in the treatment of childhood meningitis (Question 44) because they have the highest activity against the three major causes, namely, *H influenzae*, *N meningitidis*, and *S pneumoniae*. The patient in Question 45 has woolsorter's disease (inhalation anthrax) from contaminated wool on the farm where he works. Of the third-generation cephalosporins, only ceftazidime is consistently active against *Pseudomonas aeruginosa*. Finally, the patient in Question 47 has acquired a methicillin-resistant *S aureus* (MRSA) infection, against which vancomycin may be effective. However, *S aureus* strains are emerging with decreased susceptibility to vancomycin.

48 to 52. The answers are 48-e, 49-a, 50-d, 51-b, 52-c. *(Brooks, pp 174-182, 191-192, 650-651. Levinson, pp 69-84. Murray-2009, pp 199-209. Ryan, pp 195-198, 201-202, 204, 643-644.)* Trimethoprim (TMP), a diaminopyrimidine, is a folic acid antagonist. Although TMP is commonly used in combination with sulfa drugs, its mode of action is distinct. TMP is structurally similar to the pteridine portion of dihydrofolate and prevents the conversion of folic acid to tetrahydrofolic acid by inhibition of dihydrofolate reductase. Fortunately, this enzyme in humans is relatively insensitive to TMP.

The antibiotics in these questions have significantly different modes of action. Recent evidence suggests that while penicillin inhibits the final cross-linking of the cell wall, it also binds to penicillin-binding proteins and inhibits certain key enzymes involved in cell-wall synthesis. The mechanism is complex. Amdinocillin, although classified as penicillin, selectively binds to PBP-2. Binding to PBP-2 results in aberrant cell-wall elongation and spherical forms, seen when *E coli*, for example, is exposed to mecillinam.

The β-lactam drugs (penicillins, etc) are selective inhibitors of bacterial cell-wall synthesis and active against growing bacteria. These drugs bind to cell receptors (PBPs) and transpeptidation is inhibited. Lytic enzymes are activated and lysis of the bacteria occurs. Penicillin and cephalosporin drugs are similar in structure to acyl-D-alanyl-D-alanine and cause loss of D-alanine from the peptide involved in gram-positive cell wall cross-linking.

Because amphotericin binds to sterols (such as ergosterol, a compound of fungal membrane) in the cell membrane, its range of activity is predictable; that is, it is effective against microorganisms that contain sterol in the cell membrane (such as molds, yeasts, and certain amebas). These polyene antibiotics cause reorientation of sterols in the membrane, and membrane structure is altered to the extent that permeability is affected. If sterol synthesis is blocked in fungi, then amphotericin is not effective. This occurs when fungi are exposed to miconazole, another antifungal antibiotic.

Chloramphenicol can be either bacteriocidal or bacteriostatic, depending on the organism. It is bacteriostatic against organisms such as *S typhi*, but is bacteriocidal against encapsulated organisms that cause meningitis such as *H influenzae*, *S pneumoniae*, and *N meningitidis*. Bacterial ribosomes are spherical particles. Protein synthesis takes place on the ribosome by a complex process involving various ribosomal subunits, tRNA, and mRNA. Chloramphenicol, in contrast to the aminoglycosides and tetracycline, attaches to the 50S ribosome subunit. The enzyme peptidyl transferase, found in the 50S subunit, is inhibited. Removal of the inhibition—in this case, chloramphenicol—results in full activity of the enzyme.

53 to 57. The answers are 53-d, 54-c, 55-a, 56-c, 57-b. (*Brooks, pp 116-118. Murray-2009, pp 165-168. Ryan, pp 251-255.*) The process of PCR is complicated, and its steps are interrelated. A number of steps in the process can markedly affect the results of clinical testing. For example, the detection of amplified products is essential in order to determine whether target nucleic acid was present in the specimen. Product can be detected by staining of the gel that separates the products, Southern blot (a radioactive procedure), or an ELISA-like capture method. A failure of this production step prevents detection of product.

One of the essential parts of the PCR process is the thermal cycling of the reaction. If the reaction is not heated, primer DNA will not hybridize with the target sequences. Nor will the strands reanneal if the mixture is not cooled. Failure of the thermocycler could cause such a problem.

False-positive results are usually due to contamination of the reaction by foreign DNA. In such a case, the foreign DNA sequences are amplified even if the target sequences are not present.

There are a number of reasons why PCR would be falsely negative, but a prime reason is failure to choose the right primer sets. Suboptimum detection of amplified products is another reason. Ethidium bromide staining of the PCR gel is less sensitive than detection of the products by Southern blot.

58. The answer is e. *(Brooks, pp 302-303. Levinson, pp 119-123. Ryan, pp 19-20.)* At least 13 serogroups of meningococci have been identified by immunologic specificity of capsular antigens. A, B, C, Y, and W are the most important strains associated with disease. Virulence factors include capsules, endotoxin, and pili. Porin proteins are integral outer membrane proteins that form channels for nutrients to pass into the cell and waste to exit. The gene products, Por A and Por B proteins, are both expressed in *N meningitidis*, the Por A gene is silent to *N gonorrhoeae*. Por B is an important virulence factor for *N gonorrhoeae*, affecting neutrophil function, facilitating bacterial invasion into epithelial cells, and making bacteria resistant to complement-mediated serum killing. The γ-glutamyl polypeptide forms the capsule of *B anthrasis*, while hyaluronic acid provides a capsular function for streptococci. Outer membrane proteins are found in all gram-negative bacteria. *Streptococcus pneumoniae* type 3 has a capsule composed of glucose and glucuronic acid residues.

59. The answer is b. *(Brooks, pp 235-240. Levinson, pp 111-116. Ryan, p 276.)* Group A streptococci in the early stages of growth have hyaluronic acid capsules. This capsule (similar to human hyaluronic acid structure) is rapidly destroyed by the organism's own hyaluronidase. Bacteria have a variety of components; some are unique to certain genera and species, others are characteristic of all bacteria. All bacteria have peptidoglycan in their cell walls, although the peptidoglycan layer is much thinner in gram-negative than in gram-positive bacteria. In gram-positive bacteria, teichoic acids, polysaccharides, and peptid glycolipids are covalently attached to the peptidoglycans.

60. The answer is b. *(Brooks, pp 24-29. Levinson, pp 9-10, 13, 46. Ryan, pp 19-20.)* The LPS of gram-negative cell walls consists of a complex glycolipid, called Lipid A, and is attached to a polysaccharide core. Lipid A is embedded in the outer leaflet of the membrane anchoring the LPS. LPS is required for the function of many outer membrane proteins. The polysaccharide core is similar in all gram-negative species that have LPS which includes two characteristic sugars, ketodeoxyoctulonate acid and a heptose. LPS (endotoxin) is firmly bound to the cell surface and is released only when the cells are lysed. Sialic acid polymers are found in Group B *N meningitidis* and *E coli* K1.

61. The answer is a. *(Brooks, pp 320-331. Levinson, pp 161-168. Ryan, pp 439-442.)* Mycobacteria are rod-shaped, aerobic bacteria that do not form spores. While *Mycobacterium* also has peptidoglycan, up to 40% of the cell wall may be a waxy glycolipid that is responsible for the "acid fastness" of *Mycobacterium* and *Nocardia*, an aerobic actinomycete. They are neither gram-positive nor gram-negative since once stained, they resist decolorization by acid or alcohol and are called "acid-fast." Acid-fastness depends on the integrity of the waxy envelope. The Ziehl-Neelsen technique is used to identify acid-fast bacteria.

62. The answer is a. *(Brooks, pp 203-206. Levinson, pp 124-126. Ryan, pp 305-307.)* *Bacillus anthracis* produces an unusual capsule, composed of glutamic acid subunits. The capsule prevents phagocytosis of the organisms by PMNs and is an important virulence factor. Strains that do not produce capsules are nonvirulent.

63. The answer is d. *(Brooks, pp 241-242. Levinson, pp 116-118. Ryan, pp 288-293.)* Capsules are found in both gram-positive and gram-negative bacteria. With the exception of those found in *Bacteroides fragilis*, capsules are not in and of themselves toxic but rather are antiphagocytic and are immunologic (or serologic) determinants. The α-hemolytic streptococci produce capsules composed of hyaluronic acid, while *S pneumoniae* strains produce capsules of a repeating polysaccharide composed of glucose and glucuronic acid.

Virology

Questions

64. A human immunodeficiency virus (HIV)-positive patient has progressed from fatigue, rash, nausea, and night sweats to occasional but defined opportunistic infections. He inquires as to what can be done to predict his chances of developing symptomatic AIDS. Which of the following tests would be most useful?

a. CD4 lymphocyte count
b. HIV antibody test
c. HIV p24 antigen
d. HIV reverse transcriptase (RT) PCR
e. Neopterin

65. A 9-year-old male presents with fever and nonspecific symptoms followed by a distinctive rash on the cheeks (slapped cheek). Which of the following viruses is the most likely cause of this disease and has been associated with transient aplastic crises in persons with sickle cell disease?

a. *Herpes simplex*
b. Parvovirus B19
c. Rubella
d. Rubeola
e. Varicella-zoster

66. A 20-year-old female presents to her physician with a low-grade fever, headache, and painful genital lesions. Culture detects herpes simplex virus (HSV). Which of the following best describes infection with this common human pathogen?

a. Infection with type 1 virus is most common.
b. Initial infection usually occurs by intestinal absorption of the virus.
c. It can be reactivated by emotional disturbances.
d. It rarely recurs in a host who has a high antibody titer.
e. The central nervous system (CNS) and visceral organs are usually involved.

67. A 24-year-old street person, who is a known user of injection drugs, complains of a series of opportunistic infections that have recently affected him. His community health program tests him for HIV and finds him positive in the screening and confirmatory tests. He is to start on a highly active antiretroviral therapy (HAART) program, which became available in 1996, utilizing azidothymidine (AZT), dideoxyinosine (DDI), and saquinavir or similar agents. By 1997, HIV/AIDS dropped from the first to the second leading cause of death in young adults in the United States. By 2000, it was not even one of the top 10 causes of death in this group. Use of these three drugs inhibits which of the following viral processes?

a. All membrane synthesis
b. Glycoprotein (gp) 120 formation
c. Protein (p) 24 antibody expression
d. Reverse transcriptase, protease
e. RNase, DNase

68. An HIV-positive patient, prior to being treated with AZT, DDI, and saquinavir, has a CD4 lymphocyte count and an HIV RNA viral load test done. Results are as follows:

CD4: 50 CD4 lymphocytes per μL
HIV RNA: 100,000 copies per mL

Which of the following best describes this patient?

a. This patient is no longer in danger of opportunistic infection.
b. The 5-year prognosis is excellent.
c. The patient's HIV screening test is most likely negative.
d. The patient is not infectious.
e. The viral load of 100,000 copies per milliliter suggests that the patient will respond to triple therapy.

69. An HIV-positive patient with a viral load of 100,000 copies of HIV RNA per milliliter and a total CD4 count of 50 is at increased risk for a number of infectious diseases. For which of the following diseases is the patient at no more added risk than an immunocompetent host?

a. Herpes simplex virus
b. Kaposi sarcoma
c. Mycobacterial disease
d. Pneumococcal pneumonia
e. Pneumocystic pneumonia

70. A 19-year-old college student presents to the student health clinic complaining of sore throat, fever, swollen neck lymph nodes, and malaise of several days. Viral capsid antibody (IgM) tests are positive, indicating infectious mononucleosis. This potentially debilitating viral disorder is characterized by which of the following?

a. Affected persons respond to treatment with the production of heterophil antibodies.
b. It is caused by a rhabdovirus.
c. It is most prevalent in children less than 14 years old.
d. Ribavirin is the treatment of choice.
e. The causative pathogen is an Epstein-Barr virus (EBV).

71. During a medical checkup for a new insurance policy, a 60-year-old grandmother is found to be positive in the enzyme-linked immunosorbent assay (ELISA) screening test for antibodies against HIV-1. She has no known risk factors for exposure to the virus. Which of the following is the most appropriate next step?

a. Immediately begin therapy with azidothymidine.
b. Perform the screening test a second time.
c. Request that a blood culture be done by the laboratory.
d. Tell the patient that she is likely to develop AIDS.
e. Test the patient for *Pneumocystis jiroveci* infection.

72. Patients in an outbreak of arbovirus disease on a Caribbean island present with a variety of symptoms, including encephalitis, hemorrhagic fever, or fever with myalgia. Which of the following is a characteristic of arboviruses?

a. Are closely related to Parvoviruses
b. Are transmitted by insect vectors
c. Are treatable with antiviral chemotherapy
d. Are usually resistant to ether
e. Usually cause symptomatic infection in humans

73. Recombinant interferon-α (IFN-α) is the currently approved therapy for patients who are chronically infected with hepatitis B virus (HBV) or hepatitis C virus (HCV). IFN was originally described in chicken embryo cells infected with influenza viruses. Which of the following statements best describes IFN's suspected mode of action as an antiviral reagent?

a. It stimulates a cell-mediated immunity.
b. It stimulates humoral immunity.
c. Its direct antiviral action is related to the suppression of messenger RNA formation.
d. Its action is related to the synthesis of a protein that inhibits translation or transcription.
e. It alters the permeability of the cell membrane so that viruses cannot enter the cell.

74. In the severe acute respiratory syndrome (SARS) outbreak in Canada, cases progressed from mild to severe respiratory distress, requiring ventilatory support for a substantial number of cases. A death rate of 10% was experienced due to progressive respiratory failure in a number of patients. Coronaviruses have characteristic large, widely spaced spikes that form a "corona" around the virion. In 2003, over 8000 cases of SARS (severe respiratory illness and failure) occurred in 29 countries with a mortality rate of almost 10%. Which of the following is a characteristic ability of non–SARS coronaviruses?

a. Agglutinate human white blood cells
b. Cause common cold
c. Grow profusely at 50°C
d. Grow well in the usual cultured cell lines
e. Infect infants more frequently than adults

75. An elderly male patient with known chronic HBV status suddenly presents with acute hepatitis episodes. Serology confirms hepatitis D virus (HDV) coinfection. Which one of the following best describes the delta agent?

a. A hepatitis B mutant
b. A defective RNA virus
c. An incomplete hepatitis B virus
d. Hepatitis C mutant
e. Related to hepatitis A virus

76. Antiviral compounds are well known for herpes viruses and some retroviruses, but direct, specific antiviral chemotherapy for many human viruses is still being sought. Which of the following antiviral agents is a purine nucleoside analogue that has shown promise with Lassa fever, influenza A and B, and respiratory syncytial virus (RSV)?

a. Amantadine
b. Acyclovir
c. Ribavirin
d. Rimantadine
e. Vidarabine

77. A clinic associated with a medical school and located in a lower income city district documents a series of cases involving picornaviruses in school-age children. Most cases experienced complete recovery even without specific antiviral therapy. Enteric cytopathogenic human orphan viruses (echoviruses) appear worldwide and are more apt to be found in young patients. Family studies demonstrated the ease and high frequency of transmission. Which of the following body systems is the main target of echoviruses?

a. Bladder and urinary tract
b. Blood and lymphatic systems
c. Central nervous system
d. Intestinal tract
e. Respiratory system

78. A newborn infant presents with disseminated vesicular lesions and failure to thrive. Herpes simplex virus (HSV) is suspected, and laboratory confirmation is desired to justify antiviral chemotherapy. Which of the following is the most sensitive test for the diagnosis of HSV meningitis in a newborn infant?

a. Cerebrospinal fluid (CSF) protein analysis
b. HSV culture
c. HSV IgG antibody
d. HSV polymerase chain reaction
e. Tzanck smear

79. An outbreak of acute hemorrhagic conjunctivitis (AHC) was reported in school-age children in India. The infections were characterized by conjunctival congestion, vascular dilation, and onset of edema. Seroepidemiology studies of AHC patients showed that AHC is caused by which of the following viruses?

a. Coronavirus
b. Enterovirus
c. Reovirus
d. Respiratory syncytial virus
e. Rhinovirus

80. A 10-year-old boy is taken to his pediatrician after experiencing fever, malaise, and anorexia followed by tender swelling of his parotid glands. Which of the following characterizes infection by this etiologic agent?

a. Is apt to recur periodically in many affected persons
b. Is maintained in a large canine reservoir
c. Is preventable by immunization
d. Usually produces severe systemic manifestations
e. Will usually cause orchitis in postpubertal males

81. An otherwise healthy 65-year-old male was in a car accident and broke several ribs on the left side. Approximately 12 days later he develops a painful, well-circumscribed vesicular rash over the left rib cage that persists for several weeks. The rash is most likely due to which of the following?

a. Primary infection with herpes B virus
b. Primary infection with herpes simplex virus type 1
c. Primary infection with herpes simplex virus type 2
d. Reactivation of latent Epstein-Barr virus
e. Reactivation of latent varicella-zoster virus

82. A 3-year-old child presents at the physician's office with symptoms of coryza, conjunctivitis, low-grade fever, and small, bluish-white ulcerations on the buccal mucosa opposite the lower molars. The causative agent of this disease belongs to which one of the following groups of viruses?

a. Adenovirus
b. Herpesvirus
c. Paramyxovirus
d. Picornavirus
e. Orthomyxovirus

83. A young woman who has lived on the street for several years has a legal and medical history of prostitution and drug use. An examination at a public health clinic diagnoses her as having genital warts. No specific antiviral therapy is available for this condition, but it is now known that cell-mediated immunity is important for virus eradication, and an approved vaccine is available that should be given before sexual activity occurs. Which one of the following viruses is the basis for this vaccine?

a. Adenovirus
b. Cytomegalovirus
c. Epstein-Barr virus
d. Herpes simplex virus
e. Papillomavirus

84. Two siblings, ages 2 and 4, experience fever, rhinitis, and pharyngitis that result in laryngotracheo-bronchitis. Both have a harsh cough and hoarseness. Which of the following viruses is the leading cause of their syndrome?

a. Adenovirus
b. Group B coxsackievirus
c. Parainfluenza virus (RSV)
d. Rhinovirus
e. Rotavirus

85. In an area of India with poor sanitation, an outbreak of hepatitis E virus (HEV) occurs. A number of women in the area are pregnant, creating concern due to the higher mortality seen in this patient group. HEV is an RNA virus and may be classified as a calicivirus. While it presents primarily as an acute disease, there is no treatment or vaccine currently available. Which of the following statements is most accurate regarding hepatitis E virus?

a. It is not a threat to the blood supply.
b. It is a major cause of bloodborne hepatitis.
c. It is prevalent in North America.
d. It is a single-stranded DNA virus.
e. The disease resembles hepatitis C.

86. An 18-year-old man was taken to an emergency medicine department because of fever and complaints of a stiff neck. No bacterial agents appeared to be involved and an initial diagnosis of aseptic meningitis was made. During the initial 24 hours of the course of aseptic meningitis, an affected person's CSF is characterized by which of the following laboratory findings?

a. Decreased protein content
b. Elevated glucose concentration
c. Eosinophilia
d. Lymphocytosis
e. Polymorphonuclear leukocytosis

87. A street person well known to the local public health clinic appears to have acute symptoms of hepatitis and tests positive for hepatitis D virus (HDV) antigen. Knowing that HDV requires hepatitis B virus coinfection, which of the following serologic tests can be used to determine whether a patient with HDV is an HBV carrier?

a. HCVcAg
b. HBc IgM
c. HBeAg
d. HBs IgM
e. HBs IgG

88. A nurse develops clinical symptoms consistent with hepatitis. She recalls sticking herself with a needle approximately 4 months before, after drawing blood from a patient. Serologic tests for HBsAg, antibodies to HBsAg, and hepatitis A virus (HAV) are all negative; however, she is positive for IgM core antibody. Which of the following characterizes the current health state of the nurse?

a. Does not have hepatitis B
b. Has hepatitis A
c. Has hepatitis C
d. Is in the late stages of hepatitis B infection
e. Is in the "window" (after the disappearance of HBsAg and before the appearance of anti–HBsAg)

89. A 62-year-old Florida fisherman forgot his insect repellent on a recent sporting trip. A week later, he presented to his physician with fever, chills, headache, and flu-like symptoms that progressed to possible CNS involvement. Control of the etiologic agent, associated with a high (50%-70%) fatality rate, could be possible by eradication of which of the following?

a. Birds
b. Fleas
c. Horses
d. Mosquitoes
e. Ticks

90. A local school district finds large numbers of student absences, with the children presenting with mild upper respiratory symptoms. The local health department finds that rhinoviruses are the most commonly recovered agents. Very brief incubation periods were noted. These agents are primarily transmitted by which one of the following mechanisms?

a. Droplet aerosolization
b. Fecal-oral route
c. Fomites
d. Sexual activity
e. Vertical transmission (mother to child)

91. A 9-year-old schoolchild develops malaise, a low-grade fever, and a morbilliform rash that appears on the same day. The rash started on the face and spread to the extremities. Small, light-colored ulcerations appeared on the buccal mucosa right before the rash appeared. Which of the following best describes the etiologic agent causing this disease?

a. Incubation time is approximately 3 to 4 weeks.
b. Measles (rubeola) and German measles (rubella) are caused by the same virus.
c. Onset is abrupt, with cough, coryza, and fever lasting 3 days.
d. Specific antibody in the serum does not prevent disease.
e. Vesicular rashes are characteristic.

92. A biopsy specimen is collected from the skin of the neck and at the hairline of a patient from outside the United States who presents with possible encephalitis. Impression materials are stained with immunofluorescent reagents including a monoclonal antibody, currently considered the most rapid and accurate diagnostic procedure for this case. Results demonstrate host intranuclear inclusions, which are sharply demarcated, spherical, and less than 10 μm in diameter. Which of the following is the most likely diagnosis?

a. Aseptic meningitis
b. Congenital rubella
c. Infectious mononucleosis
d. Mumps
e. Rabies

93. Kuru is a fatal disease of certain New Guinea natives and is characterized by tremors and ataxia; Creutzfeldt-Jakob disease (CJD) is characterized by both ataxia and dementia. CJD has been accidentally transferred to others by contaminated growth hormone from human pituitary glands, corneal transplants, and contaminated surgical instruments. These diseases are thought to be caused by which of the following?

a. Cell wall-deficient bacteria
b. Environmental toxins
c. Flagellates
d. Prions
e. Slow viruses

94. Vaccinia virus vaccine was used to eliminate variola from the world population. Recent concerns about possible terrorist use of variola have resulted in new recommendations for use of the vaccine. According to recommendations issued by the US Public Health Service, which of the following statements regarding vaccination against smallpox is currently most accurate?

a. Children should be vaccinated before they begin school.
b. Persons traveling abroad need not be vaccinated.
c. Persons who have eczema should be vaccinated soon after diagnosis.
d. Persons who have immune deficiencies should be vaccinated every 5 years.
e. Pregnant women should be vaccinated in the first trimester.

95. A 35-year-old man developed headache, nausea, vomiting, and sore throat 8 weeks after returning from a trip abroad. He eventually refused to drink water and had episodes of profuse salivation, difficulty in breathing, and hallucinations. Two days after the patient died of cardiac arrest, it was learned that he had been bitten by a dog while on his trip. Which of the following treatments, if given immediately after the dog bite, could have helped prevent this disease?

a. Bed rest
b. Interleukin 2
c. High-dose acyclovir
d. Broad-spectrum antibiotics
e. Vaccine specific for the etiologic agent

96. A patient who works in an industrial setting presents to his ophthalmologist with acute conjunctivitis, enlarged and tender preauricular nodes, and early stages of keratitis. The differential diagnosis should include infection with which of the following viruses?

a. Adenovirus
b. Epstein-Barr virus
c. Parvovirus
d. Respiratory syncytial virus
e. Varicella-zoster virus

97. A hospital worker is found to have hepatitis B surface antigen. Subsequent tests reveal the presence of e antigen as well. Which of the following best describes the worker?

a. Is infective and has active hepatitis
b. Is infective but does not have active hepatitis
c. Is not infective
d. Is evincing a biologic false-positive test for hepatitis
e. Has both hepatitis B and hepatitis C

98. A 12-year-old boy from a rural community returned from a summer camping experience, and 1 week later had flu-like symptoms and headache. His physician was concerned about potential encephalitis and ordered serological testing. Which of the following diseases is caused by an alphavirus?

a. Dengue
b. Marburg virus disease
c. Saint Louis encephalitis
d. Western equine encephalitis
e. Yellow fever

99. A 2-month-old infant was admitted to the medical center for treatment of bronchiolitis. A virus was isolated and identified by the clinical laboratory. Ribavirin treatment was started immediately and is a purine nucleoside analog with a relatively broad antiviral spectrum in cell culture, possibly using several different mechanisms. Original FDA approval for ribavirin use was against which virus listed below?

a. Group A coxsackievirus
b. Hepatitis B virus
c. Herpes simplex virus
d. Parvovirus
e. Respiratory syncytial virus

100. An immunocompromised person with a history of seizures has an MRI that reveals a temporal lobe lesion. Brain biopsy results show multinucleated giant cells with intranuclear inclusions. Which of the following is the most probable cause of the lesion?

a. Coxsackievirus
b. Hepatitis C virus
c. Herpes simplex virus
d. *Listeria monocytogenes*
e. Parvovirus

101. A 19-year-old college freshwoman seeks medical help for symptoms of headache, malaise, fatigue, and sore throat. She admits to attending multiple parties in the dorm. Her physician notes her enlarged lymph nodes and spleen. Which of the following procedures or clinical signs is most specific for the diagnosis of infectious mononucleosis caused by the Epstein-Barr virus (EBV)?

a. B-cell lymphocyte proliferation
b. Growth in tissue culture cells
c. Heterophile antibodies in serum
d. Laboratory diagnosis based on the presence of atypical lymphocytes and EBV-specific antibody
e. Lymphadenopathy and splenomegaly on physical examination

102. A 5-month-old infant, seen in the emergency room (ER), presents with fever and persistent cough with wheezing. Physical examination and a chest x-ray suggest pneumonia. Which of the following is most likely the cause of this infection?

a. Adenovirus
b. Coxsackievirus
c. Respiratory syncytial virus
d. Rhinovirus
e. Rotavirus

103. Which one of the following groups of people may be at increased risk for HIV infection?

a. Factory workers whose coworkers are HIV-positive
b. Foreign services employees who are hospitalized in Zaire for bleeding ulcers
c. Homosexual females
d. Members of a household in which there is a person who is HIV-positive
e. Receptionists at a hospital

104. An obstetrician sees a pregnant patient who was exposed to rubella virus in the 18th week of pregnancy. She does not remember getting a rubella vaccination. Which of the following is the best immediate course of action?

a. Administer rubella immune globulin.
b. Administer rubella vaccine.
c. Order a rubella antibody titer to determine immune status.
d. Reassure the patient because rubella is not a problem until after the 30th week.
e. Terminate the pregnancy.

105. Mad cow disease emerged in Great Britain in 1986 and indications arose to indicate that humans could also be infected. Human cases showed changes in cerebral function (memory loss, confusion) and death within a few years. This disease is caused by which of the following?

a. A prion
b. A virus
c. A bacterium with a defective cell wall
d. An autoimmune reaction
e. *Rickettsia rickettsiae*

106. A traveler visited a geographic area where hepatitis A was endemic and did not remember to take γ-globulin for passive protection. Four weeks later, he experienced fever, nausea, and jaundice, with dark urine. HAV infection was suspected, but all the tests for HAV-IgG and HAV-IgM were nonreactive. Which of the following is the most likely cause of this infection?

a. Hepatitis B surface antigen
b. Hepatitis C
c. Hepatitis D
d. Hepatitis E
e. Rotavirus

107. A 70-year-old nursing home patient refused the influenza vaccine and subsequently developed influenza. She died of acute pneumonia 1 week after contracting the flu. Which of the following is the most common cause of acute post-influenza pneumonia?

a. *Escherichia coli*
b. *Klebsiella pneumoniae*
c. *Legionella pneumophila*
d. *Listeria monocytogenes*
e. *Staphylococcus aureus*

108. A 5-year-old boy was sent home from kindergarten because his left eye was red with a watery, nonpurulent discharge. Several of his classmates recently had mild sore throat but no fever. Conjunctivitis lasted 1 week with complete recovery. Which of the following organisms was the most likely cause of his infection?

a. Adenovirus
b. Herpes simplex virus
c. *Staphylococcus aureus*
d. *Chlamydia trachomatis*
e. *Hemophilus aegyptius*

109. A husband and wife performed the yearly spring cleaning of their mountain cabin, located in the southwestern part of the United States. The wife presented to her physician 2 weeks later with fever, myalgia, headache, and nausea, followed by progressive pulmonary edema. Which of the following best describes the pathogen or disease progression in this patient?

a. Hemolysis is common in infected patients.
b. Influenza-like symptoms are followed rapidly by acute respiratory failure.
c. It is acquired by inhalation of aerosols of the urine and feces of deer.
d. Transmission from human to human is common.
e. There is effective antiviral therapy available.

110. A 27-year-old professional businesswoman was diagnosed as having a mild case of genital warts. A laboratory test was able to identify papillomavirus type 16 being present in the tissue. It was decided that removal by means of liquid nitrogen would be utilized. Which of the following best applies to the oncogenes of DNA viruses?

a. They are early viral genes that perform essential viral functions.
b. They are cell genes that are expressed during embryonic development.
c. They encode a protein that has tyrosine kinase–like activity.
d. They are virtually identical to the oncogenes of RNA tumor viruses.
e. They are cell genes accidentally incorporated into the viral genome.

111. A 32-year-old gay male went to his community STD clinic, where it was found that he had perianal condyloma acuminatum. No antiviral chemotherapy was considered because of noncompliance of the patient. Physical removal was recommended. Which of the following viruses may be a definitive human tumor virus?

a. Epstein-Barr virus (EBV)
b. Herpes simplex virus type 2 (HSV-2)
c. Human immunodeficiency virus (HIV)
d. Papillomavirus
e. Varicella-zoster virus (VZV)

112. A young, elementary school student who was reported to have had recent mild flu-like symptoms was taken to his family physician because of the appearance of an erythematous facial rash. The physician told the parents that the rash would fade in 2 to 4 days and was caused by circulating IgM-virus complexes. Which of the diseases listed below is caused by Parvovirus B19 and presents as a highly significant medical problem?

a. Aplastic crisis in chronic anemia
b. Epidemic acute respiratory disease
c. Gastroenteritis
d. Keratoconjunctivitis
e. Whooping cough–like disease

113. Within the first year of life, an infant exhibited severe hearing loss, ocular abnormalities, and apparent mental retardation. Standard peripheral blood smears demonstrated multinucleated cells with giant nuclei and intranuclear inclusions. Which of the following best describes the etiologic agent?

a. It can be transmitted across the placental barrier.
b. While a common infection, CMV is almost always symptomatic.
c. The CMV can be cultured from red blood cells of infected patients.
d. Unlike other viral infections, CMV is not activated by immunosuppressive therapy.
e. There is no specific therapy for CMV.

114. An outbreak of acute viral gastroenteritis occurred in a child-care center, with several very young children exhibiting nausea, vomiting, and watery, nonbloody diarrhea. Which of the following characterizes routine human rotavirus infections?

a. They produce an infection that is seen primarily in adults.
b. They produce cytopathic effects in many conventional tissue culture systems.
c. They are lipid-containing RNA viruses possessing a double-shelled capsid.
d. They can be sensitively and rapidly detected in stools by the ELISA technique.
e. They have been implicated as a major etiologic agent of infantile respiratory disease.

115. Subacute sclerosing panencephalitis (SSPE) is characterized by inflammatory lesions and begins with mild changes in personality, ending with dementia and death. Which of the following best describes the disease characteristics?

a. Demyelination is characteristic.
b. It is a common event occurring in 1 of 300,000 cases of mumps.
c. It is a late CNS manifestation of mumps.
d. It is a progressive disease involving both white and gray matter.
e. Viral DNA can be demonstrated in brain cells.

116. The virus shown below contains double-stranded RNA within a double-walled capsid. It was obtained from a 9-month old child in rural India who had been brought to a village clinic suffering from severe dehydration and general failure to thrive. No specific antiviral therapy was available. Which of the following best describes this agent?

(Reproduced, with permission, from Bhushan et al. First Aid for the USMLE Step 1. New York, NY: McGraw-Hill; 2006: 155.)

a. Early breast-feeding offers no protection to neonates against it.
b. It is a major cause of neonatal diarrhea.
c. It is readily cultured from the stool of infected persons.
d. Maternal antibody does not appear to be protective.
e. There are no related animal viruses.

117. A young child was taken to the family physician with a barking cough and difficult breathing. Laboratory tests identified a helical virus with a negative sense linear RNA genome as the etiologic agent. Which disease listed below is most commonly associated with this virus?

a. Croup
b. Fifth disease
c. Otitis media
d. Rubella
e. Tonsillitis

118. A transplant patient taking high levels of immunosuppressive medications becomes infected with Epstein-Barr virus (EBV) and develops a lymphoma. The dosage of immunosuppressive drugs given to the patient is decreased, and the tumor regresses. Which of the following properties of EBV infection is related to the patient's tumor development?

a. Immortalization of B cells
b. Increased white blood cell count
c. Presence of atypical lymphocytes
d. Production of heterophile antibodies

119. A 39-year old man volunteering his assistance in a refugee camp in central Africa was injured in an auto accident and received several units of blood as part of his medical treatment. Six months later, he experienced fatigue, nausea, and night sweats. Plasma HIV RNA tests were positive and appropriate anti-HIV treatment was started. Reverse transcriptase is an enzyme found in retroviruses and hepadnaviruses. Which of the following is a function of the enzyme reverse transcriptase?

a. DNAse activity
b. DNA-dependent RNA polymerase activity
c. RNA-dependent DNA polymerase activity
d. RNA-dependent RNA polymerase activity
e. RNA isomerase activity

120. Several young adults camped in a wilderness area and received multiple mosquito bites. Ten days later, one had a sudden onset of headache, chills, and fever, and became stuporous 48 hours later. He was diagnosed with Saint Louis encephalitis (SLE) and recovered completely. Which of the following best describes SLE?

a. It is transmitted to humans by the bite of an infected tick.
b. It is caused by a togavirus.
c. It is the major arboviral cause of central nervous system infection in the United States.
d. It always presents initially with influenza-like symptoms.
e. Laboratory diagnosis is routinely made by cultural methods.

121. There is considerable overlap of signs and symptoms seen in congenital and perinatal infections. In a neonate with classic symptoms of congenital cytomegalovirus (CMV) infection, which of the following tests would be most useful in establishing a diagnosis?

a. CMV IgG titer on neonate's serum at birth
b. CMV IgG titer on mother's serum at birth of infant
c. CMV IgM titer on neonate's serum at birth and at 1 month of age
d. Culture of mother's urine
e. Total IgM on neonate's serum at birth

122. A middle-aged man with a long history of multiple operations and blood transfusions was diagnosed with chronic hepatitis C. He was then treated with pegylated interferon (IFN) and ribavirin. Such treatments became available because of early studies that showed polyethylene glycol (PEG) causes the IFN to remain in the body longer and prolong the effects of the material. Interferons are host-coded proteins that are cytokines and are produced within hours of microbial infection. IFNs then modulate humoral and cellular immunity. Which of the following stimulates IFN production in patients and cells in tissue culture?

a. Botulinum toxin
b. Chlamydiae
c. Gram-positive bacteria
d. Synthetic polypeptides
e. Viruses

123. A 35-year-old man presents with symptoms of jaundice, right upper quadrant pain, and vomiting. His ALT is elevated. He is diagnosed with HAV infection after eating at a restaurant where others were also infected. Which of the following should be done to protect his family members?

a. A series of three vaccinations at 0, 1, and 6 months.
b. Administer α-interferon.
c. Quarantine household contacts and observe.
d. No treatment is necessary.
e. One dose of γ-globulin administered intramuscularly.

124. A 17-year-old girl presents with cervical lymphadenopathy, fever, and pharyngitis. Which of the following is the most rapid and clinically useful test to make a diagnosis?

a. Antibody to Epstein-Barr nuclear antigen (EBNA)
b. C-reactive protein (CRP)
c. Culture
d. IgG antibody to viral core antigen (VCA)
e. IgM antibody to viral core antigen

125. A latent infection is usually manifested by persistence of viral genomes, expression of none or a few viral genes, and survival of the infected cells. Reactivation may occur sporadically or not at all, usually dependent upon immune competence. Which of the following viruses would be most likely to establish a latent infection?

a. Adenovirus
b. Coxsackievirus group B
c. Influenza virus
d. Measles virus
e. Poliovirus

126. On November 6, a patient had the onset of an illness characterized by fever, chills, headache, cough, and chest pain. The illness lasted 1 week. On December 5, she had another illness very similar to the first, which lasted 6 days. She had no flu immunization during this period. Her hemagglutination inhibition (HI) antibody titer to swine flu virus was as follows:

November 6: 10
November 30: 10
December 20: 160
(There was no laboratory error.)

Which of the following is the best conclusion from these data?

a. The patient was ill with swine flu on November 6.
b. The patient was ill with swine flu later, and the November 6 illness was due to another pathogen.
c. The patient was ill with swine flu on December 20.
d. It is impossible to relate either illness with the specific virus.

127. A college freshman went to the student health service with a fever and sore throat. The staff noted enlarged lymph nodes and unusual blood cell results. This person is most likely to have which disease listed below?

a. Encephalitis caused by herpes simplex virus (HSV)
b. Chronic hepatitis C
c. Mononucleosis induced by Epstein-Barr virus
d. Parvovirus infection
e. Rotavirus gastroenteritis

128. A tourist who recently returned from a Caribbean cruise suddenly develops arthralgia, a maculopapular rash, and lymphadenopathy with back and bone pain. Which of the following is the most likely diagnosis?

a. Dengue fever
b. Hepatitis infection
c. HIV infection
d. Infectious mononucleosis
e. Saint Louis encephalitis

129. A 30-year-old female with a recent history of serious illness requiring surgery and necessary blood products developed fever, nausea, and jaundice. Her condition continued as a clinically mild disease, with AST = 552, ALT = 712, and the HBV panel was negative. Which of the following best characterizes the illness?

a. Blood products are not tested for antibody to HCV.
b. Few cases progress to chronic liver disease.
c. HBV but not HCV infections occur in IV drug abusers.
d. HCV is a DNA virus.
e. HCV is the most common cause of posttransfusion hepatitis.

Questions 130-133

130. An IV-drug user discovered that a friend with whom he shared needles for injections was diagnosed with viral hepatitis. He had his blood drawn at the local public health clinic and tested for hepatitis B virus (HBV). Which of the following markers is usually the first viral marker detected after hepatitis B infection?

a. HBcAg (core)
b. HBeAg
c. HBsAg (surface)
d. HBeAb
e. Anti–HBc (core)

131. The individual in Question 130 had negative serological tests for hepatitis B virus (HBV) initially, but his symptoms for hepatitis infections continued. Which of the following may be the only detectable serological marker during the early convalescent phase of HBV infection (window phase)?

a. HBcAg (core)
b. HBeAg
c. HBsAg (surface)
d. HBeAb
e. Anti–HBc (core)

132. As the individual in Questions 130-131 continues to wonder if he is infected with hepatitis B virus (HBV), which of the following markers is closely associated with HBV infectivity and DNA polymerase activity?

a. HBcAg (core)
b. HBeAg
c. HBsAg (surface)
d. HBeAb
e. Anti–HBc (core)

133. The IV-drug user (Questions 130-132) was diagnosed as definitely infected with hepatitis B virus by serological testing. Which of the following is found within the nuclei of infected hepatocytes and not usually in the peripheral circulation?

a. HBcAg (core)
b. HBeAg
c. HBsAg (surface)
d. HBeAb
e. Anti–HBc (core)

134. An infant was born and presented with intrauterine growth retardation, jaundice, hepatosplenomegaly, microcephaly, and retinitis. Which one of the following viruses most likely caused these congenital malformations?

a. Cytomegalovirus (CMV)
b. Mumps
c. Human immunodeficiency virus (HIV)
d. Respiratory syncytial virus (RSV)
e. Rubeola

135. A 20-year-old male who had not received the normal and usual pediatric vaccinations experienced a paramyxovirus infection and developed a high fever at the end of the first week of illness. This was accompanied by swelling, tenderness, and severe pain in the testes that lasted 5 days. This infection was a manifestation of which of the following viruses?

a. Cytomegalovirus
b. Mumps
c. Rabies
d. Respiratory syncytial virus
e. Rubeola

136. Worldwide 3 to 5 million cases of severe influenza illnesses and 250,000 to 500,000 deaths occur annually. It is significant that virologists know the exact stains of viruses involved to include in the killed virus vaccines, such as the recent H1N1 cases that were reported in the media and the scientific literature. These can be monitored by detecting antigenic drift and shift. Which of the following describes events that would most likely lead to a new influenza epidemic?

a. Antigenic drift represents the sudden appearance of new subtypes of hemeagglutinin (HA) and/or neuraminidase (NA).
b. Antigenic drift represents a gradual change in the HA and/or NA antigens.
c. Antigenic shift represents the sudden appearance of new subtypes of HA and/or NA.
d. Antigenic shift represents a gradual change in HA and/or NA antigens.
e. Antigenic shift results in the inactivation of interferons.

137. A visitor from rural Mexico visited the United States and was admitted to a hospital after being diagnosed of probable encephalitis of an unknown cause. A number of human viruses are known to be able to invade the human central nervous system (CNS) by a variety of mechanisms. Differences and similarities of such entry need to be well understood to be able to plan protective measures. Which of the following viruses may enter the CNS at neuromuscular junctions or directly into the CNS without replication, resulting in fatal encephalitis, and may be prevented by a vaccine?

a. Cytomegalovirus
b. Mumps
c. Rabies
d. Respiratory syncytial virus
e. Rhinovirus

138. Although vaccination with live, attenuated, or killed viral vaccines has been the most effective way of controlling viral disease in the population, common colds remain widespread because of the multiple serotypes identified. Which of the following viruses represents this problem?

a. Cytomegalovirus
b. Mumps
c. Rabies
d. Respiratory syncytial virus
e. Rhinovirus

139. Seven people of various ages ate at a local restaurant and developed nausea, vomiting, and mild fever within 24 to 48 hours. Hepatitis A virus (HAV) was found to be the cause of the outbreak and contains RNA. It principally infects children in lower socioeconomic conditions, although outbreaks in commercial eating establishments may involve all age groups as in this episode. Which of the following is available and effective for HAV control?

a. Acyclovir
b. Interferons
c. Killed virus vaccine
d. Live virus vaccine
e. Recombinant viral vaccine

140. Uncomplicated influenza appears abruptly, with chills, headache, and dry cough, followed by high fever, muscle aches, malaise, and anorexia, lasting around 3 to 5 days. All age groups may be affected during the yearly flu season. In order to prevent infections and frequent complications, individuals should be vaccinated annually with which of the following vaccines?

a. Immune serum globulin
b. Inactivated/killed virus vaccine
c. Purified hemagglutinin/neuraminidase preparations
d. Live virus vaccine
e. Recombinant viral vaccine

141. Typical measles can occur at any age. A 2- to 4-day incubation (fever, malaise, conjunctivitis, and pharyngitis) is followed by a maculopapular rash (face to distal extremities). Which of the following best characterizes the vaccine that has dramatically reduced the incidence of this disease in the United States?

a. Interferons
b. Inactivated virus vaccine
c. Killed virus vaccine
d. Live virus vaccine
e. Recombinant viral vaccine

142. A newlywed couple was surprised to find that both experienced genital herpes lesions in their first year of marriage. Both also denied prior evidence of infection. One apparently contracted the virus from the partner's subclinical infection. HSV incidence remains high in the population, although control measures are available. Which of the following is the treatment of choice for HSV infection?

a. Acyclovir
b. Azythromycin
c. Herpes immune globulin
d. Killed virus vaccine
e. Recombinant viral vaccine

143. Viral vaccines continue to be the most effective mechanism of controlling disease in the population, even though chemotherapy and IFNs are available. Which of the following best describes the presently available vaccine for hepatitis B?

a. Inactivated virus vaccine
b. Killed virus vaccine
c. Live virus vaccine
d. Recombinant viral vaccine
e. Synthetic peptide vaccine

144. Two weeks after contact with an individual with an acute disease presentation, a 12-year-old girl has fever and malaise, followed by a rash composed of crops of vesicles which lasts 5 days. This common childhood disease is caused by which of the following viruses?

a. Adenovirus
b. Cytomegalovirus
c. Papillomavirus
d. Rubeola
e. Varicella virus

145. New military recruits undergoing basic training experienced an acute respiratory disease outbreak in their second month of camp. The symptoms ranged from fever and sore throats with coughing to several who developed pneumonia. A small number also developed acute conjunctivitis. All eventually recovered and successfully completed this stage of their training. Which of the following agents is the most likely cause of this outbreak?

a. Adenovirus
b. Cytomegalovirus
c. Papillomavirus
d. Rotavirus
e. Varicella virus

146. Cervical cancer is the second most frequent cancer in women worldwide. Such cancer develops slowly and multiple factors are involved in progression to malignancy. Persistent infection of which virus listed below is a necessary component to this process?

a. Adenovirus
b. Cytomegalovirus
c. Papillomavirus
d. Rotavirus
e. Varicella virus

147. An outbreak of infant diarrheal illness occurred. Watery diarrhea, fever, abdominal pain, and vomiting, resulting in dehydration was observed. No virus was isolated by standard laboratory techniques, but a medium-sized round virus was observed by electron microscopy. Which virus listed below could cause this disease and recently had an approved vaccine recalled?

a. Adenovirus
b. Cytomegalovirus
c. Papillomavirus
d. Rotavirus
e. Varicella virus

148. A young adult presented himself to the local emergency medicine department complaining of headache, fever, and malaise for 2 weeks and now a sore throat. The physician noted enlarged lymph nodes. Laboratory tests found increased number of atypical lymphocytes and a reactive heterophile antibody test. Which organism listed below is responsible for this infection?

a. Adenovirus
b. Coxsackievirus
c. Cytomegalovirus
d. Herpes simplex virus
e. Varicella-zoster virus

149. A college couple dated for several weeks and both went to the campus health center complaining of headache, fatigue, and sore throats. Their diagnostic tests demonstrated that both had increased atypical lymphocyte levels and reactive heterophile antibody tests. Which of the agents listed below was responsible for these illnesses?

a. *Borrelia burgdorferi*
b. Epstein-Barr virus
c. Parvovirus
d. Rubella virus
e. *Toxoplasma*

150. A patient has complement fixation antibody titers against measles virus as follows: acute = 40, convalescent = 80. Which of the following is the correct conclusion concerning this patient?

a. The patient has a recurrent, acute infection.
b. Infection occurred sometime in the past.
c. The antibodies could only have been made due to vaccination.
d. The patient would be incompletely immune to measles due to lack of CMI immunity.
e. An immediate booster shot would be necessary to enhance the patient's protection against measles.

151. A 10-year-old boy in a malarial area of Africa was diagnosed with a poorly differentiated B-cell tumor of the jaw that was characterized by elevated "early antigen" tests with a restricted pattern of fluorescence. This disease is caused by which of the following?

a. *Borrelia burgdorferi*
b. Cytomegalovirus
c. Epstein-Barr virus
d. Herpes simplex virus
e. Lymphogranuloma venereum

152. A 55-year-old Chinese man in southern China sought medical help due to a serious otitis media, which was related to obstruction of his eustachian tubes. Medical examination and laboratory testing resulted in a diagnosis of nasopharyngeal carcinoma. This is a cancer of epithelial cells that appears to be generated by genetic and environmental factors. Which of the following viruses may be detected by the polymerase chain reaction (PCR) in a variety of cells of patients with this type of carcinoma?

a. Epstein-Barr virus
b. Measles
c. Mumps
d. Parvovirus
e. Rubella

153. A 2-day-old newborn with a mononucleosis-like syndrome has microcephaly, cataracts, and "owl eye" cytopathic effects in biopsy tissue cells. Which of the following viruses is the most likely cause of this infection?

a. Cytomegalovirus
b. Epstein-Barr virus
c. Human herpesvirus-6
d. Norwalk virus
e. Parvovirus

154. An estimated 6.2 million new human papillomavirus (HPV) infections occur annually in the United States. The peak incidence occurs in adolescents and young adults under 25 years of age. Which of the following specimens is best for detection of HPV?

a. Blood
b. Cervical tissue
c. Skin
d. Synovial fluid

155. A mother who did not have prenatal care gave birth to an infant with growth retardation, retinitis, jaundice and hepatosplenomegaly. Cytomegalovirus (CMV) was isolated and identified. This virus is ubiquitous, and worldwide, with 1% of infants excreting CMV in urine at delivery. About 90% of these infants appear normal, but up to 20% of these develop hearing loss, mental retardation, or both. Ganciclovir is available for treatment. Which of the following specimens is best for detection of CMV?

a. Blood
b. Cerebrospinal fluid
c. Cervical tissue
d. Skin
e. Synovial fluid

156. An outbreak of aseptic meningitis occurred in an orphanage where public health facilities were not readily available. The children presented with fever, headache, and mild muscle weakness, but all recovered fully. Enteroviruses appear to be clinically significant in causing a wide range of clinical syndromes, including skin, cardiac, ocular, respiratory, gastrointestinal, neurologic, and other generalized disease of infants. Which of the following specimens is best for detection of enterovirus?

a. Blood
b. Cerebrospinal fluid
c. Cervical tissue
d. Skin
e. Synovial fluid

157. Varicella-zoster virus (VZV) is a mild, highly contagious disease of children, but may be severe in adults or immunocompromised individuals. Acyclovir (and similar products) can prevent the development of systemic disease in immunosuppressed individuals, making laboratory diagnosis significant. Which of the following specimens is best for detection of VZV?

a. Blood
b. Cerebrospinal fluid
c. Cervical tissue
d. Skin
e. Synovial fluid

158. Children at an elementary school experienced cough, nasal congestion, fever, and sore throats. Adenoviruses were shown to be the cause of the infections and have been shown to replicate in epithelial cells of the respiratory tract, eye, GI tract, urinary bladder, and liver. About one-third of known serotypes cause different clinical diseases. Which of the following specimens is best for detection of adenoviruses?

a. Blood
b. Cerebrospinal fluid
c. Cervical tissue
d. Stool
e. Synovial fluid

159. Twenty-five days following consumption of shellfish, a 35-year-old man presents with acute jaundice and liver function abnormalities. Which of the following is the most likely cause of his infection?

a. Adenovirus 40/41
b. Astrovirus
c. Hepatitis A virus
d. Norwalk virus
e. Rotavirus

160. Key signs and symptoms of infectious diarrhea include increased frequency and/or the presence of unformed or watery stools. Abdominal cramping/pain, fever, and nausea and vomiting are common. Which of the following viruses causes only gastroenteritis and is the *second* most common cause of pediatric diarrhea?

a. Adenovirus 40/41
b. Astrovirus
c. Hepatitis A virus
d. Norwalk virus
e. Rotavirus

161. Diarrheal illnesses remain a major cause of morbidity and mortality throughout the world. Given the ubiquitous nature of infectious diarrhea, primary care physicians must have a firm understanding of the diagnosis and treatment of these diverse illnesses. Which of the following is difficult to grow in cell culture but can be detected easily using ELISA, and is the most common cause of pediatric diarrhea?

a. Adenovirus 40/41
b. Astrovirus
c. Hepatitis A virus
d. Norwalk virus
e. Rotavirus

162. Adults and older children experienced an outbreak of diarrhea with nausea and vomiting while aboard a cruise ship in the Caribbean. Which virus listed below was responsible for this episode and had to be diagnosed using ELISA and electron microscopy?

a. Adenovirus 40/41
b. Astrovirus
c. Hepatitis A virus
d. Norwalk virus
e. Rotavirus

163. An outbreak of diarrhea occurred among elderly patients in an assisted care facility, which had been repeatedly cited by the public health department for poor hygiene practices. The agents that caused the infections had a starlike morphology in electron micrographs. No specific antiviral treatments exist for these viruses. Which of the following etiologic agents caused these infections and are difficult to isolate in the diagnostic laboratory?

a. Adenovirus 40/41
b. Astrovirus
c. Hepatitis A virus
d. Norwalk virus
e. Rotavirus

164. A group of elementary school-aged children living in a lower economic community developed an acute febrile illness accompanied by a maculopapular rash. Medical histories found that almost none of them had received the usual pediatric vaccinations one would normally expect to have been given. Rubella is a common cause of exanthems in children and is best described by which of the following statements?

a. Incubation time is approximately 3 to 4 weeks.
b. Infections routinely fail to generate an immune response.
c. It can be diagnosed by the presence of Koplik spots.
d. Rubeola and rubella are caused by the same virus.
e. Specific antibody in the serum does prevent disease.

165. A recent immigrant from Africa to the United States had been injured in his home country and received blood transfusions there. In the United States, he was examined for a clinically mild disease that presented with jaundice. Enzyme immunoassay (EIA) testing revealed antibody to a flavivirus. Which of the following viruses listed below caused this illness?

a. Hepatitis A virus
b. Hepatitis B virus
c. Hepatitis C virus
d. Hepatitis D virus
e. Hepatitis E virus

166. Control of viral hepatitis in individuals who have injection drug problems became easier when specific vaccines were available. Vaccines made of surface antigen isolated from chronic viral carriers and from yeasts containing the surface antigen gene are able to provide immunity to which of the following viruses?

a. Hepatitis A virus
b. Hepatitis B virus
c. Hepatitis C virus
d. Hepatitis D virus
e. Hepatitis E virus

167. In an outbreak of hepatitis in New Delhi in 1955, over 29,000 cases of icteric hepatitis occurred when the city's drinking water supply was contaminated with sewage. Pregnant women experienced a 20% mortality rate due to severe liver damage. The virus that caused this outbreak was classified as a calicivirus. The reservoir is in pigs, and humans acquire it via the fecal-oral route. Which of the following is this virus?

a. Hepatitis A virus
b. Hepatitis B virus
c. Hepatitis C virus
d. Hepatitis D virus
e. Hepatitis E virus

168. Acute hepatitis symptoms appeared in a 40-year-old man known to be chronically infected with another hepatitis virus. This unclassified RNA virus is capable of causing acute or chronic hepatitis. It is also known to be defective in its growth ability. Which of the following is the virus?

a. Hepatitis A virus
b. Hepatitis B virus
c. Hepatitis C virus
d. Hepatitis D virus
e. Hepatitis E virus

169. Viruses have various ways of entering the human body and producing disease. Which of the following descriptions accurately describes the route and mechanism for the virus indicated?

a. Coronaviruses enter the gastrointestinal tract through the mouth and move into the stomach, where they proliferate within mucosal cells to produce peptic ulcers.

b. Enteroviruses enter through the mouth, replicate in the pharynx and bowel, and move via the blood to distant target organs (central nervous system).

c. HIV is directly injected into the bloodstream by insects requiring blood for egg development.

d. Influenza viruses enter through the respiratory tract, replicate within lymphocytes in the lung, and move via the lymphatic vessels to joints and the CNS to produce muscle aches, stiff joints, and fever.

e. Mumps virus enters through abraded skin in the genital area and moves into the testicles of males to produce swelling and sterility.

170. A flavivirus recently appeared in the United States with birds as the primary hosts. The virus produces viremia in humans and is currently the leading cause of arboviral encephalitis in older patients. Which of the following is this virus?

a. Human papillomavirus
b. *Polyomavirus*
c. Subacute sclerosing panencephalitis virus
d. Tick-borne encephalitis virus
e. West Nile virus

171. An immunocompromised patient presented with a progressive cerebral deterioration that led to paralysis. An MRI revealed lesions in the white matter, and virions were visible on brain biopsy. Normal CSF findings (cell count, glucose, protein) were present, but viral DNA was found in the CSF by PCR. Which of the following viruses causes the diagnosed progressive multifocal leukoencephalopathy?

a. Human papillomavirus
b. *Polyomavirus*
c. Subacute sclerosing panencephalitis virus
d. Tick-borne encephalitis virus
e. West Nile virus

172. An irritable 18-month-old toddler with fever and blister-like ulcerations on mucous membranes of the oral cavity refuses to eat. The symptoms worsen and then slowly resolve over a period of 2 weeks. Which of the following statements would be most likely to occur, assuming that the etiological agent was the herpes simplex type 1 virus?

a. Antivirals do not provide any benefit.
b. The virus remains latent in the trigeminal ganglia.
c. Recurrence is likely to result in a generalized rash.
d. Polyclonal B cell activation is a prominent feature.
e. The child is at high risk for developing cancer later in life.

173. A sexually active 17-year-old man presents to the local free clinic to check some small papules that appeared on his penis. The papules are small, white lesions with a central depression. There is no discharge or pain on urination. What group listed below does this etiologic agent belong to?

a. Adenoviridae
b. Arenaviridae
c. Papovaviridae
d. Parvoviridae
e. Poxviridae

174. A fifth-grade student with a maculopapular rash attended class and was sent home at noontime. Two weeks later, three classmates developed fever, coughing, running nose, and white ulcerations on the buccal mucosa before developing a similar rash. Which of the following viruses caused these infections?

a. Adenovirus
b. Influenza virus
c. Measles virus
d. Parainfluenza virus
e. Respiratory syncytial virus

175. Newborn to 12-month-old infants are at risk of picking up dangerous germs from siblings and others, but have limited immune capacity. With narrow airways, bronchiolitis and community-acquired pneumonias are especially dangerous. Which of the following viruses is the leading cause of bronchiolitis and community-acquired pneumonia in infants?

a. Adenovirus
b. Influenza virus
c. Measles virus
d. Parainfluenza virus
e. Respiratory syncytial virus

176. A 3-month old infant was seen at the emergency medicine department for treatment of severe lower respiratory disease. This was diagnosed as bronchiolitis and treatment was started immediately since symptoms progression may be very rapid in these situations. Which of the following viral infections is localized, lacking a viremic stage, and chiefly dependent on secretory IgA for viral neutralization?

a. Coronavirus
b. Measles virus
c. Mumps virus
d. Respiratory syncytial virus
e. Variola major virus

177. A respiratory outbreak occurred at a school, with the children coughing, having nasal congestion, fever, and sore throat. Many of the children's siblings experienced conjunctivitis or some gastrointestinal distress. Depending on the clinical disease, a double-stranded DNA virus was recovered from stool samples or from throat, conjunctival, or rectal swabs. Which virus listed below was responsible for this outbreak?

a. Adenovirus
b. Influenza virus
c. Measles virus
d. Parainfluenza virus
e. Respiratory syncytial virus

178. An elderly man had been in several military conflicts during the early 1980s and received blood transfusions for injuries. He recently consulted his physician for what was diagnosed as cryoglobulinemia and glomeru-lonephritis. Additional testing revealed that he was infected by a flavivirus whose transmission was bloodborne. Which of the following viruses was involved in this infection?

a. Hepatitis A virus
b. Hepatitis B virus
c. Hepatitis C virus
d. Hepatitis D virus
e. Hepatitis E virus

179. An outbreak of influenza occurred in a rural community, with abrupt onset of chills, headache, and dry cough. Most patients had fever for 3 to 5 days. Influenza can be treated; therefore, specific detection of the virus becomes much more important. Which of the following is best for detection of influenza?

a. Cold agglutinin test
b. Culture of respiratory secretions on monkey kidney cells
c. Detection of antigen in respiratory secretions
d. Detection of specific antigen in urine
e. Electron microscopy of sputum

Virology

Answers

64. The answer is d. *(Brooks, pp 611-612. Murray, pp 1271-1272. Murray, pp 494, 633-639. Ryan, pp 614-615. Toy, p 214.)* RT PCR, a nucleic acid amplification test for HIV RNA, has recently been shown to be the most valuable test for (a) monitoring a patient's progress during triple drug therapy and (b) determining the chances of progression to AIDS. A viral load of 100,000 to 750,000 copies per milliliter significantly increases the chance of progression to AIDS within 5 years. The amount of HIV in the blood (viral load) is of significant prognostic value. The steady-state level of virus (virus replication vs viral killing) reflects the number of infected cells and the average burst size. Plasma HIV quantitative RNA levels can be determined by the RT PCR and appears to be the best predictor of long-term clinical outcome. CD4 counts appear to be the best predictor of

The location of the envelope glycoproteins (gp 120 and gp 41) is shown, as are the major viral core proteins (p 25, p 17, p 9, and p 7). The core protein, p 17, is found outside the viral nucleoid and forms the matrix of the virion. RT indicates reverse transcriptase.

short-term risk of developing an opportunistic infection. Effectiveness of antiretroviral drug therapy is most often assessed by RT PCR assays. The other tests listed (CD4 count, HIV Ab test, HIV p24 Ag, neopterin) do not accurately predict progression to AIDS. Neopterin belongs to the pteridine chemical group. It is synthesized by macrophages and activated T cells by γ-interferon and is a marker of cellular immune system activation. The following figure shows the basic structure of HIV, including the enzyme reverse transcriptase.

65. The answer is b. *(Brooks, pp 413-417. Murray, pp 547-550. Ryan, pp 522-523. Toy, pp 242.)* Parvovirus B19 is the causative agent of erythema infectiosum (fifth disease). It is associated with transient aplastic crisis in persons with hereditary hemolytic anemia. In adults, it is also associated with polyarthralgia (and fetal loss in pregnant women). Serology detects specific IgM antibody to Parvovirus. The "slapped cheek" rash appearance and term is generally referring only to parvovirus B19 infections. These symptoms and associated aplastic crises are not generally related to herpes simplex or zoster, rubella or rubeola infections.

66. The answer is c. *(Brooks, pp 431-436. Murray, pp 518-525. Ryan, pp 558. Toy, pp 208.)* The initial infection by HSV is often inapparent and occurs through a break in the skin or mucous membranes, such as in the eye, throat, or genitals. Latent infection often persists at the initial site despite high antibody titers. Recurrent disease can be triggered by temperature change, emotional distress, and hormonal factors. Type 1 HSV is usually, but not exclusively, associated with ocular and oral lesions; type 2 is usually, but not exclusively, associated with genital and anal lesions. Type 2 infection is more common. In addition to mucocutaneous infections, the CNS and occasionally visceral organs can be involved. Both HSV-1 and HSV-2 are widely spread in the population and appear to be equally common. Intestinal absorption of the virus would be highly unlikely and probably impossible to verify. Individuals without symptoms may possess high Ab titers due to prior infection. The viruses generally move cell to cell and would not be affected by circulating antibodies. The CNS may well be affected by the virus, but the visceral organs are usually not.

(Reproduced, with permission, from Cunningham FG, et al. William's Obstetrics. 21st ed. New York, NY: McGraw-Hill; 2001:1495.)

67 to 69. The answers are 67-d, 68-e, 69-d. (*Brooks, pp 609-615. Levinson, pp 329-330. Murray, pp 484-486, 633, 640. Ryan, pp 615-616. Toy, pp 214.*) The advent of triple therapy, or a therapeutic "cocktail," has had a marked effect on AIDS patients. The combination of drugs works together as reverse transcriptive inhibitors and a protease inhibitor. If RT and protease activities are prevented, membrane synthesis, glycoprotein synthesis, P24 synthesis, and nuclease activities would, by definition, be essentially eliminated. Patients improve rapidly, their CD4 lymphocyte counts increase, and their HIV viral loads are drastically reduced, often to less than 50 copies per milliliter. On the other hand, an untreated HIV-positive patient with a low CD4 and a high viral load (a) is at increased risk of opportunistic infection and (b) has a much greater chance of developing AIDS than if the viral load was less than 10,000. The patient is infectious and his HIV antibody screening test will be positive. The high viral load, however, is not a predictor of response to therapy. Many patients with high viral loads do very well on triple therapy, although resistance to one or more of the agents may subsequently occur. A low CD4 count does not predict progression to AIDS but does indicate increased chance of opportunistic infection such as those listed. Kaposi sarcoma, which has been linked to herpesvirus type 8, pneumocystis, and mycobacterial disease are three of the most prevalent opportunistic infections. While HIV-positive patients contract pneumococcal pneumonia, they are probably at no more risk than the general population, as protection against pneumococcal disease is linked to the presence of anticapsular antibody. Early-stage infection with HIV usually finds some immune competence, and antibodies to pneumococcus would most likely be produced. HSV, mycobacterial and pneumocystic diseases, and Kaposi sarcoma would probably be difficult to fight in an AIDS patient when compared to the responses that could be seen in immunocompetent hosts.

70. The answer is e. *(Brooks, pp 446-447. Murray, pp 529-533. Ryan, pp 571-573. Toy, p 190.)* All of Koch postulates have been verified for the relationship between infectious mononucleosis and EBV, a herpesvirus.

PROPERTIES OF HERPES VIRUSES			
Virus	**Target Cell**	**Site of Latency**	**Transmission**
Herpes simplex virus type 1	Epithelial cells of the mucosa	Neurons	Close contact
Herpes simplex virus type 2	Epithelial cells of the mucosa	Neurons	Close contact (sexually transmitted)
Varicella-zoster virus	Epithelial cells of the mucosa	Neurons	Respiratory and close contact
Epstein-Barr virus	B cells and epithelial cells	B cell	Person to person via saliva
Kaposi sarcoma-related virus	Lymphocytes	Unknown	Close contact (sexually transmitted)
Cytomegalovirus	Monocytes, lymphocytes, epithelial cells	Monocytes, lymphocytes	Close contact, blood, and tissue transplantation, and congenital

(Reproduced, with permission, from Toy EC, DeBord C, Wanger A, et al. Case Files: Microbiology. 2nd ed. New York: McGraw-Hill; 2008:191.)

However, the relationship between this virus and Burkitt lymphoma, sarcoid, and systemic lupus erythematosus (SLE) is less clear. Infectious mononucleosis is most common in young adults (14-18 years of age) and is very rare in young children. There is no specific treatment. Heterophil antibody titer is helpful in diagnosis, but is not expressed as a function of clinical recovery.

71. The answer is b. *(Brooks, pp 614-615. Levinson, pp 328. Murray, pp 638-639. Ryan, pp 614-615. Toy, pp 214.)* The standard screening test for HIV antibody detection is the ELISA. It is well standardized and available in kit format for relative ease of use in laboratories. As a screening test, however, some false-positive and false-negative results may occasionally be obtained. The standard practice, therefore, is to always perform a second ELISA test before reporting any test result. In fact, before any final report in HIV diagnosis is sent out, a confirming test (Western blot test, in most cases) will need to be performed. HIV culture is not routinely done. No evidence of *P jiroveci* was noted in the history. Until confirmed, no AZT use is justified and, certainly, no suggestion of AIDS development would be made on the basis of screening test results.

72. The answer is b. *(Brooks, pp 511-515. Murray, pp 609-614. Ryan, pp 587-593.)* Arboviruses (arthropod [insects]-borne viruses) may or may not be surrounded by a lipid envelope, although most are inactivated by lipid solvents such as ether and may contain either double-stranded or single-stranded RNA. Physicochemical studies have demonstrated a great heterogeneity among these viruses. Arboviruses cause disease in vertebrates; in humans, encephalitis is a frequent arbovirus illness. Most human infections with arbovirus, however, are asymptomatic. Parvoviruses are single-stranded DNA viruses. No antiviral chemotherapy is currently available to modify arbovirus infections, while prevention by vaccine immunization is available for some.

73. The answer is d. *(Brooks, pp 127, 405-407. Levinson, pp 228-229, 241. Murray, pp 132-134, 482. Ryan, pp 104.)* IFN is a protein produced by cells in response to a viral infection or certain other agents. Entering uninfected cells, IFN causes production of a second protein (AVP-antiviral protein) that alters protein synthesis. As a result of inhibition of either translation or transcription, new viruses are not assembled following infection of IFN-protected cells. Host cell-mediated and humoral immunity is not directly affected by IFNs regarding direct antiviral activity, nor is direct suppression of host or viral mRNA formation observed. IFNs do not alter the host's cell membrane in any way that would prevent viral attachment and/or penetration.

74. The answer is b. (*Brooks, pp 567-570. Murray, pp 565-567. Ryan, pp 511.*) Coronaviruses, discovered in 1965, are thought to be a major agent of the common cold, especially in older children and adults. The virion is known to contain RNA, but other elements of its structure are unclear. At 34°C, viral multiplication is profuse; however, infectivity is greatly reduced at higher temperatures or following extended incubation. Rhinoviruses (picornaviruses) are the other major cause of common cold. There is no common connection between the SARS agent and those causing colds. Coronaviruses may also cause gastroenteritis in humans, although these agents have not been isolated. Coronavirus OC43 can cause hemeagglunti-nation of RBCs, but not WBCs. Human coronaviruses do not grow well in cell culture, making details of virus replication uncertain.

75. The answer is b. (*Brooks, pp 467-471. Levinson, pp 300-301. Murray, pp 657-658. Ryan, pp 550-551.*) The delta agent was first described in 1977 and has recently been shown to be a defective RNA virus that requires HBsAg for replication. It is found most often in persons, who have multiple parenteral exposures—for example, intravenous (IV) drug abusers, hemophiliacs, and multiply transfused patients. HDV may cause acute or chronic infection, and HDV remains unclassified as to virus group-ing but is not a variant of HAV, HBV, or HCV.

76. The answer is c. (*Brooks, pp 404. Murray, pp 480-485, 581, 626. Ryan, pp 209-210.*) As an IV agent, ribavirin is effective against Lassa fever in the first week of onset of the disease. It may also be administered as an aerosol that is quite useful in infants with RSV. Unlike amantadine, which is effica-cious only with influenza A, ribavirin has activity against both influenza A and influenza B if administered by aerosol in the first 24 hours of onset. Amantadine and rimantadine are used in influenza A infections by blocking viral uncoating. Acyclovir is used in herpesvirus infections where it acts as a viral polymerase inhibitor. Vidarabine is also a viral polymerase inhibitor and has been used in herpesvirus, vaccinia virus, and HBV infections.

77. The answer is d. *(Brooks, pp 496-498. Murray, pp 554-557. Ryan, pp 537-539.)* Echoviruses were discovered accidentally during studies on poliomyelitis. They were named echoviruses because, at the time, they had not been linked to human disease and thus were considered "orphans." Echoviruses now are known to infect the intestinal tract of humans; they also can cause aseptic meningitis, febrile illnesses, and the common cold. Echoviruses range in size from 24 to 30 nm in diameter and contain a core of RNA. Bladder and urinary tracts, as well as blood and lymphatic systems are not usually affected by echoviruses. CNS and respiratory systems involvement are usually secondary to intestinal tract infection.

78. The answer is d. *(Brooks, pp 431-437. Murray, pp 522-525. Ryan, pp 559-562.)* HSV meningitis or encephalitis is difficult to diagnose by laboratory tests, as there is a low titer of virus present in the CSF. Neonatal HSV infects the child during the birth process. While culture, Tzanck smear, and even antibody tests may be useful in adults, particularly those with HSV-rich lesions, they are not useful for CSF testing. Only PCR is sensitive enough to detect HSV DNA in the CSF. Once diagnosed rapidly, HSV encephalitis or meningitis can be treated with acyclovir.

79. The answer is b. *(Brooks, pp 378, 487-495. Levinson, pp 290-294. Murray, pp 554-560.)* Enterovirus and coxsackievirus A can be recovered from conjunctival scrapings of patients with AHC during the first 3 days of illness. Isolation rates are somewhat higher for enterovirus than for coxsackievirus. Less than 5% of throat swab or fecal specimens have been positive for either virus. Echovirus 70 is the chief cause of this disease. Coronaviruses in humans remain limited to the upper respiratory tract. Reoviruses in the United States are responsible for acute respiratory and gastroenteritis infections. RSV is a paramyxovirus involved primarily in respiratory illnesses. Rhinoviruses are common cold viruses.

80. The answer is c. *(Brooks, pp 557-559. Levinson, pp 274-275. Murray, pp 578-579. Ryan, pp 514-515. Toy, p 236.)* Much of the public's understanding of mumps is based on suppositions that are without any scientific basis. For example, natural mumps infection confers immunity after a single infection, even if the infection was a unilateral, not a bilateral, parotitis.

Also, sterility from mumps orchitis is not ensured; only 20% of males older than 13 years of age develop orchitis. The majority of patients with mumps do not develop systemic manifestations. In fact, some do not develop parotitis. Last, the virus is maintained exclusively in human populations; canine reservoirs are not known. The mumps vaccine is a live, attenuated virus vaccine derived from chick-embryo tissue culture.

81. The answer is e. (*Brooks, pp 437-441. Levinson, pp 256-257. Murray, pp 526-528. Ryan, pp 563-565.*) This is a classic description for a reactivation of varicella-zoster viral latent infection. Many initial infections with VZV are subclinical and result in latent infections in sensory ganglion nerve tissue. Varicella (chicken pox) is mild and highly contagious in children. Zoster (shingles) is a sporadic, incapacitating illness seen in adults. Treatment may include acyclovir or famciclovir. Herpes B virus infections occur primarily in monkeys. HSV primary infections are most often subclinical and occur primarily in children. EBV (infectious mononucleosis) persists in latent infections in B lymphocytes.

82. The answer is c. (*Brooks, pp 559-562. Levinson, pp 273-274. Murray, pp 573-576. Ryan, pp 517-518.*) Koplik spots are pathognomonic for measles. The measles virus is a paramyxovirus. In industrialized countries, vaccination has reduced the importance of this childhood infection (although US incidence increased in 1989 and 1990). In developing countries, however, measles is a major killer of young children. In America, most states now require proof of immunity before school enrollment, and this has reduced the incidence of disease. While many of the initial symptoms may be seen in the child, only rubeola (measles) will produce the Koplik spots. Adenoviruses, herpesviruses, picornaviruses, and the flu viruses (orthomyxoviruses) do not.

83. The answer is e. (*Brooks, pp 597-600. Levinson, pp 264-265. Murray, pp 499-504. Ryan, pp 619. Toy, pp 178, 190, 222.*) HPV is the cause of genital warts. It is one of the most pervasive of all the sexually transmitted diseases. There is no specific cure, but a quadrivalent vaccine has recently been approved. There are multiple serotypes of papillomavirus, and some serotypes are linked to cervical cancer. New techniques for molecular diagnosis of HPV show promise for rapid and sensitive detection and perhaps more aggressive treatment. HSV-2 was originally thought to be etiologically involved, but is now not considered so. HSV-2 evidence came primarily from serological data. HSV-1, HSV-2, and CMV can all be transmitted sexually and have DS DNA. However, all herpesvirus DNA molecules are linear, not circular. EBV infections occur via infected saliva and in the oropharynx. No vaccines are currently approved for herpesviruses, except for an approved live, attenuated varicella vaccine, or adenoviruses. Adenoviruses also contain linear, double-stranded DNA genomes.

84. The answer is c. *(Brooks, pp 551-554. Levinson, pp 275-277. Murray, pp 577-579. Ryan, pp 506-507.)* Parainfluenza viruses are important causes of respiratory diseases in infants and young children. The spectrum of disease caused by these viruses ranges from a mild febrile cold to croup, bronchiolitis, and pneumonia. Parainfluenza viruses contain RNA in a nucleocapsid encased within an envelope derived from the host cell membrane. Infected mammalian cell cultures will hemeabsorb red blood cells owing to viral hemagglutinin on the surface of the cell. Adenoviruses, coxsackie B viruses, and rhinoviruses (common cold) can routinely infect the upper respiratory tract and cause less serious illnesses than that described. Rotaviruses (reoviruses) are a major cause of diarrheal illness in human infants, as well as calves and piglets. Rotavirus infection in humans is not uncommon.

85. The answer is a. *(Brooks, pp 472. Levinson, pp 301. Murray, pp 658. Toy, pp 196.)* Hepatitis E is a newly recognized single-stranded RNA virus in the calicivirus family. Epidemics have been observed in Asia, Africa, India, and Mexico. Like HAV, it is enterically transmitted, but there is no vaccine available nor is there a routine detection test. Chronic liver disease does not occur, and because it is not bloodborne, it is of no threat to the blood supply.

86. The answer is e. *(Brooks, pp 733. Murray, pp 671-672.)* Aseptic meningitis is characterized by a pleocytosis of mononuclear cells in the CSF; polymorphonuclear cells predominate during the first 24 hours, but a shift to lymphocytes occurs thereafter. The CSF of affected persons is free of culturable bacteria and contains normal glucose and slightly elevated protein levels. Peripheral white blood cell counts usually are normal. Although viruses are the most common cause of aseptic meningitis, spirochetes, chlamydiae, and other microorganisms also can produce the disease.

CSF findings

Bacterial: pressure ↑, polys ↑, proteins ↑, glucose ↓.

Viral: pressure normal / ↑, lymphs ↑, proteins normal, glucose normal.

TB/fungal: pressure ↑, lymphs ↑, proteins ↑, glucose ↓.

87. The answer is c. *(Brooks, pp 467-468. Murray, pp 653-654, 657-658.)* In coinfection with HBV and HDV, antibody to HDVcAg develops late in the acute phase of infection, usually of low titer. Assays for HDVcAg or HDRNA in the serum or for IgM-anti-HDV are preferable. HDV markers and antibody disappear during convalescence, but superinfection of HDV usually results in high levels of HDV antibodies and RNA. Although HBc IgM is present in acute stages, in a chronic HBV carrier, there would be no HB core IgM antibody, whereas it would be present in a new HBV infection. The HBe antigen could be present in either an HBV carrier or in acute infection. HBsAg would be present in either a new infection or in the carrier state, while HBsAb would not be present in either case. There is no specific diagnostic test available for HCV (Option A).

88. The answer is e. *(Brooks, pp 476-477. Levinson, pp 294-298. Murray, pp 648-654. Ryan, p 549. Toy, p 196.)* In a small number of patients with acute hepatitis B infection, HBsAg can never be detected. In others, HBsAg becomes negative before the onset of the disease or before the end of the clinical illness. In such patients with acute hepatitis, hepatitis B virus infection may be established only by the presence of anti–hepatitis B core IgM (anti–HBc IgM), a rising titer of anti–HBc, or the subsequent appearance of anti–HBsAg.

HBsAg positive, anti–HBs, and anti–HBc negative would identify an early acute HBV infection. HBsAg and anti–HBc positive could indicate an acute or chronic HBV infection. IgM anti–HBc could differentiate between these conditions. HBsAg negative and anti–HBs positive tests indicate immunity due to natural infection or vaccination. Hepatitis symptoms and negative HBsAg, anti–HBs, and anti–HBc test would indicate another infectious agent, toxic injury to the liver, or possible disease of the biliary tract.

INTERPRETATION OF HBV SEROLOGIC MARKERS IN PATIENTS WITH HEPATITIS

Assay Results			
HBsAg	Anti-HBs	Anti-HBc	Interpretation
Positive	Negative	Negative	Early acute HBV infection. Confirmation is required to exclude nonspecific reactivity.
Positive	(±)	Positive	HBV infection, either acute or chronic. Differentiate with IgM anti–HBc. Determine level of replicative activity (infectivity) with HBeAg or HBV DNA.
Negative	Positive	Positive	Indicates previous HBV infection and immunity to hepatitis B.
Negative	Negative	Positive	Possibilities include: HBV infection in remote past; "low-level" HBV carrier; "window" between disappearance of HBsAg and appearance of anti–HBs; or false-positive or nonspecific reaction. Investigate with IgM anti–HBc, challenge with HBsAg vaccine, or both. When present, anti–HBe helps validate the anti–HBc reactivity.
Negative	Negative	Negative	Another infectious agent, toxic injury to liver, disorder of immunity, hereditary disease of the liver, or disease of the biliary tract.
Negative	Positive	Negative	Vaccine-type response.

(Modified, with permission, from Hollinger FB. Hepatitis B virus. In: Fields BN, et al (ed). Fields Virology. 3rd ed. Philadelphia, PA: Lippincott-Raven; 1996.)

89. The answer is d. (Brooks, pp 511-519. Levinson, pp 303-304. Murray, pp 610-616.) Eastern equine encephalitis (EEE) is a severe disease usually seen in the summer months when *Aedes* mosquitoes are prevalent. In 1996 and 1997, there were several outbreaks in the northeastern United States. Control of EEE is a function of mosquito eradication. Horses and humans are accidental hosts. If the patient survives, the CNS sequelae are usually severe. While draining of swamps helps, other measures to eliminate mosquitoes, such as spraying, are the most effective. Birds appear to be natural hosts of the equine encephalitic viruses. As mentioned, horses and humans are accidental hosts when they are bitten by infected mosquito vectors. Horses may be protected by vaccines, but these vaccines are not approved for human use. Fleas and ticks are not considered to be vectors for transmission of the encephalitic viruses.

90. The answer is c. *(Brooks, pp 497-499. Levinson, pp 288. Murray, pp 561-563.)* Rhinovirus is a major cause of the common cold. The primary mode of transmission is the contact of contaminated hands, fingers, or fomites (fomites are objects such as clothing or utensils that can harbor or transmit a disease) with the conjunctiva or nasal epithelium. While several studies have shown no evidence of aerosol transmission, a study by Dick and associates in 1986 did show aerosol transmission can occur. This is not, however, the main mode of transmission. Additional studies showed that rhinoviruses can be recovered from the hands of 40% to 90% of persons with colds and only 6% to 15% of inanimate objects around them. These viruses can survive on these objects for many hours. Transmission by the fecal-oral route, vertical transmission, and sexual activity have not been shown to be important mechanisms in rhinovirus transmission.

91. The answer is c. *(Brooks, pp 559-562. Levinson, pp 273-275. Murray, pp 573-576. Ryan, pp 519-520.)* Measles (rubeola) caused by a paramyxovirus is an acute, highly infectious disease characterized by a maculopapular rash. German measles (rubella—a togavirus) is an acute, febrile illness characterized by a rash as well as suboccipital lymphadenopathy. Incubation time for measles is 9 full days after exposure. Onset is abrupt and symptoms mostly catarrhal. Koplik spots, pale, bluish-white spots in red areolas, can frequently be observed on the mucous membranes of the mouth and are pathognomonic for measles. Incubation times are measured in days (8-12), not weeks. Specific serum antibodies, whether from prior vaccination or illness, prevent the disease from occurring. The characteristic rash is maculopapular, not vesicular (fluid-containing).

92. The answer is e. (*Brooks, pp 573-579. Levinson, pp 279-281. Murray, pp 593-597. Ryan, pp 599.*) The definitive diagnosis of rabies in humans is based on the finding of Negri bodies, which are cytoplasmic inclusions in the nerve cells of the spinal cord and brain, especially in the hippocampus. Negri bodies are eosinophilic and generally spherical in shape; several may appear in a given cell. Negri bodies, although pathognomonic for rabies, are not found in all cases of the disease. In addition to CNS specimens, skin from the neck and at the hairline may be collected for microscopic examination. Tissues infected with rabies virus are currently identified most rapidly and accurately, using fluorescence or immunoperoxidase staining with antirabies monoclonal antibodies. Rabies should be considered in any case of encephalitis or myelitis (spinal cord) of unknown cause, especially in a person who has lived or traveled outside the United States. Negri bodies (inclusions) would not be found in cases of aseptic meningitis, congenital rubella, infectious mono, or mumps.

93. The answer is d. (*Brooks, pp 2-3, 581-582. Levinson, pp 196-197. Murray, pp 661-664. Ryan, pp 625-627.*) Kuru and CJD are similar but not identical diseases with very different epidemiology. Kuru was prevalent among certain tribes in New Guinea who practiced ritual cannibalism by eating the brains of the departed. CJD is found worldwide and has been transmitted by corneal transplants and in pituitary hormone preparations. There is some association between CJD and mad cow disease in England. Prions are unconventional self-replicating proteins, sometimes called *amyloid*. It is now thought that CJD, Kuru, and animal diseases such as scrapie, visna, and bovine spongiform encephalopathy (mad cow disease) are caused by prions. Prions do not contain DNA or RNA. Bacteria, flagellates (parasites), and viruses all contain nucleic acid genomes. No apparent evidence of environmental toxins able to cause Kuru/CJD have been reported.

94. The answer is b. (*Brooks, pp 455-460. Levinson, pp 246, 261. Murray, pp 541-544. Toy, p 266.*) Routine vaccination of infants and children for smallpox has been discontinued in the United States, both because the risk of contracting the disease is so low and because the complications of smallpox vaccination, including generalized vaccinia eruption, postvaccinal encephalitis, and fetal vaccinia, are significant. Owing to the extremely effective eradication of smallpox worldwide by the World Health Organization, US citizens traveling abroad no longer require vaccination. Pregnancy, immune deficiencies, and eczema and other chronic dermatitides are contraindications to smallpox vaccination. Recent concerns about a possible terrorist attack involving smallpox have resulted in recommendations for using vaccinia vaccine on a limited scale, probably starting with health care workers.

95. The answer is e. (Brooks, pp 573-579. Levinson, pp 279-281. Murray, pp 593-597. Ryan pp 597-600.) Rabies is caused by a rhabdovirus (contains negative sense RNA, helical structure). The virus has a wide host of warm-blooded animals, including humans. The virus is widely distributed in the infected animals, with high levels in saliva. Street viruses (freshly isolated strains) have long incubation periods, leading to eventual viral infection of the CNS. Essentially, all organs are infected, giving rise to the described symptoms. Fixed (mutant) virus strains do not grow in neural tissue. Because of the long incubation period (weeks), active treatment (inactivated vaccine) and passive treatment (human or horse immune globulin) are used to prevent disease. If symptoms appear, essentially 100% fatality results. All other answer options are ineffective against rabies disease.

96. The answer is a. (Brooks, pp 419-425. Levinson, pp 263-264. Murray, pp 512-515. Toy, p 178.) Mild ocular involvement occurs as part of the respiratory-pharyngeal syndromes caused by adenoviruses. Industrial accidents leading to eye infections in the past were due to examinations using nonsterile medical equipment. The described disease episode above usually resolves in 2 weeks. Adenovirus type 8 is associated with epidemic keratoconjunctivitis, while adenovirus types 3 and 4 are often associated with "swimming pool conjunctivitis." There are also reports of nosocomial conjunctivitis with adenovirus. EBV, RSV, VZV, and parvoviruses are not routinely reported as causing this type of illness. HSV-1 can infect the conjunctiva, causing keratoconjunctivitis and keratitis.

97. The answer is a. (Brooks, pp 476-478. Levinson, pp 294-298. Murray, pp 649-653. Ryan, pp 547-549. Toy, p 196.) The e antigen is related to the hepatitis B virus and is associated with viral replication (Dane particle). Possession of the e antigen suggests active disease and thus an increased risk of transmission of hepatitis to others. HBsAg and e antigen are components of hepatitis B only and are not shared by other hepatitis viruses. HBV e antigen and antibody to e antigen have been shown to specifically be related to HBV infection and growth, with no evidence offered to suggest that e antigen gives a false positive test result in the laboratory.

98. The answer is d. *(Brooks, pp 511-519. Levinson, pp 303-305. Murray, pp 609-615. Ryan, p 586.)* Saint Louis encephalitis, yellow fever, and dengue are caused by flaviviruses. Western equine encephalitis is caused by an alphavirus. Laboratory diagnosis is usually made by demonstration of a fourfold rise in specific antibody titer in paired sera, although viruses may be isolated in specialist laboratories. Marburg virus is a filovirus, distantly related to the Ebola virus. These both cause systemic diseases with internal and external bleeding, leading to shock and death.

99. The answer is e. *(Brooks, pp 404, 554. Levinson, p 240. Murray, pp 480, 482, 485. Ryan, pp 209-210.)* Ribavirin is effective to varying degrees against several RNA- and DNA-containing viruses in vitro. It has been approved for aerosol treatment of respiratory syncytial virus infections in infants. Currently, aerosol treatment of children is no longer standard treatment. IV administration has proved effective in treating Lassa fever. Ribavirin also remains useful as an adjunct to pegylated IFN for the treatment of HCV infections. Ribavirin is not FDA-approved for treatment of coxsackieviruses, HBV, HSV, or parvovirus infections.

100. The answer is c. *(Brooks, pp 431-436. Murray, pp 518-525. Ryan, pp 559-560.)* HSV causes primary and recurrent disease. The typical skin lesion is a vesicle that contains virus particles in serous fluid. Giant multinucleated cells are typically found at the base of the herpesvirus lesion. Encephalitis, which usually involves the temporal lobe, has a high mortality rate. Severe neurologic sequelae are seen in surviving patients. PCR amplification of viral DNA from CSF has replaced viral isolation. Coxsackeviruses strains may cause self-limited neurologic symptoms. DNA parvoviruses are primarily known for causing "fifth disease" in children. HCV is primarily involved in liver disease. *Listeria monocytogenes* can cause meningoencephalitis primarily in immunocompromised patients and is a bacterium that can be isolated in the laboratory. Interestingly, *L monocytogenes* can move from cell to cell, similar to many viruses, without being exposed to antibodies, complement or polymorphonuclear (PMN).

101. The answer is d. *(Brooks, pp 446-448. Levinson, pp 258-259, 314. Murray, pp 529-533. Ryan, pp 571-572. Toy, p 190.)* Contact with infected secretions such as saliva can result in infection with EBV, thus the term *kissing disease.* Laboratory diagnosis of EBV-induced infectious mononucleosis is usually determined by presence of atypical lymphocytes, heterophile antibodies, or specific antiviral antibodies such as VCA (viral capsid antibody). B-cell lymphocyte proliferation can be induced by exposure to a variety of chemicals and thus, would be considered nonspecific. EBV does not grow in normal or usual cell cultures used in viral diagnosis. If inoculated into a B-cell culture, those cells would be altered or immortalized by the virus, but no virus progeny would be produced. Heterophile antibodies are those that nonspecifically agglutinate sheep RBCs. These do not measure anything specific regarding EBV, but are useful as a nonspecific screening test. Changes in lymph nodes and the spleen can be induced by EBV but also by a number of other microbial agents.

102. The answer is c. *(Brooks, pp 554-556. Levinson, p 276. Murray, pp 579-581. Ryan, pp 504-506.)* RSV is the most important cause of pneumonia and bronchiolitis in infants. The infection is localized to the respiratory tract. The virus can be detected rapidly by immunofluorescence on smears of respiratory epithelium. In older children, the infection resembles the common cold. Aerosolized ribavirin is recommended for severely ill hospitalized infants. Wheezing symptoms observed in an RSV infection are most likely due to increased IgE antibodies. Adenoviruses and picornaviruses most often infect older children, not infants in this age range. Rotaviruses primarily affect the gastrointestinal tract, producing diarrhea.

103. The answer is b. *(Brooks, pp 609-616. Levinson, pp 322-330. Murray, pp 632-640. Ryan, pp 609-610. Toy, p 214.)* Because a substantial portion of the blood supply in Central African countries is HIV infected, hospitalization is risky, particularly if transfusion is necessary. Many believe that casual contact with patients who are HIV-positive increases the risk of acquiring the disease. This is not the case. It is also clear that homosexual females have a low rate of HIV acquisition. Factory workers, household members, and hospital receptionists have little to no risk for contracting HIV in their normal and usual interactions with people around them.

104. The answer is c. (*Brooks, pp 562-565. Levinson, pp 278-279. Murray, pp 617-620. Ryan, pp 519-520.*) The highest risk of fetal infection with rubella occurs during the first trimester. In seronegative patients, the risk of infection exceeds 90%. However, before other measures (such as termination of pregnancy) are considered, a rubella immune status must be performed. A rubella titer of 1:10 is protective. Immune globulin intravenous (IV) injected into the mother does not protect the fetus against rubella because it is usually not given early enough to prevent viremia. The same is likely to be true of using the live vaccine, and in general, use of a live, attenuated vaccine to a pregnant female is generally not recommended. Termination of the pregnancy would probably not be recommended due to the lowered risk of fetal injury at 18 weeks versus the first 1 or 2 months of the pregnancy.

105. The answer is a. (*Brooks, pp 581-582. Levinson, pp 196-197, 317-321. Murray, pp 661-665. Ryan, pp 627-628.*) Mad cow disease is related to both scrapie in sheep and bovine spongiform encephalopathy virus. The fear in Great Britain is the potential for acquiring CJD, which is a slowly progressive neurodegenerative disease. Theoretically, such acquisition could be through ingestion of beef from infected cows. A prion consists of protein material without nucleic acid. While related to a virus, a prion is a proteinaceous infectious particle that replicates within cells. Viruses, bacteria with or without cell walls and *R rickettsiae* all have genetic nucleic acid molecules and can thus be eliminated as etiological agents for CJD or mad cow disease. Prions (PrP) produce disease by altering affected cells, especially the formation of amyloid-containing plaques. Such changes to the cells would not be caused by any known autoimmune reactions.

106. The answer is d. (*Brooks, pp 467. Levinson, pp 301. Murray, pp 658. Ryan, pp 552-553. Toy, pp 196.*) HEV is a single-stranded RNA virus. It is transmitted enterically, and the disease is often referred to as *enteric hepatitis C*. There is no test for HEV routinely available. Diagnosis is clinical and is also one of exclusion. Diagnostic laboratory tests do exist for HAV, HBV, HCV, and HDV. Rotavirus primarily affects children and not adults.

107. The answer is e. (*Brooks, pp 227, 711. Murray, pp 586-589. Ryan, pp 501.*) *Staphylococcus aureus* is the most common cause of postinfluenzal secondary bacterial pneumonia. It most often affects the elderly, although patients of any age may be afflicted. The pneumococcus as well as group A streptococci and *Haemophilus influenzae* may also cause pneumonia, but are not isolated from these cases as much as *S aureus*. *Escherichia coli* and *Klebsiella pneumoniae* are significant opportunists, but reported numbers of opportunistic pneumonias are also lower than for *S aureus*. *Legionella* organisms primarily found in warm, moist environments are usually the primary cause of disease, especially in patients with risk factors. Human *Listeria* infections are usually derived from in utero infections or the GI tract by ingestion of contaminated foods.

108. The answer is a. *(Brooks, pp 419-425. Murray, pp 512-515. Toy, pp 178, 208.)* Conjunctivitis is inflammation of the eye tissue and is seen in many childhood infections. The most common cause, however, is infection with Adenoviruses. These also routinely cause URT and GI infections as well. Adenoviruses are easily spread between children, especially in community settings. Herpes simplex in the eye usually presents as a kerititis (corneal ulcer), with HSV-1 occurring in adults and HSV-2 in neonates. HSV most often occurs as a reactivation from a latent infection. *Staphylococcus aureus* usually presents with a purulent discharge. *Haemophilus aegyptius* may cause epidemic conjunctivitis but is usually seen in tropic climates. Trachoma (*Chlamydia trachomatis*) is most often seen in Africa, the Middle East, and nothern India. Transmitted by flies, fingers, and fomites, repeated *C trachomatis* infections may lead to blindness, although treatment with tetracycline or azithromycin can be curative.

109. The answer is b. *(Brooks, pp 525-526. Levinson, pp 222-223. Murray, pp 621-624.)* In 1993, an outbreak of a fatal respiratory disease occurred in the southwestern United States. This disease is caused by a hantavirus endemic in deer mice. The mortality rate is 60%. Ribavirin has been used but is not effective. A vaccine is not available. Transmission among rodents seems to occur horizontally, and transmission to humans occurs by inhaling aerosols of rodent excreta (urine, feces, or saliva). Person-to-person transmission has been reported in South American outbreaks but is uncommon. Hemorrhagic fever with a renal syndrome is an acute disease, which may lead to renal failure. Hantavirus pulmonary syndrome (HPS) is uncommon but may be severe enough to cause death by severe respiratory compromise. HPS involves the functional impairment of vascular endothelium. Hemolysis of blood cells is not significant. Deer do not maintain the disease in nature, but deer mice do. Person-to-person transmission is uncommon but reports from South America have been published. Ribavirin has been used for treatment with uncertain beneficial results.

110. The answer is a. (*Brooks, pp 585-602. Levinson, pp 309-310. Murray, p 627. Ryan, pp 110-112.*) "Oncogene" is the general term given to genes involved in cancer causations. Normal versions of those transforming genes are present in normal cells and have been called proto-oncogenes. Transforming genes of DNA viruses encode functions for viral replication and do not have normal analogs in cells. DNA virus transforming proteins complex with normal cell proteins and alter their function. Most RNA tumor viruses belong to the retrovirus family, carrying a reverse transcriptase enzyme (RNA-dependent DNA polymerase) that is responsible for constructing a DNA copy of the viral RNA genome. Direct-transforming RNA oncoviruses carry an oncogene of cellular origin, whereas weakly oncogenic RNA viruses have no oncogene and produce leukemias after long incubation periods by indirect mechanisms.

ASSOCIATION OF VIRUSES WITH HUMAN CANCERS*

Virus Family	Virus	Human Cancer
Papovaviridae	Human papillomaviruses	Genital tumors Squamous cell carcinoma Oropharyngeal carcinoma
Herpesviridae	EB virus	Nasopharyngeal carcinoma African Burkitt lymphoma B-cell lymphoma
Hepadnaviridae	Hepatitis B virus	Hepatocellular carcinoma
Retroviridae	HTL virus	Adult T-cell leukemia
Flaviviridae	Hepatitis C virus	Hepatocellular carcinoma

*Candidate human tumor viruses include human herpesvirus 8, additional types of papillomaviruses, and human and simian polyomaviruses.

(*Reprinted, with permission, from Brooks GF, et al. Jawetz's Medical Microbiology. 22nd ed. New York, NY: McGraw-Hill; 2001.*)

111. The answer is d. (*Brooks, pp 585-602. Levinson, pp 281-283. Murray, pp 499-504. Toy, p 222.*) Only two human viruses have been confirmed as human tumor viruses. They include human T-cell lymphotrophic/leukemia virus (HTLV) and papillomavirus. Others, such as EBV, HSV, and hepatitis B and C, have been implicated as tumor viruses. The virus that causes chicken pox and shingles (VZV) is not known to be oncogenic.

112. The answer is a. (*Brooks, pp 413-418. Levinson, pp 265-266. Murray, pp 547-551. Ryan, pp 522-523. Toy, pp 178, 242.*) Parvovirus B19, not adenovirus, causes acute hemolytic anemia, and is most often the cause of transient aplastic crisis that may complicate chronic hemolytic anemia. Such crisis is associated with bone marrow transplantation where there is an abrupt cessation of RBC synthesis in the bone marrow and is reflected by the absence of erythroid precursors in the marrow. Parvoviruses are not involved in acute respiratory disease, gastroenteritis, keratoconjunctivitis, or whooping cough, a bacterial disease. Adenoviruses are widespread and cause a variety of respiratory and gastrointestinal clinical problems. Many of the "viral sore throats" among young people living in close quarters are due to adenovirus.

113. The answer is a. (*Brooks, pp 441-446. Levinson, pp 257-258. Murray, pp 534-537. Ryan, pp 567-568.*) Although infection with CMV is common, it only rarely causes clinically apparent disease. Lesions characteristic of infection with CMV are found in up to 10% of stillborn babies; however, CMV, which can be transmitted transplacentally, usually is not the cause of death. Children and adults with immunosuppressive problems are susceptible to active disease. In severely immunodeficient patients such as those with AIDS, CMV ocular disease may occur. The patient suffers blurring of vision or vision loss, and ophthalmic examination reveals large yellowish-white areas with flame-shaped hemorrhages. Ganciclovir is now licensed for treatment of CMV retinitis in AIDS patients. CMV was one of the first viruses shown to be capable of causing in utero infection. It is not cultured from RBCs, but can be isolated from and grown in nucleated cells. CMV can be activated from a latent-type infection by use of immunosuppressive therapy, with numerous reports available from organ transplantation studies.

114. The answer is d. (*Brooks, pp 501-505. Levinson, p 290. Murray, pp 601-604. Ryan, pp 578-580. Toy, p 254.*) Rotaviruses were initially identified by direct electron microscopy (EM) of duodenal mucosa of infants with gastroenteritis. Subsequent studies in several countries have shown them to be the cause of 30% to 40% of cases of acute diarrhea in infants. They are nonlipid-containing RNA viruses with a double-shelled capsid. Although the virus has been serially propagated in human fetal intestinal organ cultures, cytopathic changes are minimal or absent; multiplication is detected by immunofluorescence. Numerous methods for rotavirus antigen detection, including radioimmunoassay, counterimmunoelectrophoresis, and ELISA, have been developed and found to be about as effective as EM. Rotaviruses do not appear to be a significant cause of infant respiratory disease.

115. The answer is d. *(Brooks, pp 559-561. Levinson, pp 269-273. Murray, p 576. Ryan, pp 517-518.)* SSPE is a late and rare manifestation of measles. It is a progressive encephalitis involving both white and gray matter. Demyelination is seen only at an advanced stage of the disease in a few cases. In 1985, viral RNA was demonstrated in brain cells from a patient with SSPE by the use of in situ hybridization. This is a rare disease of young adults, with slowly progressing demyelination in the CNS, ending in death. There are large numbers of measles nucleocapsid structures in neurons and glial cells, but no envelope gene expression, which does not allow virion maturation. Mumps virus, also a paramyxovirus, does not cause SSPE. Paramyxoviruses contain RNA, not DNA genomes.

116. The answer is b. *(Brooks, pp 503-506. Levinson, p 290. Murray, pp 601-604. Ryan, pp 578-580. Toy, p 254.)* Rotavirus is a viral entity that is similar to Nebraska calf diarrhea virus and is thought to be a major cause of acute diarrhea in newborn infants. Three-quarters of all adults have antibodies against rotavirus; passive transfer of these antibodies to the baby, especially through the colostrum, seems to be protective. Although vaccination would be expected to be of little use to the neonate, it might effectively immunize pregnant mothers. Rotaviruses are extremely difficult to culture. Viruses in stools are demonstrated by immune electron microscopy (IEM), agglutination tests, or ELISA.

117. The answer is a. *(Brooks, pp 551-554. Levinson, pp 273-277. Murray, pp 577-579. Ryan, pp 506-507. Toy, p 236.)* Both mumps and measles are well-recognized paramyxovirus infections. This group also includes parainfluenza virus, which causes laryngotracheobronchitis (croup) in children, and respiratory syncytial virus, which can cause bronchiolitis in infants. Paramyxoviruses have glycoprotein spikes that extend their lipid membrane and are responsible for hemagglutination activities. Fifth disease is caused by B19 parvovirus. Otitis media and tonsillitis are infections that may be caused by a variety of bacteria or viruses, but not specifically by paramyxoviruses. Rubella produces German measles (3-day measles).

118. The answer is a. (*Brooks, pp 446-447. Murray, pp 529-532.*) Aggressive monoclonal B-cell lymphomas can develop in patients with reduced T-cell function. The immortalization of B cells in the absence of functional T-cell immunity can give rise to lymphoproliferative disease such as Hodgkin lymphoma, Burkitt lymphoma, and nasopharyngeal carcinoma. Increased numbers of circulating WBCs, with a predominance of large, atypical T lymphocytes, are seen in infectious mononucleosis. Heterophile antibodies are nonspecific Abs that agglutinate sheep RBCs and may be used as a screening test for EBV infection.

119. The answer is c. (*Brooks, p 372. Levinson, pp 203, 281. Murray, pp 628-631. Ryan, p 545.*) The replication of a retroviral genome is dependent on the reverse transcriptase enzyme, which performs a variety of functions. It builds a complementary strand of DNA from the viral RNA template; it builds a second DNA strand complementary to the previous DNA; it degrades the original RNA, leaving a DNA–DNA duplex; and, finally, it is responsible for integrating the new viral DNA hybrid into the host genome. It is, therefore, an RNA-dependent DNA polymerase. It has RNase activity, not DNase function. Human cells have DNA-dependent RNA polymerases to produce mRNA and DNA-dependent DNA polymerases to replicate DNA. Reverse transcriptase does not catalyze the isomerization of any RNA being used as a template.

120. The answer is c. (*Brooks, pp 514-519. Levinson, pp 303-304. Murray, pp 610-616. Ryan, p 591.*) Saint Louis encephalitis virus has structural and biologic characteristics in common with other Flaviviruses. It is the most important arboviral disease in North America. Saint Louis encephalitis virus was first isolated from mosquitoes in California. Patients who contract the disease usually present with one of three clinical manifestations: febrile headache, aseptic meningitis, or clinical encephalitis. Mosquitoes are the only insect vector that can transmit SLE, not ticks. Inapparent infections are common and a few persons may develop mild flu-like illness whereas others develop encephalitis. Diagnosis routinely uses HI and ELISA testing since it is so difficult and dangerous to isolate these viruses.

121. The answer is c. (*Brooks, pp 441-446. Levinson, pp 257-258. Murray, pp 534-537. Ryan, p 568.*) (See figure.) Presently, cytomegalovirus (CMV) is the most common cause of congenital and perinatal viral infections. Culture of the virus is a sensitive diagnostic technique; in the case of a neonate with classic symptoms, serum samples from the mother and neonate are obtained at birth. The IgM antibody titer in the infant's serum should be higher than the mother's titer, but they may be similar. For this reason, another sample from the infant at 1 month of age is tested simultaneously with the initial sample. The results should indicate a rise in IgM titer. Measurement of total IgM in the infant's sera at birth is nonspecific and may show false-negative and false-positive reactions. IgG titer in the infant's serum at birth could easily be maternal immunoglobulins. The mother would likely possess IgG anti-CMV Abs since the virus is so widespread in the population. The mother's urine may or may not yield a CMV isolate, depending on whether or not she would be shedding virus.

Cytomegalovirus-infected human embryonic fibroblasts stained with fluorescein-labeled monoclonal antibody to early nuclear antigen (×1000).

122. The answer is e. *(Brooks, pp 405-407. Levinson, pp 228-229, 241. Murray, pp 87-89. Ryan, pp 104, 212.)* IFN is a protein that alters cell metabolism to inhibit viral replication. It induces the formation of a second protein that interferes with the translation of viral messenger RNA. Production of IFN has been demonstrated when cells in tissue culture are challenged with viruses, rickettsiae, endotoxin, or synthetic double-stranded polynucleotides. IFN confers species-specific, not virus-specific, protection for cells. Botulism toxins, chlamydiae, gram-positive bacteria, and synthetic peptides do not induce interferons (IFNs).

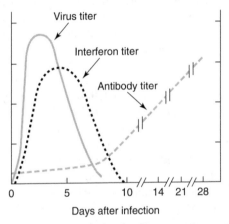

Illustration of kinetics of interferon and antibody synthesis after respiratory viral infection. The temporal relationships suggest that interferons are involved in the recovery process.
(Reproduced, with permission, from Brooks GF, et al. Jawetz's Medical Microbiology. 22nd ed. New York, NY: McGraw-Hill: 2001.)

123. The answer is e. *(Brooks, pp 466-468. Murray, pp 645-648. Toy, p 196.)* Since this was diagnosed and confirmed as a Hepatitis A infection, there is little likelihood of long-term sequelae. One dose of standard γ-globulin, which contains antibodies from a series of normal population individuals, will provide passive protection to the family members for several weeks due to the presence of antibodies against HAV. Vaccination with the killed HAV vaccine might be considered, but for immediate protection, the preformed anti–HAV antibodies will provide immediate and excellent protection. HAV transmits readily, so the no-treatment option could not guarantee no transmission might occur within the family. IFN treatment is approved only for HBV and HCV infections.

124. The answer is e. (*Brooks, pp 446-448. Levinson, pp 258-259, 314. Murray, pp 529-533. Ryan, p 472. Toy, p 190.*) With an acute case of primary infection by EBV, such as infectious mononucleosis, IgM antibodies to VCA should be present. Antibodies to EBNA should be absent, as they usually appear 2 to 3 months after onset of illness. Culture is not clinically useful because it (1) requires freshly fractionated cord blood lymphocytes, (2) takes 3 to 4 weeks for completion, and (3) is reactive in the majority of seropositive patients. IgG antibodies to VCA would appear after the IgM.

125. The answer is a. (*Brooks, pp 419-425. Levinson, pp 216-217, 263. Murray, pp 513-515. Ryan, p 508. Toy, p 178.*) While the herpesviruses (HSV, CMV, and VZV) are all well known for latency, adenovirus can also form a latent infection in the lymphoid tissue. In 50% to 80% of surgically removed tonsils or adenoids, adenovirus can be cultured. The virus has also been cultured from mesenteric lymph nodes, and, in rare cases, viral DNA has been detected in peripheral lymphocytes. Recurrent illness usually does not arise from these latent infections; however, activation can occur in the immunosuppressed. SSPE is a rare disease caused by latent altered measles viruses unable to produce mature virions. Picornaviruses and influenza do not form latent infections.

126. The answer is b. (*Brooks, pp 539-543. Levinson, pp 267-272. Murray, pp 588-590. Ryan, p 501.*) The symptoms described are consistent with influenza virus infection. The titers of antibody on November 6 and 30 show low levels of antibody against swine influenza, but indicate at least a measurable amount. The 160 titer on December 20 reflects a definitive diagnostic rise in antibody against swine influenza (>1:4 rise between acute and convalescent sera). The previous titers (10 or 1:10) most likely represent cross-reacting antibodies from a non-swine influenza virus hemagglutinin or neuraminidase enzymes, which could account for cross-reacting antibodies.

127. The answer is c. *(Brooks, pp 446-448. Levinson, pp 258-259, 314. Murray, pp 529-533. Ryan, p 572. Toy, p 190.)* EBV replication initially occurs in epithelial cells of the pharynx and salivary glands. Infected B cells spread the infection systematically. Most virus-infected cells are eliminated in healthy hosts, but small numbers may persist for a lifetime. Atypical lymphocytes are the hematologic hallmark of infectious mononucleosis with 90% or more of the circulating lymphocytes being atypical in some cases. These abnormal lymphocytes are not pathognomonic for infectious mononucleosis. They are also seen in other diseases, including CMV infection, viral hepatitis, toxoplasmosis, rubella, mumps, and roseola.

128. The answer is a. *(Brooks, pp 511-519, 522. Levinson, pp 218-222, 306. Murray, p 616. Ryan, p 592.)* Dengue (breakbone fever) is caused by a group B togavirus that is transmitted by mosquitoes. The clinical syndrome usually consists of a mild systemic disease characterized by severe joint and muscle pain, headache, fever, lymphadenopathy, and a maculopapular rash. Hemorrhagic dengue, a more severe syndrome, may be prominent during some epidemics; shock and, occasionally, death result. Hepatitis virus infections will primarily affect liver function. HIV infection involves T cells but most likely would not show any alterations in T cell concentrations until AIDS develops and produces a loss of T-cell numbers. Infectious mononucleosis (EBV) produces an increase in circulating WBCs but would not produce the arthralgia and rash as described. SLE would invade the CNS primarily.

129. The answer is e. *(Brooks, pp 468-475. Levinson, pp 298-300. Murray, pp 655-656. Ryan, pp 551-552. Toy, p 196.)* The assumption here is that blood transfusion was done. HCV is a positive-stranded RNA virus, classified as a flavivirus. About half of HCV patients develop chronic hepatitis. A large number of infections appear among IV drug abusers. About 90% of the cases of transfusion-associated hepatitis are thought to be caused by HCV. Blood products are rigorously screened for potential pathogens, including HCV. IV drug users could be at risk for HCV (and HBV) infection if they shared a used needle which was contaminated with blood containing these viruses. HCV is an RNA virus.

130 to 133. The answers are 130-c, 131-e, 132-b, 133-a. *(Brooks, pp 474-478. Levinson, pp 294-298. Murray, pp 645-654. Ryan, pp 548-549.)*

Advances in the serodiagnosis of viral hepatitis have been dramatic, and the findings of specific viral antigens have led to further elucidation of the course of infections. The "Australia antigen," discovered in 1960, was first renamed hepatitis-associated antigen (HAA) and then, finally, hepatitis B surface antigen (HBsAg). It appears in the blood early after infection, before onset of acute illness, and persists through early convalescence. HBsAg usually disappears within 4 to 6 months after the start of clinical illness, except in the case of chronic carriers.

HBeAg appears during the early acute phase and disappears before HBsAg is gone, although it may persist in the chronic carrier. Persons who are HBeAg-positive have higher titers of HBV and therefore are at a higher risk of transmitting the disease. HBeAg has a high correlation with DNA polymerase activity.

The HBcAg is found within the nuclei of infected hepatocytes and not generally in the peripheral circulation, except as an integral component of the Dane particle. The antibody to this antigen, anti–HBc, is present at the beginning of clinical illness. As long as there is ongoing HBV replication, there will be high titers of anti–HBc. During the early convalescent phase of an HBV infection, anti–HBc may be the only detectable serologic marker (window phase) if HBsAg is negative and anti–HBsAg has not appeared. The DNA polymerase found in HBV is actually a reverse transcriptase (RNA-dependent DNA polymerase). In HBV-infected cells, the viral core Ag stays in the cells (hepatocytes) and antibodies to the antigens would be found in the patient's serum. See the Table "Interpretation of HBV Serologic Markers in Patients with Hepatitis."

134. The answer is a. (*Brooks, pp 441-445. Levinson, pp 257-258. Murray, pp 534-538. Ryan, pp 566-569.*) CMV causes cytomegalic inclusion disease (CID), especially congenital abnormalities, in neonates. Malformations include microencephaly. Seizures, deafness, jaundice, and purpura can also occur. CID is also one of the leading causes of mental retardation in the United States. Mumps virus does not cross the placenta and cannot cause an infection in utero. HIV, on the other hand, does cross the placenta. This virus grows in T cells, macrophages, and monocytes. HIV infection in utero would not produce the condition described for the newborn infant. RSV and rubeola (measles) also do not cross the placenta.

135. The answer is b. (*Brooks, pp 557-559. Levinson, pp 274-275. Murray, pp 578-579. Ryan, pp 513-515. Toy, p 236.*) Orchitis, a complication of mumps virus infection in postpubertal males, can cause sterility if bilateral. While HIV can cross the placenta, it results in infection with no malformations as described. Rubeola (measles) does not cross the placenta, while Rubella (German measles) can. Rubella is also responsible for a wide range of in utero malformations. Rubeola (measles) is also a paramyxovirus, but does not cause complications with the testes or ovaries. None of the other viral options can cause the complication of testes infection and orchitis. CMV is a herpesvirus and rabies is an RNA rhabdovirus. While RSV and measles (rubeola) are paramyxoviruses, RSV is primarily seen in infants as a respiratory infection, and measles is a systemic disease characterized by a maculopapular rash.

136. The answer is c. (*Brooks, pp 533-543. Levinson, pp 268-272. Murray, pp 585-590. Ryan, pp 495-503.*) Antigenic drift and antigenic shift account for antigenic changes in the two surface glycoproteins (HA-hemeagglutin and NA-neuraminidase) of influenza viruses. Antigenic drift is a gradual change in antigenicity due to point mutations that affect major antigenic sites on the glycoprotein. Antigenic shift is an abrupt change due to genetic reassortment with an unrelated strain of virus. Changes in HA and NA occur independently. Internal proteins of the virus (eg, NP) do not undergo antigenic changes.

137. The answer is c. (*Brooks, pp 573-578. Levinson, pp 279-281. Murray, pp 593-597. Ryan, pp 597-600.*) The rabies virus is transmitted by the bite of a rabid animal. It almost always causes fatal encephalitis if untreated. Postexposure treatment includes use of a killed vaccine and human rabies globulin (HIG). Rabies virus multiplies in muscle or CT at the site of inoculation and then enters peripheral nerves at neuromuscular junctions. It spreads up the nerves to the CNS. It multiplies in the CNS and progressive encephalitis develops. The virus then spreads to the salivary glands and other tissues via peripheral nerves. Rabies virus has not been isolated from the blood. RSV and rhinoviruses do not infect the CNS. CMV may infect the CNS in utero and may cause aseptic meningitis (10%-30% of cases).

138. The answer is e. (*Brooks, pp 497-498. Levinson, pp 250, 288. Murray, pp 561-563. Ryan, p 510.*) Rhinoviruses are the common cold viruses. They can be recovered from people with mild upper respiratory illness. More than 100 species (100-120) are known, making vaccine development difficult, if not impossible. Viruses enter the upper respiratory tract, invade the surface epithelium of the nasal mucosa, and produce cold symptoms in 1 to 2 days. Neutralizing antibodies form but do not last long. No specific prevention or treatment is available, although intranasal α-interferon looks promising. Mumps and rabies have excellent vaccines available. RSV had one vaccine that looked promising, but recipients developed more severe symptoms if they contracted RSV in the next season. CMV has no vaccine available.

139. The answer is c. (*Brooks, pp 446, 478. Levinson, pp 292-293. Murray, pp 645-648. Ryan, pp 541-544.*) HAV is widespread throughout the world. Transmission occurs through the fecal-oral route through close personal contact. The vaccine for HAV is prepared from virus grown in culture and inactivated with formalin. Passive immunization with immune serum globulin confers passive protection in 90% of those exposed when given within 1 to 2 weeks after exposure. In the United States, hepatitis A infections dropped 10-fold after the vaccine was approved for use. Acyclovir does not inhibit HAV growth. IFNs do not appear to be useful. Live virus vaccines or recombinant viral vaccines have not been successfully developed.

140. The answer is b. (*Brooks, pp 533-543. Levinson, pp 268-272. Murray, pp 583-590. Ryan, pp 495-503.*) Influenza usually occurs in successive waves of infection with peak incidences during the winter months. If only minor antigenic drift is expected for the next influenza season, then the most recent strains of A and B viruses representative of the main antigens are included in the vaccine. Influenza vaccine consists of killed viruses. Immune globulin is not an efficient mechanism for controlling influenza spread due to the short incubation time frame and difficulty in treating the population. Purified NA/HA preparations as well as killed whole virus preparations do not appear to immunize. Live virus vaccines or recombinant viral vaccines have not been successfully developed.

141. The answer is d. (*Brooks, pp 559-561. Levinson, pp 273-274, 482. Murray, pp 573-576. Ryan, pp 515-518.*) Live, attenuated measles virus vaccine effectively prevents measles. Protection is provided if given before or within 2 days of exposure. Vaccination confers immunity for at least 15 years. Interferons are not an effective mechanism to control measles within the population due to difficulties in treating potential patients and cost of the product. The live, attenuated vaccine gave higher levels of population protection than killed/inactivated or recombinant vaccines.

142. The answer is a. (*Brooks, pp 403-409. Levinson, pp 236, 238. Murray, pp 481-483, 525. Ryan, p 208.*) Acyclovir is an analogue of guanosine or deoxyguanosine that strongly inhibits HSV but has little effect on other DNA viruses. When employed for the treatment of primary genital infection by HSV, both oral and IV formulations have reduced viral shedding and shortened the duration of symptoms. Such treatment, however, does not appear to cure the infection due to viral latency in host cells. Azithromycin is an antibacterial antibiotic and does not act against HSV. Passive immunity (globulin) is also ineffective in controlling latent infections and recurrences since the virus moves cell to cell. No effective vaccines have been developed for HSV control.

143. The answer is d. (*Brooks, pp 466-468, 475. Levinson, pp 294-298. Murray, pp 649-654. Ryan, pp 544-549. Toy, p 196.*) The original vaccine for hepatitis B was prepared by purifying hepatitis B surface antigen (HBsAg) from healthy HBsAg-positive carriers and treating it with viral-inactivating agents. The second-generation vaccine for hepatitis B is produced by recombinant DNA in yeast cells containing a plasmid into which the gene for HBsAg has been incorporated. The other vaccine strategies (killed/inactivated, live virus, or synthetic peptides) were not as effective as purified HBsAg or the recombinant HBsAg. Live vaccines for viruses capable of going latent are especially hard to engineer.

144. The answer is e. (*Brooks, pp 437-440. Levinson, pp 256-257. Murray, pp 526-528. Ryan, pp 562-565.*) Varicella-zoster virus is a herpesvirus. Chicken pox is a highly contagious disease of childhood that occurs in the late winter and early spring. It is characterized by a generalized vesicular eruption with relatively insignificant systemic manifestations. Rubeola (measles) produces a maculopapular rash. Adenovirus, CMV, and papillomaviruses do not produce maculopular or vesicular rashes.

145. The answer is a. (*Brooks, pp 419-425. Levinson, pp 216-218, 263. Murray, pp 512-515. Ryan, pp 507-510. Toy, p 178.*) Adenovirus has been associated with adult respiratory disease among newly enlisted military troops. Crowded conditions and strenuous exercise may account for the severe infections seen in this otherwise healthy group. CMV, papillomaviruses, rotaviruses, and VZV do not usually cause acute conjunctivitis. Zoster reactivation may affect the ophthalmic division of the trigeminal nerve in 10% to 15% of cases. The typical crop of VZV vesicles (usually in persons immunocompromised by disease, therapy or aging) would usually be present as an aid to diagnosis.

146. The answer is c. (*Brooks, pp 597-600. Levinson, pp 264-265. Murray, pp 499-504. Ryan, pp 617-620. Toy, p 222.*) Papillomavirus is one of two members of the family Papovaviridae, which includes viruses that produce human warts. These viruses are host-specific and produce benign epithelial tumors that vary in location and clinical appearance. The warts usually occur in children and young adults and are limited to the skin and mucous membranes. Cervical cancer is a major cause of death in developing countries. Integrated copies of HPV DNA are usually present in cervical cancer cells. HPV types 16 and 18 are considered to be high cancer risk. Viral early proteins E6 and E7 are synthesized in cancer tissue with cellular proteins. Cell-mediated immunity is important to control the behavior of HPV lesions, and a quadrivalent HPV vaccine was approved in the United States in 2006. Adenoviruses, CMV, rotaviruses, and VZV do not produce wart lesions.

147. The answer is d. (*Brooks, pp 501-505. Levinson, pp 285-290. Murray, pp 149, 601-604. Ryan, pp 578-581. Toy, p 254.*) Rotaviruses cause the major portion of diarrheal illness in infants and children worldwide but not in adults. These are medium-sized viruses with 11 segments of RNA genome. Rotaviruses, like influenza with a segmented genome, can lead to genetic reassortment. They are fastidious agents to culture and would not be recovered in standard diagnostic laboratories. A live oral vaccine was approved in the United States in 1998 but was withdrawn a year later due to bowel blockages in vaccinated infants. Adenoviruses, CMV, papillomaviruses, and VZV do not cause these symptoms in infected infants.

148. The answer is c. (*Brooks, pp 446-448. Levinson, pp 257-258. Murray, pp 534-537. Ryan, pp 566-569. Toy, pp 184, 190.*) Infectious mononucleosis caused by CMV is clinically difficult to distinguish from that caused by EBV. Lymphocytosis is usually present, with an abundance of atypical lymphocytes. CMV-induced mononucleosis should be considered in any case of mononucleosis that is heterophil-negative and in patients with fever of unknown origin. Adenoviruses, coxsackieviruses, HSV, and VZV do not cause these symptoms in such patients.

149. The answer is b. (*Brooks, pp 446-448. Levinson, pp 258-259. Murray, pp 529-533. Ryan, pp 569-573. Toy, p 190.*) EBV is a herpesvirus that causes a number of syndromes; the most common is infectious mononucleosis. It is a ubiquitous enveloped DNA virus. Only one serotype of EBV has been recognized, although molecular methods have reorganized a number of genotypes of EBV.

Infectious mononucleosis is an acute disease most commonly seen in younger people. It is characterized by a proliferation of lymphocytes, lymph node enlargement, pharyngitis, fatigue, and fever. Infection in young children is usually either asymptomatic or characteristic of an acute upper respiratory infection. Diagnosis is usually made by a positive heterophil test. Heterophil antibodies are those that occur in one species (human) and react with antigens of a different species. The heterophil test may be insensitive (30% to 60%) in children. Definitive diagnosis is made by detection of antibodies to EBV components.

Similar mononucleosis-like diseases are caused by CMV and Toxoplasma gondii, a parasite. CMV causes fewer than 10% of infectious mononucleosis-like diseases. CMV "mono" is primarily characterized by fatigue. Congenital infection with CMV almost always causes serious sequelae, such as retardation and hearing loss. T gondii also causes a variety of clinical problems, among them are encephalitis in AIDS patients and food poisoning from the ingestion of raw meat. Although CMV and T gondii are relatively rare causes of infectious mononucleosis, they must be ruled out, particularly when EBV tests are nonreactive. Borrelia burgdorferi causes Lyme disease, and Toxoplasma is a parasite. Neither affects the heterophile antibody test. Neither do parvoviruses or rubella (German measles) affect that test.

150. The answer is b. (*Brooks, p 727. Levinson, pp 453-455. Murray, pp 173-174, 447. Ryan, p 245.*) Complement fixation antibody measurements against viruses may be a useful diagnostic tool if two serum samples are collected from the patient. The acute serum is collected as early in the illness as possible, and the convalescent serum is collected 7 to 10 days later. Both are included in the same test run against measles CF antigen. A positive diagnostic test occurs in the antibody titer when the convalescent serum is fourfold or greater than the acute sample. The sera are diluted in a twofold manner (1:2, 1:4, 1:8, and so on) for quantitation. The measures given above (40 and 80) are considered essentially the same level of antibodies in both samples. This patient must have had measles in the past and has the same amount of antibody in both serum samples.

151 and 152. The answers are 151-c, 152-a. (*Brooks, pp 446-448. Levinson, pp, 258-259. Murray, pp 529-533. Ryan, pp 569-573. Toy, p 190.*) EBV causes a variety of other syndromes including Burkitt lymphoma, the most common childhood cancer in Africa, and nasopharyngeal carcinoma, commonly seen in China. Most African tumors contain EBV DNA. Malaria may enlarge the pool of EBV-infected cells in some manner. There are chromosome translocations that involve immunoglobulin genes, perhaps promoting cancer development. No associations with Burkitt lymphoma have ever been suggested for *B burgdorferi*, CMV, HSV, or LGV. EBV components have been detected in cells from patients with NPC by PCR. No such evidence of measles or mumps viruses, nor parvoviruses or rubella virus has been observed.

153. The answer is a. (*Brooks, pp 441-445. Levinson, pp 257-258. Murray, pp 534-537. Ryan, pp 566-569. Toy, p 184.*) Cytomegaloviruses are ubiquitous viruses that commonly cause a variety of human diseases. Cytomegalic inclusion disease is a generalized infection of infants by intrauterine or early postnatal infection by CMV. Such infections may lead to severe congenital anomalies. CMV produces a characteristic cytopathic effect. Perinuclear cytoplasmic inclusions form in addition to the intranuclear inclusions typical of herpes viruses. These have been referred to as "owl eye" CPE. In addition, many infected cells become greatly enlarged. The other viruses listed (EBV, HHV6, Norwalk virus, and parvoviruses) do not produce this characteristic CPE.

154 to 158. The answers are 154-b, 155-a, 156-b, 157-d, 158-d. (*Brooks, pp 431-437, 441, 487, 597. Murray, pp 489-496. Ryan, p 231. Toy, p 272.*) The diagnosis of a viral infection is made easier by the creation of a greater number of diagnostic virology laboratories during the past few decades. In order for viral diagnosis to be successful, the most appropriate specimen must be collected for the disease in question.

HPV is often detected microscopically in cervical biopsies. Alternatively, there are methods to detect HPV DNA in such tissues as well as to serotype the virus. Evidence suggests that some HPV serotypes are more likely than others to cause cervical cancer.

Many viruses have a viremic phase, but only a few, such as CMV, persist after the patient becomes symptomatic. CMV can be isolated from lymphocytes and polymorphonuclear leukocytes. This usually requires special separation procedures, particularly in those compromised patients who may be neutropenic.

Enteroviruses such as echoviruses and coxsackieviruses are the predominant cause of aseptic viral meningitis. While enterovirus infections are often diagnosed by specific antibody response, it is possible to isolate the virus from CSF. HSV can also be isolated from CSF in cases of herpes encephalitis or meningitis.

VZV and HSV are most often recovered from skin lesions, although varicella IgM antibody detection may be the most rapid way to diagnose acute VZV infection. Detection and identification of these viruses is essential because of the availability of antiviral agents such as acyclovir. Other viruses, such as enteroviruses and paramyxoviruses, cause skin lesions.

Many viruses can be isolated from feces. Of the viral groups in these questions, adenovirus 40/41 is the most common stool isolate. Norwalk agent and other caliciviruses may also be isolated or detected from stools, but usually only in specialized laboratories.

159 to 163. The answers are 159-c, 160-a, 161-e, 162-d, 163-b. (*Brooks, pp 503-509. Murray, pp 669-670. Ryan, p 578.*) A number of viruses that cause gastroenteritis are now being recognized. The following table summarizes the characteristics of rotavirus, Norwalk virus, adenovirus, calicivirus, and astrovirus (See table below.).

	Norwalk and Norwalk-like Viruses	Rotavirus	Adenovirus	Others Calicivirus	Astrovirus
Size (nm) diameter	27-35	70	70-90	35-39	
Nucleic acid	RNA (single-stranded)	RNA (double-stranded)	DNA	RNA	RNA
Minimum number of serotypes	3	4 (3 groups, A, B, C)	2	3-5	5
Seasonality (temperate climate)	Winter	Winter	All seasons	—	—
Epidemicity	Epidemic	Sporadic, epidemic	Sporadic	Epidemic	Sporadic
Age with clinical disease	≤ 6 years	6 to 24 months most common	≤ 2 years	≤ 2 years	≤ 7 years
Transmission	Fecal-oral, water, food	Fecal-oral, water, food	Fecal-oral	Fecal-oral	Fecal-oral

(Adapted, with permission, from Howard BJ, Keiser JF, Smith TF, Weissfeld AS, Tilton RC. Clinical and Pathogenic Microbiology. 2nd ed. St. Louis, MO: Mosby-Year Book Inc.; 1993.)

164. The answer is e. (*Brooks, pp 562-564. Murray, pp 617-620.*) Rubella (German measles, 3-day measles) is an acute febrile illness characterized by a rash and lymphadenopathy that affects children and young adults. It is the mildest of the viral examthems. Problems arise from in utero infections, especially within the first trimester of pregnancy, when serious and permanent damage, including fatalities, may occur in the fetus. The incubation period is average for viral infections, approximately 1 week. The infections are controlled within the population by using an excellent live, attenuated vaccine. Rubella is an excellent antigen, giving rise to antibodies that provide essentially lifelong protection against the wild-type virus. These preexisting antibodies have been shown to be the main mechanism of protection. Koplik spots are characteristic of rubeola (hard measles) infection. Rubella is classified as part of the Togavirus group, while rubeola is a paramyxovirus.

165 to 168. The answers are 165-c, 166-b, 167-e, 168-d. (*Brooks, pp 466-483. Levinson, pp 292-301. Murray, pp 645-658. Ryan, p 542. Toy, p 196.*) Hepatitis A virus (HAV) possesses a single-stranded linear RNA genome, while hepatitis B virus (HBV) contains a double-stranded DNA genome. Detection of anti–HAV IgM in a single serum specimen obtained in the acute or convalescent stage is the quickest and most reliable method to diagnose hepatitis A infection. This antibody is usually present at onset of symptoms and may persist for 3 to 6 months. Demonstration of hepatitis B surface antigen (HBsAg) in serum is the most common method of diagnosing HBV infection. Other serologic markers helpful in characterizing infection with HBV include hepatitis B surface antibody (anti–HBs), anti–hepatitis B core (anti–HBc), anti–hepatitis B e antigen (anti–HBe), and hepatitis B e antigen (HBeAg). Several epidemiologic studies have demonstrated that immune serum globulin (ISG) can prevent clinical hepatitis A even when given up to 10 days after exposure. Similar studies have shown that ISG was able to decrease the incidence of hepatitis B infection in exposed persons. Purified, noninfectious HBsAg derived from healthy HBsAg carriers has been used as a vaccine for active immunization for HBV infection. Hepatitis C is a single-stranded RNA virus belonging to the family Flaviviridae. The viral reservoir is human. Recent retrospective "lookbacks" suggest that many people were infected with HCV before testing of the blood supply was initiated in the early 1990s. The HCV is treatable with combinations of drugs. The genotype of the virus plays an important role in the determination of length of therapy. Hepatitis D virus is an incomplete or defective virus that requires HBsAg as a cofactor. Both coinfection and secondary delta infection exist, with secondary infection being the most serious. Hepatitis E virus is an RNA virus. Transmission is by the fecal-oral route, although maternal-fetal transmission has recently been described. Prognosis is usually favorable with rare cases of fulminant HEV reported.

169. The answer is b. *(Brooks, p 487. Levinson, pp 290-294. Murray, pp 553-561. Ryan, pp 532-535.)* Enteroviruses (poliovirus, Coxsackie virus, and echoviruse) are ingested through contaminated water and/or food. Their main replication occurs in the intestinal tract, and virus progeny may get into the blood. From blood, distant target organs (eg, the CNS) may become involved. Most enterovirus CNS infections are self-limited, but some may progress to a life-threatening stage. Mumps virus and coronaviruses are inhaled initially. Influenza does not replicate in lymphocytes and does not involve the CNS. HIV has not been shown to be transmitted by any type of insect vector.

170 to 172. The answers are 170-e, 171-b, 172-b. *(Brooks, pp 431-436, 518, 595-597. Levinson, pp 264-265, 252-260, 305. Murray, pp 499-504, 518-525, 604-606. Ryan, pp 559-561.)* West Nile virus (WNV) is an arbovirus. Although prevalent in Europe, Africa, and the Middle East, it was not seen in the United States until the summer of 1999. It is transmitted by mosquitoes and birds, especially crows; these animals are a reservoir. WNV causes mild encephalitis in humans, the exception being older patients or those who may be immunocompromised.

Although most infections by HPV are benign, some undergo malignant transformation into in situ and invasive squamous cell carcinoma. Both HPV and polyomavirus have icosahedral capsids and DNA genomes. JC virus, a polyomavirus, was first isolated from the diseased brain of a patient with Hodgkin lymphoma who was dying of progressive multifocal PML. This demyelinating disease occurs usually in immunosuppressed persons and is the result of oligodendrocyte infection by JC virus. JC virus has also been isolated from the urine of patients suffering from demyelinating disease. Cryotherapy and laser treatments are the most popular therapies for warts, although surgery may be indicated in some cases. At the present time, there is no effective antiviral therapy for treatment of infection with polyomavirus or HPV.

Primary HSV-1 infections are usually asymptomatic. Symptomatic disease occurs most frequently in small children (1-5 years old). Buccal and gingival mucosa are most often involved, and lesions, if untreated, may last 2 to 3 weeks. Acyclovir treatment is effective therapy and should be started immediately. The classic location of latent HSV-1 infection is the trigeminal ganglia. Reactivation results in sporadic vesicular lesions and may also be treated with acyclovir. B-cell activation would be unusual, and there appears to be no greater risk for cancer development than that seen in the general population.

173. The answer is e. *(Brooks, pp 461-462. Levinson, pp 261, 506. Murray, p 546. Toy, p 230.)* The disease is caused by Molluscum contagiosum, a Poxvirus. It is characterized by small, white papules with a central depression and usually found in the genital region. HPV cause genital warts but differ in the type of lesions described in the clinical situation. Adenoviruses cause a variety of infections, including respiratory, ocular, and GI diseases. Parvoviruses and arenaviruses do not produce lesions described in the question.

174 to 177. The answers are 174-c, 175-e, 176-d, 177-a. *(Brooks, pp 419-425, 554, 559-561. Levinson, pp 273-277. Murray, pp 573-576, 579-581. Ryan, pp 499-511. Toy, p 260.)* The paramyxoviruses include several important human pathogens (mumps virus, measles virus, respiratory syncytial virus, and parainfluenza virus). Both paramyxoviruses and orthomyxoviruses possess an RNA-dependent RNA polymerase that is a structural component of the virion and produces the initial RNA. They are 150-nm, single-stranded RNA viruses. There are two antigen groups, A and B, which play no role in diagnosis and treatment. While the overall mortality rate is 0.5%, for at-risk groups mortality may be 25% to 35% if untreated. Some parainfluenza virus infections (type 3) may be indistinguishable from RSV, but most parainfluenza infections produce a laryngotracheobronchitis known as croup. Mumps, measles, variola (smallpox), and coronaviruses all exhibit definite viremic stages in their infections. RSV, on the other hand, is the most important cause of lower respiratory tract illness in infants. RSV is inhaled and viral replication occurs initially in the epithelial cells of the nasopharynx. From there, it may spread to the lower respiratory tract, causing bronchiolitis or pneumonia. The virus remains localized and is isolated from bronchial wash materials or identified in exfoliated epithelial cells, indicating the relative lack of a viremic stage. Current treatment, in fact, consists of ribovirin being delivered in an aerosol format.

178. The answer is c. (*Brooks, pp 468-469. Levinson, pp 298-300. Murray, pp 655-656. Ryan, p 542. Toy, p 196.*) Most new HCV infections are sub-clinical, and 70% to 90% develop into chronic hepatitis. Most HCV chronic cases remain without symptoms but 10% to 20% may develop to chronic active hepatitis and cirrhosis or hepatocellular carcinoma. Mixed cryoglobulinemia and glomerulonephritis complications are not uncommon. Hepatitis A virus (HAV) possesses a single-stranded linear RNA genome and produce only acute disease, while hepatitis B virus (HBV) contains a double-stranded DNA genome. HBV can produce acute or chronic infections. HDV can only occur in HBV-infected individuals. No diagnostic tests or treatment exists for HEV infections.

179. The answer is b. (*Brooks, pp 533-543. Levinson, pp 267-272. Murray, pp 583-592.*) Particularly in the winter months, influenza must be ruled out. In the early stages of an epidemic, viral isolation in primary monkey cells is used. However, as the epidemic proceeds, diagnosis is usually made clinically or by an increase in antibody titer.

Bacteriology

Questions

180. A patient with a burning epigastric pain is admitted to the hospital, and a gastric biopsy is performed. The tissue is cultured on chocolate agar incubated in a microaerophilic environment at 98.6°F (37°C) for 5 to 7 days. At fifth day of incubation, colonies appear on the plate and curved, gram-negative, oxidase-positive rods are observed. Which of the following is the most likely identity of this organism?

a. *Campylobacter fetus*
b. *Campylobacter jejuni*
c. *Haemophilus influenzae*
d. *Helicobacter pylori*
e. *Vibrio parahaemolyticus*

181. A 2-year-old boy who missed several scheduled immunizations presents to the emergency room with a high fever, irritability, and a stiff neck. Fluid from a spinal tap reveals 20,000 white blood cells per milliliter with 85% polymorphonuclear cells. Gram stain evaluation of the fluid reveals small pleomorphic gram-negative rods that grow on chocolate agar. If an inhibitor is designed to block its major virulence, which of the following would be the most likely major virulence factor?

a. Capsule formation
b. Endotoxin assembly
c. Exotoxin liberator
d. Flagella synthesis
e. IgA protease synthesis

182. A local community is in distress due to a natural disaster. After consuming contaminated water, many individuals experience nausea, vomiting, and diarrhea that produce stools resembling rice water. An experimental compound is discovered that prevents the activation of adenylate cyclase and the resulting increase in cyclic AMP. The toxic effects of which of the following bacteria would most likely be prevented with the use of this experimental compound?

a. *Brucella abortus*
b. *Corynebacterium diphtheriae*
c. *Listeria monocytogenes*
d. *Pseudomonas aeruginosa*
e. *Vibrio cholerae*

183. A single, 30-year-old woman presents to her physician with vaginitis. She complains of a slightly increased, malodorous discharge that is gray-white in color, thin, and homogenous. Clue cells are discovered when the discharge is examined microscopically. Which of the following organisms is the most likely cause of her infection?

a. *Candida albicans*
b. *Trichomonas vaginalis*
c. *Escherichia coli*
d. *Gardnerella vaginalis*
e. *Staphylococcus aureus*

184. A 12-year-old girl begins to limp while playing soccer. She has pain in her right leg and upper right thigh. Her temperature is 102°F. X-ray of the femur reveals that the periosteum is eroded. Assuming that this case is managed as an infectious disease, which of the following is the most likely etiologic agent?

a. *Listeria monocytogenes*
b. *Salmonella enteritidis*
c. *Staphylococcus saprophyticus*
d. *Staphylococcus aureus*
e. *Streptococcus pneumoniae*

185. A scraping from a painful, inflamed wound is found to contain numerous gram-negative bacteria. Upon questioning, the feverish patient states that he was bitten by a cat while trying to rescue it from a storm drain earlier in the day. Given these observations, which of the following organisms is the most likely cause of infection?

a. *Aeromonas* species
b. *Campylobacter jejuni*
c. *Pasteurella multocida*
d. *Pseudomonas aeruginosa*
e. *Yersinia enterocolitica*

Questions 186 to 188

A 21-year-old college student complains of malaise, low-grade fever, and a harsh cough. He does not have any muscle aches or pains. An x-ray reveals a diffuse interstitial pneumonia in the left lobes of the lung. The WBC count is normal. The student has been ill for a week.

186. Which of the following is the most likely diagnosis?

a. Influenza
b. Legionellosis
c. Mycoplasma pneumonia
d. Pneumococcal pneumonia
e. Staphylococcal pneumonia

187. Which of the following laboratory tests would most rapidly assist the physician in making the diagnosis?

a. Cold agglutinins
b. Complement fixation (CF) test
c. Culture of sputum
d. Gram stain of sputum
e. Viral culture

188. The following laboratory data are available within 2 days: cold agglutinins—negative; complement fixation (*Mycoplasma pneumoniae*)—1:64; viral culture—pending, but negative to date; bacterial culture of sputum on blood agar and MacConkey agar—normal oral flora. In order to confirm the diagnosis, which of the following procedures should be ordered to achieve a specific and sensitive diagnosis?

a. A DNA probe to the 16S ribosomal RNA of an organism lacking a cell wall
b. Another viral culture in 1 week
c. A repeat complement fixation (CF) test in 5 days
d. A repeat cold agglutinin test
e. Culture of the sputum on charcoal yeast extract

189. A 40-year-old male, who was in good health earlier, begins experiencing a chronic cough. Over the following 6 weeks, the cough gradually worsens and becomes productive. He is also coughing up blood, and notes weight loss, fever, and night sweats. A sputum sample is positive for acid-fast bacilli. Which of the following pathogenic mechanisms can be primarily attributed to the etiologic agent involved in this disease?

a. Cell-mediated hypersensitivity
b. Clogging of alveoli by large numbers of acid-fast mycobacteria
c. Humoral immunity
d. Specific cell adhesion sites
e. Toxin production by the mycobacteria

190. A person living on streets is infected with an invasive salmonella organism that is resistant to most of the antibiotics that could be considered for treatment. It did show sensitivity to quinolones which are bactericidal. Which of the following is the best explanation of their mode of action on growing bacteria?

a. Inactivation of penicillin-binding protein II
b. Inhibition of β-lactamase
c. Inhibition of DNA gyrase
d. Inhibition of reverse transcriptase
e. Prevention of the cross-linking of glycine

191. A high school student with a natural immunodeficiency is treated aggressively with a variety of potent antibiotics to overcome several bacterial infections. The most recent problem is caused by *S aureus*, which is reported to be vancomycin-indeterminate (VISA). Which of the following statements concerning VISA is correct?

a. Patients with VISA isolates need not be isolated.
b. Minimum inhibitory concentration (MIC) for vancomycin is at least 1.0 mcg/mL.
c. VISAs have emerged because of the extended use of vancomycin for methicillin-resistant *Staphylococcus aureus* (MRSAs).
d. VISA isolates are infrequent, so surveillance at the present time is not warranted.
e. VISA isolates are usually methicillin susceptible.

192. A 3-year-old girl, who has missed several scheduled immunizations, presents to the emergency room with a fever and troubled breathing. A sputum sample is brought to the laboratory for analysis. Gram stain reveals the following: rare epithelial cells, 8 to 10 polymorphonuclear leukocytes per high-power field, and pleomorphic gram-negative rods. As a laboratory consultant, which of the following interpretations is correct?

a. The appearance of the sputum is suggestive of *H influenzae*.
b. The patient has pneumococcal pneumonia.
c. The patient has Vincent disease.
d. The sputum specimen is too contaminated by saliva to be useful.
e. There is no evidence of an inflammatory response.

193. A 25-year-old medical student presents with a ruptured appendix. A peritoneal infection develops, despite prompt removal of the organ and extensive flushing of the peritoneal cavity. An isolate from a pus culture reveals a gram-negative rod identified as *Bacteroides fragilis*. Anaerobic infection with *B fragilis* is best characterized by which of the following?

a. A black exudate in the wound
b. A foul-smelling discharge
c. A heme-pigmented colony formation
d. An exquisite susceptibility to penicillin
e. Severe neurologic symptoms

194. Several days after an unprotected sexual encounter, a healthy 21-year-old male develops pain and pus on urination. A Gram stain reveals gram-negative diplococci. Which of the following structures is responsible for adherence of the offending microbe to the urethral mucosa?

a. Capsule
b. Fimbriae
c. Flagella
d. The F pili
e. The peptidoglycan
f. The lipopolysaccharide (LPS)

195. A 1-week-old newborn develops meningitis. Short, gram-positive rods are isolated. History reveals that the mother had eaten unpasteurized cheese from Mexico during pregnancy, and she recalled having a flu-like illness. Which of the following is the most likely etiologic microorganism?

a. *Corynebacterium diphtheriae*
b. *Escherichia coli*
c. Group B streptococci
d. *Listeria monocytogenes*
e. *Streptococcus pneumoniae*

Questions 196 to 199

196. A 30-year-old male patient is seen by the emergency service and reports a 2-week history of a penile ulcer. He notes that this ulcer did not hurt. Which of the following conclusions/actions is most valid?

a. Draw blood for a herpes antibody test.
b. Even if treated, the lesion will remain for months.
c. Failure to treat the patient will have no untoward effect, as this is a self-limiting infection.
d. Perform a dark-field examination of the lesion.
e. Prescribe acyclovir for primary genital herpes.

197. The laboratory reports that the Venereal Disease Research Laboratory (VDRL) test performed on the above patient is reactive at a dilution of 1:4 (4 dils). The patient also reports to you that he has recently been diagnosed with hepatitis A. Which one of the following is most appropriate next step in management?

a. Order a confirmatory test such as the fluorescent treponemal antibody (FTA) test.
b. Order a rapid plasma reagin (RPR) test.
c. Perform a spinal tap to rule out central nervous system (CNS) syphilis.
d. Repeat the VDRL test.
e. Report this patient to the health department, as he has syphilis.

198. In the same patient from the previous vignette, which of the following test combinations for syphilis is most appropriate?

a. FTA-Abs (IgG)/FTA-Abs (IgM)
b. RPR/culture of the lesion
c. RPR/FTA-Abs
d. *Treponema pallidum* hemagglutination (TPHA)/microhemagglutination—*Treponema pallidum* (MHTP) tests
e. VDRL/RPR

199. Assume that the same patient from the previous vignette absolutely denies any contact, sexual or otherwise, with a person who had syphilis. Also assume that both the RPR and the FTA-Abs are positive on this patient. Which of the following tests could be used to show that this patient probably does not have syphilis?

a. Frei test
b. MHTP test
c. Quantitative RPR
d. *Treponema pallidum* immobilization (TPI) test
e. VDRL

200. A 55-year-old man who is being treated for adenocarcinoma of the lung is admitted to a hospital because of a temperature of 102°F (38.9°C), chest pain, and a dry cough. Sputum is collected. Gram stain of the sputum is unremarkable, and culture reveals many small, gram-negative rods able to grow only on a charcoal yeast extract agar. Which of the following is the most likely organism?

a. *Chlamydia trachomatis*
b. *Klebsiella pneumoniae*
c. *Legionella pneumophila*
d. *Mycoplasma pneumoniae*
e. *Staphylococcus aureus*

201. A patient is hospitalized after an automobile accident. The wounds become infected, and the patient is treated with tobramycin, carbenicillin, and clindamycin. Five days after antibiotic therapy was initiated, the patient develops severe diarrhea and pseudomembranous enterocolitis. Antibiotic-associated diarrhea and the more serious pseudomembranous enterocolitis can be caused by which of the following organisms?

a. *Bacteroides fragilis*
b. *Clostridium difficile*
c. *Clostridium perfringens*
d. *Clostridium sordellii*
e. *Staphylococcus aureus*

202. A premature neonate suffers from pneumonia and sepsis. Sputum swab culture on blood agar plate yields pinpointed β-hemolytic colonies. Which of the following is a simple test to determine whether the organism is *S agalactiae* or *L monocytogenes* (both important neonatal pathogens)?

a. Bacitracin sensitivity test
b. Catalase test
c. Coagulase test
d. Polymerase chain reaction (PCR)
e. Sugar fermentation test

203. A 2-year-old child has a fever, stiff neck, and is irritable. Gram stain smear of spinal fluid reveals gram-negative, small pleomorphic coccobacillary organisms. What is the most appropriate procedure to follow in order to reach an etiological diagnosis?

a. Culture the spinal fluid in chocolate agar, and identify the organism by growth factors.
b. Culture the spinal fluid in mannitol-salt agar.
c. Perform a catalase test of the isolated organism.
d. Perform a coagulase test with the isolate.
e. Perform a latex agglutination (LA) test to detect the specific antibody in the spinal fluid.

204. A patient complains to his dentist about a draining lesion in his mouth. A Gram stain of the pus shows a few gram-positive cocci, leukocytes, and many-branched gram-positive rods. Branched yellow sulfur granules are observed by microscope. Which of the following is the most likely cause of the disease?

a. *Actinomyces israelii*
b. *Actinomyces viscosus*
c. *Corynebacterium diphtheriae*
d. *Propionibacterium acnes*
e. *Staphylococcus aureus*

205. A female infant, born prematurely after rupture of membranes, develops fever within 1 day of birth and dies. The pregnant mother had been cultured just prior to the birth of her child, and her vaginal culture revealed group B streptococci (GBS, *S agalactiae*). Which of the tests shown in the following figure would provide the most rapid and useful information?

a. Direct Gram stain demonstrating *Streptococcus agalactiae* in CSF of infected neonate (μ1000).
b. Blood agar plate demonstrating diffuse β-hemolysis due to group B streptococci from CSF.
c. Brain at autopsy demonstrating acute hemorrhagic response to *S agalactiae*.
d. Brain section with blood vessel occluded by group B streptococci.

206. A 39-year-old primigravid Caucasian female lawyer develops premature rupture of membranes at 35 weeks of gestation. She develops fever up to 103°F, and the amniotic fluid reveals a group B *Streptococcus*. Which of the following is the best option to reduce Group B streptococcal infection in her fetus?

a. Identification of possible high-risk births
b. Intravenous penicillin administered at least 4 hours before delivery
c. Screening of pregnant female at the first office visit, usually during the first trimester
d. Screening of pregnant female in the last trimester
e. Use of a polysaccharide vaccine

207. A 1-week-old neonate presents to the pediatric emergency room with fever, irritability, poor feeding, and a bulging anterior fontanelle. Lumbar puncture is performed, and the cerebrospinal fluid (CSF) grows group B *Streptococcus*. Which of the following is the most likely pathogenic mechanism?

a. Complement C5a, a potent chemoattractant, activates polymorphonuclear neutrophils (PMNs).
b. In the absence of a specific antibody, opsonization, phagocyte recognition, and killing do not proceed normally.
c. The alternative complement pathway is activated.
d. The streptococci are resistant to penicillin.

208. A man who has a penile chancre appears in a hospital's emergency service. The VDRL test is negative. Which of the following is the most appropriate course of action?

a. Perform dark-field microscopy for treponemes.
b. Perform a Gram stain on the chancre fluid.
c. Repeat the VDRL test in 10 days.
d. Send the patient home untreated.
e. Swab the chancre and culture on Thayer-Martin agar.

209. A clinically depressed farmer complains of extreme weakness, a daily rise and fall in fever, and night sweats. Small gram-negative rods are isolated from blood cultures after a 2-week incubation period. Which of the following organisms is the most likely etiologic agent?

a. *Brucella melitensis*
b. *Campylobacter jejuni*
c. *Francisella tularensis*
d. *Salmonella enteritidis*
e. *Serratia marcescens*

210. An outbreak occurs in a community where the water supply is contaminated. Multiple patients experience nausea and vomiting as well as profuse diarrhea with abdominal cramps; stools are described as "rice water." Curved, gram-negative rods are isolated on a sulfate-citrate-bile-sucrose agar. In the treatment of patients who have cholera, the use of a drug that inhibits adenyl cyclase would be expected to have which of the following characteristics?

a. Block the action of cholera toxin.
b. Eradicate the organism.
c. Increase fluid secretion.
d. Kill the patient immediately.
e. Reduce intestinal motility.

211. A box of ham sandwiches with mayonnaise, prepared by a person with a boil on his neck, is left out of the refrigerator for the on-call interns. Three doctors become violently ill approximately 2 hours after eating the sandwiches. Which of the following is the most likely cause?

a. *Clostridium perfringens* toxin
b. Coagulase from *S aureus* in the ham
c. Penicillinase given to inactivate penicillin in the pork
d. *Staphylococcus aureus* enterotoxin
e. *Staphylococcus aureus* leukocidin

212. A 34-year-old diabetic truck driver notices maceration of the web space of his toes on the right foot. Two days later he has a temperature of up to 100°F, exquisite tenderness, erythema, and swelling of the right leg. Culture exudate from the foot yields *S aureus*. Which of the following often complicates treatment of *S aureus* infection with penicillin?

a. Allergic reaction caused by staphylococcal protein
b. Inability of penicillin to penetrate the membrane of *S aureus*
c. Lack of penicillin-binding sites on *S aureus*
d. Production of penicillin acetylase by *S aureus*
e. Production of penicillinase by *S aureus*

213. Two of three family members have dinner at a local restaurant and, within 48 hours, start experiencing double vision, difficulty in swallowing and speaking, and breathing problems. These symptoms are consistent with which of the following?

a. Activation of cyclic AMP
b. Endotoxin shock
c. Ingestion of a neurotoxin
d. Invasion of the gut epithelium by an organism
e. Secretion of an enterotoxin

214. A clinical research group attempting to develop an improved *Neisseria meningitidis* vaccine is granted approval to gather volunteers for a clinical trial. Part of the volunteer evaluation is to sample bacteriologically for normal oral flora *Neisseria*. They find that almost all of the participants have several commensal species as part of their URT flora. Which of the following statements accurately describes the significance of these bacteria?

a. As a part of the normal flora, *Neisseria* provide a natural immunity in local host defense.
b. As a part of the respiratory flora, they are the most common cause of acute bronchitis and pneumonia.
c. Commensal bacteria stimulate a cell-mediated immunity (CMI).
d. Commensal *Neisseria* in the upper respiratory tract impede phagocytosis by means of lipoteichoic acid.
e. Normal flora, such as nonpathogenic *Neisseria*, provides effective nonspecific B-cell-mediated humoral immunity.

215. A family routinely consumes unpasteurized milk, claiming "better taste." Several members experience a sudden onset of crampy abdominal pain, fever, and profuse bloody diarrhea. *Campylobacter jejuni* is isolated and identified from all patients. Which of the following is the treatment of choice for this type of enterocolitis?

a. Ampicillin
b. *Campylobacter* antitoxin
c. Ciprofloxacin
d. Erythromycin
e. Pepto-Bismol

216. An unimmunized, 2-year-old boy presents with drooling from the mouth, elevated temperature, and enlarged tonsils. During attempts at intubation, no grey-white membrane is observed but the epiglottis appears "beefy" red and edematous. Which of the following is the most likely organism?

a. *Haemophilus haemolyticus*
b. *Haemophilus influenzae*
c. *Klebsiella pneumoniae*
d. *Mycoplasma pneumoniae*
e. *Neisseria meningitidis*

Questions 217 to 219

217. A 70-year-old female patient is readmitted to a local hospital with fever and chills following cardiac surgery at a major teaching institution. A gram-positive coccus grows within 24 hours from blood taken from the patient. Initial tests indicate that this isolate is resistant to penicillin. Which of the following is the most likely identification?

a. *Enterococcus species*
b. Group A *Streptococcus*
c. Group B *Streptococcus*
d. *Neisseria species*
e. *Streptococcus pneumoniae*

218. Further testing of the patient in the previous question reveals that the isolate possesses the group D antigen, and is not β-lactamase-positive, but is resistant to vancomycin. Which of the following is the most likely identification of this isolate?

a. *Enterococcus cassiflavus*
b. *Enterococcus durans*
c. *Enterococcus faecalis*
d. *Enterococcus faecium*
e. *Streptococcus pneumoniae*

219. Which of the following is the treatment of choice for the isolate in Question 218?

a. Ciprofloxacin
b. Gentamicin
c. Gentamicin and ampicillin
d. Rifampin
e. No available treatment

220. A young man crashes his bicycle, injuring one leg. Bacteria from the wound and a subsequent blood culture are isolated and identified, and an acute hematogenous osteomyelitis is diagnosed. Which organism listed below most often causes this type of infection?

a. *Escherichia coli*
b. *Proteus mirabilis*
c. *Staphylococcus aureus*
d. *Staphylococcus epidermidis*
e. *Streptococcus faecalis*

221. A 3-year-old girl, with no history of vaccination, is brought to the hospital with a sore throat, fever, malaise, and difficulty in breathing. Physical examination reveals a gray membrane covering the pharynx. Growth of the etiologic agent on cysteine-tellurite agar forms gray-to-black colonies with a brown halo. The major virulence factor of this organism is only produced by those strains that will most likely have which of the following characteristics?

a. Encapsulated
b. Endotoxin
c. Glucose fermenters
d. Lysogenic for β-prophage
e. Sucrose fermenters

Questions 222 to 224

A 28-year-old menstruating woman appears in the emergency room with the following signs and symptoms: fever, 104°F (40°C); WBC, 16,000/μL; blood pressure, 90/65 mm Hg; a scarlatiniform rash on her trunk, palms, and soles; extreme fatigue; vomiting; and diarrhea.

222. Which of the following is the most likely diagnosis?

a. Chicken pox
b. Guillain-Barré syndrome
c. Scalded skin syndrome
d. Staphylococcal food poisoning
e. Toxic shock syndrome (TSS)

223. Culture of the menstrual fluid in this case cited would most likely reveal a predominance of which of the following?

a. *Clostridium difficile*
b. *Clostridium perfringens*
c. *Gardnerilla vaginalis*
d. *Staphylococcus aureus*
e. No organisms isolated

224. Which of the following is the most likely source and characteristic finding not yet revealed in the case just presented?

a. A meal of chicken in a fast-food restaurant
b. A retained tampon
c. Heavy menstrual flow
d. Recent exposure to rubella
e. Travel to Vermont

Questions 225 and 226

A severe URT outbreak occurs in the residence of students of a private school, resulting in several cases of otitis media and acute sinusitis. Some students do not have any clinical evidence of infection. The state public health laboratory receives and evaluates a new latex agglutination (LA) reagent for *H influenzae* polysaccharide capsular antigen in urine (intact antigen elimination). Results, shown below, are compared with the isolation of *H influenzae* from pharyngeal swabs.

LA POS, CULT POS: 25
LA POS, CULT NEG: 5
LA NEG, CULT POS: 5
LA NEG, CULT NEG: 95

	LA +ve	LA –ve	total
Cul +ve	25	5	30
Cul –ve	5	95	100
total	30	100	130

225. Which of the following best indicates the sensitivity of LA?

a. 0%
b. 30%
c. 85%
d. 95%
e. 100%

226. Which of the following best indicates the specificity of LA?

a. 0%
b. 30%
c. 80%
d. 95%
e. 100%

227. A severely burned firefighter develops a rapidly disseminating bacterial infection while hospitalized. "Green pus" is noted in the burned tissue, and cultures of both the tissue and blood yield small, oxidase-positive, gram-negative rods. Which of the following statements best describes this organism?

a. Endotoxin is the only virulence factor known to be produced by these bacteria.
b. Humans are the only known reservoir hosts for these bacteria.
c. The bacteria are difficult to culture because they have numerous growth requirements.
d. These are among the most antibiotic resistant of all clinically relevant bacteria.
e. These highly motile bacteria can "swarm" over the surface of culture media.

228. Several hours after dining on sweet and sour chicken and pork fried rice at the home of an Asian friend, a 34-year-old car salesman exhibits abdominal discomfort, nausea, and vomiting. In the middle of the night he awakens with watery diarrhea. Which of the following pairs of organisms is routinely responsible for food poisoning?

a. *Clostridium botulinum* and *Bacillus anthracis*
b. *Clostridium difficile* and *C botulinum*
c. *Clostridium perfringens* and *B cereus*
d. *Clostridium tetani* and *B anthracis*
e. *Clostridium tetani* and *B cereus*

229. MRSA is isolated from seven patients in a 14-bed intensive care unit. All patients are isolated and the unit closed to any more admissions. Which of the following best explains these rigorous methods to control MRSA?

a. MRSA causes TSS.
b. MRSA is inherently more virulent than other staphylococci.
c. MRSA is resistant to penicillin.
d. MRSA spreads more rapidly from patient to patient than antibiotic-susceptible staphylococci do.
e. The alternative for treatment of MRSA is vancomycin, an expensive and potentially toxic antibiotic.

230. A 2-year-old infant is brought to the emergency room with hematuria, fever, and thrombocytopenia. Which one of the following bacteria would most likely be isolated from a stool specimen?

a. *Aeromonas* species
b. *Enterobacter aerogenes*
c. *Escherichia coli* O157/H7
d. *Salmonella enteriditis*
e. *Shigella flexneri*

231. A 65-year-old healthy, retired female executive goes to Mexico on her yearly vacation. Unlike her previous trips, she decides to use the local water to make her favorite punch. Thirty-six hours later she develops profuse watery diarrhea, severe cramping, and abdominal pain. She is diagnosed with *Escherichia coli*-related diarrhea. Which of the following *E coli* types is characterized by the presence of heat-labile (LT) and heat-stable (ST) toxin proteins?

a. Enteroinvasive (EIEC)
b. Enterotoxigenic (ETEC)
c. Enterohemorrhagic (EHEC)
d. Enteropathogenic (EPEC)

232. A 48-year-old farmer in New Mexico is bitten by a flea and, 5 days later, develops a sudden onset of fever, chills, weakness, and headache. A few hours later he develops swollen, necrotic lymph nodes (buboes) in the right axilla and groin, which are intensely painful. This patient is subsequently diagnosed with bubonic plague and does not develop any pneumonic features of the disease. Human plague can be bubonic or pneumonic. Which of the following is the primary epidemiologic difference between the two clinical forms of plague?

a. Age of the patient
b. Geographic location of the animal vector
c. Health of the animal vector
d. Route of infection
e. Season of the year

233. A 9-year-old child is brought to the emergency room with the chief complaint of enlarged, painful axillary lymph nodes. The resident physician also notes a small, inflamed, dime-sized lesion surrounding what appears to be a small scratch on the forearm. The lymph node is aspirated and some pus is sent to the laboratory for examination. A Warthin-Starry silver impregnation stain reveals many highly pleomorphic, rod-shaped bacteria. Which of the following is the most likely cause of this infection?

a. *Bartonella henselae*
b. *Brucella canis*
c. *Mycobacterium scrofulaceum*
d. *Yersinia enterocolitica*
e. *Yersinia pestis*

234. A sixth-grade boy returns from summer camp with several minor cuts and abrasions. Within a week, extensive cellulitis develops, and it is apparent that subcutaneous tissue is involved, requiring surgical removal of nonviable tissue. Antibiotics are used aggressively. Cellulitis is usually caused by which of the following?

a. *Bacillus cereus*
b. *Clostridium tetani*
c. Group A streptococci
d. *Micrococcus species*
e. *Staphylococcus aureus*

235. A 40-year-old female reports chronic gastritis. She tests positive for *H pylori*. After a course of the appropriate antibiotic therapy, her symptoms subside. Which of the following is the most effective noninvasive test for the diagnosis of *Helicobacter*-associated gastric ulcers?

a. Culture of stomach contents for *H pylori*
b. Detection of *H pylori* antigen in stool
c. Growth of *H pylori* from a stomach biopsy
d. Growth of *H pylori* in the stool
e. IgM antibodies to *H pylori*

236. The following examination and test results are observed in a woman tested in November who reports being in the woods in Pennsylvania during the past summer. While there, she was bitten by a tick, and now has a flattened red area near the bite with central clearing. She also has flu-like illness with fever, myalgia, and headache. Which of the following is the most appropriate course of action?

a. Ask the patient if she has a severe headache.
b. Do a spinal tap for CSF.
c. Observe the lesion.
d. Order a Lyme disease antibody titer.
e. Start treatment with tetracycline.

237. Several white male patients, over 50 years of age and suffering from cavitary pulmonary disease, being followed and treated at a university AIDS clinic are found to be infected by *Mycobacterium avium*, a major opportunist pathogen. *Mycobacterium avium* from these patients is best characterized by which one of the following statements

a. Few isolates from AIDS patients are acid-fast.
b. Most isolates from AIDS patients are sensitive to isoniazid and streptomycin.
c. *Mycobacterium avium* can be isolated from the blood of many AIDS patients.
d. *Mycobacterium avium* isolates from AIDS patients are of multiple serovars.
e. The majority of *M avium* isolates from AIDS patients are nonpigmented.

238. A 12-year-old girl experiences a group A streptococcus pharyngitis and within 3 weeks has chest pain and develops new murmurs of mitral regurgitation. Which of the following statements best typifies the disease she is suffering from?

a. It is a complication of group A streptococcal skin disease but usually not of pharyngitis.
b. It is characterized by inflammatory lesions that may involve the heart, joints, subcutaneous tissues, and CNS.
c. It is very common in developing countries but extremely rare and decreasing in incidence in the United States.
d. Prophylaxis with benzathine penicillin is of little value.
e. The pathogenesis is related to the similarity between a staphylococcal antigen and a human cardiac antigen.

239. After extraction of a wisdom tooth, an 18-year-old male student is diagnosed with subacute bacterial endocarditis. He has a congenital heart disease that has been under control. Which of the following is the most likely organism causing the infection?

a. *Staphylococcus aureus*
b. *Staphylococcus epidermidis*
c. *Streptococcus pneumoniae*
d. *Streptococcus viridians*
e. *Enterococcus faecalis*

240. A 70-year-old male is taken to the emergency room with a history of "cold-like" symptoms for at least 3 days. At the time of the visit, his temperature is 102°F and he experienced shaking, chills, chest pain, and a productive cough with bloody sputum. Blood agar culture reveals gram-positive α-hemolytic colonies. If a quellung test was done on the colonies, which of the following bacteria would most likely be positive?

a. *Corynebacterium diphtheriae*
b. *Enterobacter* species
c. *Haemophilus parainfluenzae*
d. *Neisseria gonorrhoeae*
e. *Streptococcus pneumoniae*

241. A 6-month-old infant is admitted to the hospital with acute meningitis. The Gram stain reveals gram-positive, short rods, and the mother indicates that the child has received "all" of the meningitis vaccinations. Which of the following is the most likely cause of the disease?

a. *Haemophilus influenzae*
b. *Listeria monocytogenes*
c. *Neisseria meningitidis*, group A
d. *Neisseria meningitidis*, group C
e. *Streptococcus pneumoniae*

242. A 40-year-old man presents to the emergency medicine department 1 week following a foot injury. He is experiencing intense pain in the area of injury and the muscles of the jaw. Which of the following is the most common portal of entry for the etiologic organism?

a. Gastrointestinal tract
b. Genital tract
c. Nasal tract
d. Respiratory tract
e. Skin

243. A 22-year-old homeless person with a known drug abuse problem and multiple opportunistic infections has a positive PPD (purified protein) test. Which of the following is the most common way this infection is acquired?

a. Gastrointestinal tract
b. Genital tract
c. Nasal tract
d. Respiratory tract
e. Skin

244. A 31-year-old school teacher returns from foreign travel and experiences a sudden (1-2 days) onset of abdominal pain, fever, and watery diarrhea, caused by a heat-labile exotoxin that affects both the gut and the central nervous system (CNS). This infection is caused by an etiologic agent commonly acquired through which of the following routes?

a. Gastrointestinal tract
b. Genital tract
c. Nasal tract
d. Respiratory tract
e. Skin

245. A college student is surprised one morning by painful urination and a cream-colored exudate. Any person who acquires the gram-negative microbe that causes this infection is most likely to have acquired it via which of the following?

a. Gastrointestinal tract
b. Genitourinary tract
c. Nasal tract
d. Respiratory tract
e. Skin

246. A 25-year-old college student with no history of allergic rhinitis has a 12-day history of facial pain, clear rhinorrhea, fever, headache, and back pain. Her symptoms do not respond to over-the-counter medication. Culture of the fluid from the sinus reveals *Moraxella (Branhamella) catarrhalis.* Which of the following best characterizes *M catarrhalis?*

a. A gram-negative, pleomorphic rod that can cause endocarditis
b. A gram-negative rod, fusiform-shaped, that is associated with periodontal disease but may cause sepsis
c. The causative agent of rat-bite fever
d. The gram-negative diplococcus which is the causative agent of sinusitis, bronchitis, and pneumonia
e. The causative agent of trench fever

247. A 16-year-old Hispanic female with poor oral hygiene and severe gingivitis presents with a temperature of 103.5°F and hypotension. Blood culture is positive for *Capnocytophaga.* Which of the following best characterizes *Capnocytophaga?*

a. A gram-negative, pleomorphic rod that can cause endocarditis
b. A gram-negative rod, fusiform-shaped, that is associated with periodontal disease but may cause sepsis
c. The causative agent of rat-bite fever
d. The causative agent of sinusitis, bronchitis, and pneumonia
e. The causative agent of trench fever

248. Several employees in a veterinary facility experience a mild influenza-like infection after working on six sheep with an undiagnosed illness. The etiologic agent causing the human disease is most often transmitted to humans by which of the following methods?

a. Fecal contamination from flea deposits on the skin
b. Inhalation of infected particles or aerosols from the suspected animal urine and feces
c. Lice feces scratched into the broken skin during the louse's blood feeding
d. Tick saliva during feeding on human blood
e. Urethral discharge from infected humans

249. An endocarditis patient under a physician's care develops a urinary tract infection (UTI). A group D enterococcus (*Enterococcus faecium*) is isolated but the UTI does not respond to ampicillin and gentamicin treatments. Which of the following options would be considered the most clinically appropriate action?

a. Consider vancomycin as an alternative drug.
b. Determine if fluorescent microscopy is available for the diagnosis of actinomycosis.
c. Do no further clinical workup.
d. Suggest to the laboratory that low colony counts may reflect infection.
e. Suggest a repeat antibiotic susceptibility test.

250. A patient with symptoms of a urinary tract infection has a culture taken, which grows 5×10^3 *E coli*. The laboratory reports it as "insignificant." Which of the following is the most appropriate next step in management?

a. Consider vancomycin as an alternative drug.
b. Determine if fluorescent microscopy is available for the diagnosis of actinomycosis.
c. Do no further clinical workup.
d. Suggest to the laboratory that low colony counts may reflect infection; follow up with culture.
e. Suggest a repeat antibiotic susceptibility test.

251. A patient appears in the emergency room with a submandibular mass. A smear is made of the drainage and a bewildering variety of bacteria are seen, including branched, gram-positive rods. Which of the following is the most clinically appropriate action?

a. Consider vancomycin as an alternative drug.
b. Determine if fluorescent microscopy is available for the diagnosis of actinomycosis.
c. Do no further clinical workup.
d. Suggest to the laboratory that low colony counts may reflect infection.
e. Suggest a repeat antibiotic susceptibility test.

252. A 55-year-old male develops malaise, fever up to 103.5°F, nonproductive cough, headache, and shortness of breath a few days after he repaired the cooling system of an old hotel. A chest x-ray reveals fluid in his lungs. From a sputum sample, a gram-negative rod grew slowly on a buffered cysteine containing charcoal-yeast agar. Which of the following antibiotic therapies is most appropriate for treating this patient?

a. Ampicillin
b. Ceftriaxone
c. Erythromycin
d. Penicillin
e. Vancomycin

253. A 60-year-old male resident from a nursing home presents to the emergency room with a fever of 105.8°F (41°C), shaking chills, severe pain to the right side of his chest that worsens with breathing, and a productive cough with blood-tinged sputum. During the previous 3 days, he noted cold-like symptoms. Gram stain evaluation of the sputum reveals gram-positive diplococci that grow into α-hemolytic colonies on blood agar. Which of the following antibiotic therapies is the most appropriate treatment for this patient?

a. Ampicillin
b. Ceftriaxone
c. Erythromycin
d. Penicillin
e. Vancomycin

254. A 12-year-old boy, after a camping trip near a wooded area in Northern California, is taken to the emergency room after complaining of a headache. He has an erythema migrans rash around what appears to be a tick bite. Which of the following is the antibiotic of choice for treating this patient?

a. Ampicillin
b. Ceftriaxone
c. Erythromycin
d. Penicillin
e. Vancomycin

255. A 6-year-old girl presents to her pediatrician with fever, headache, and a sore throat. She has swollen tender cervical lymph nodes, and her oropharynx is red with a gray-white exudate covering both her tonsils. A rapid strep test of her throat swab is positive, and the culture subsequently grows β-hemolytic *Streptococcus*. Which of the following antibiotic therapies is most appropriate for treating this patient?

a. Ampicillin
b. Ceftriaxone
c. Erythromycin
d. Penicillin
e. Vancomycin

256. A young woman being treated with a broad-spectrum antimicrobial develops endoscopically observed microabscesses and diarrhea. Which of the following is the therapy of choice for this form of enterocolitis?

a. Ampicillin
b. Ceftriaxone
c. Erythromycin
d. Penicillin
e. Vancomycin

257. Although cholera, a *Vibrio* infection, has rarely been seen in the United States, there have been recent outbreaks of classic cholera associated with shellfish harvested from the Gulf of Mexico. Vibrios are shaped like curved rods, and infections more common than cholera may be caused by a variety of curved-rod bacteria. Which of the following best describes *C jejuni*?

a. Cause of gastroenteritis; reservoir in birds and mammals, optimal growth at 107.6°F (42°C).
b. Human pathogen, halophilic, lactose-negative, sucrose-negative; causes gastrointestinal diseases primarily from ingestion of under-cooked seafood.
c. Human pathogen, halophilic, lactose-positive; produces heat-labile, extracellular toxin wound infections.
d. Organisms are susceptible to acid; not an invasive organism.
e. Urease-positive; cause of fetal distress in cattle.

258. *Vibrio cholerae* is worldwide in distribution and continues to expand as water sources become polluted. Which of the following best describes this organism?

a. Cause of gastroenteritis; reservoir in birds and mammals, optimal growth at 107.6°F (42°C)
b. Human pathogen, halophilic, lactose-negative, sucrose-negative; causes gastrointestinal diseases primarily from ingestion of under-cooked seafood
c. Human pathogen, halophilic, lactose-positive; produces heat-labile, extracellular toxin, wound infections
d. Organisms susceptible to acid; not an invasive organism
e. Urease-positive; cause of fetal distress in cattle

259. A 20-year-old female in post-Katrina New Orleans eats poorly cooked seafood (oysters, clams, and mollusks) for her birthday dinner. Twenty-four hours later, she develops explosive watery diarrhea and abdominal cramps. She is positive for *V parahaemolyticus*. Which of the following best describes this organism?

a. Cause of gastroenteritis; reservoir in birds and mammals, optimal growth at 107.6°F (42°C)
b. Human pathogen, halophilic, lactose-negative, sucrose-negative; causes gastrointestinal diseases primarily from ingestion of under-cooked seafood
c. Human pathogen, halophilic, lactose-positive; produces heat-labile, extracellular toxin, wound infections
d. Organisms susceptible to acid; not an invasive organism
e. Urease-positive; cause of fetal distress in cattle

260. A 25-year-old male, with a history of hepatitis C, has to wade through brackish water in post-Katrina New Orleans. He develops worsening abdominal pain and jaundice. Regarding *Vibrio vulnificus*, which of the following best describes this organism?

a. Cause of gastroenteritis; reservoir in birds and mammals, optimal growth at 107.6°F (42°C)
b. Human pathogen, halophilic, lactose-negative, sucrose-negative; causes gastrointestinal diseases primarily from ingestion of under-cooked seafood
c. Human pathogen, halophilic, lactose-positive; produces heat-labile, extracellular toxin, wound infections
d. Organisms susceptible to acids; not an invasive organism
e. Urease-positive; cause of fetal distress in cattle

261. *Yersinia enterocolitica*, formerly a *Pasteurella*, has more than 50 serotypes which can be isolated from rodents, sheep, cattle, swine, dogs, and cats and water contaminated by them, and is best described by which of the following?

a.   Commonly inhabits the canine respiratory tract and is an occasional pathogen for humans; strongly urease-positive
b.   Gram-negative bipolar stained bacilli that cause diarrhea by means of a heat-stable enterotoxin, with abdominal pain that may be mistaken for appendicitis
c.   Pits agar, grows both in carbon dioxide and under anaerobic conditions, and is part of the normal oral cavity flora
d.   Typically infects cattle, requires 5% to 10% carbon dioxide for growth, and is inhibited by the dye thionine
e.   Typically is found in infected animal bites in humans and can cause hemorrhagic septicemia in animals

262. Four weeks after assisting in several calf deliveries, a farmer develops fever, weakness, muscle aches, and sweats. The fever rises in the afternoon and falls during the night. *Brucella abortus* is isolated. Which one of the three *Brucella* species is a possible bioterrorism agent and is best described by one of the following?

a.   Commonly inhabits the canine respiratory tract and is an occasional pathogen for humans; strongly urease-positive
b.   Gram-negative bipolar stained bacilli that cause diarrhea by means of a heat-stable enterotoxin, with abdominal pain that may be mistaken for appendicitis
c.   Pits agar, grows both in carbon dioxide and under anaerobic conditions, and is part of the normal oral cavity flora
d.   Typically infects cattle, requires 5% to 10% carbon dioxide for growth, and is inhibited by the dye thionine
e.   Typically is found in infected animal bites in humans and can cause hemorrhagic septicemia in animals

263. *Bordetella bronchiseptica* could be confused with the agent of whooping cough since it occasionally causes chronic respiratory tract infections in humans, but has less intensive symptoms (rhinitis and cough). It is best described by which of the following?

a. Commonly inhabits the canine respiratory tract and is an occasional pathogen for humans; strongly urease-positive
b. Gram-negative bipolar stained bacilli that cause diarrhea by means of a heat-stable enterotoxin, with abdominal pain that may be mistaken for appendicitis
c. Pits agar, grows both in carbon dioxide and under anaerobic conditions, and is part of the normal oral cavity flora
d. Typically infects cattle, requires 5% to 10% carbon dioxide for growth, and is inhibited by the dye thionine
e. Typically is found in infected animal bites in humans and can cause hemorrhagic septicemia in animals

264. *Pasteurella* species can produce a range of human diseases and formerly included all *yersiniae* and *francisellae* organisms. *Pasteurella multocida* occurs worldwide in the URT and GI tracts of domestic and wild animals. It is best described by which of the following?

a. Commonly inhabits the canine respiratory tract and is an occasional pathogen for humans; strongly urease-positive
b. Gram-negative bipolar stained bacilli that cause diarrhea by means of a heat-stable enterotoxin, with abdominal pain that may be mistaken for appendicitis
c. Pits agar, grows both in carbon dioxide and under anaerobic conditions, and is part of the normal oral cavity flora
d. Typically infects cattle, requires 5% to 10% carbon dioxide for growth, and is inhibited by the dye thionine
e. Typically is found in infected animal bites in humans and can cause hemorrhagic septicemia in animals

265. A 26-year-old male presents to his family physician with complaints of painful burning during urination and a milky discharge. The purulent discharge reveals many neutrophils with intracellular gram-negative diplococci. Which of the following mediums would most likely be used for isolating *Neisseria gonorrhoeae*, the suspected organism?

a. Löffler medium
b. Löwenstein-Jensen medium
c. Sheep blood agar
d. Thayer-Martin agar
e. Thiosulfate citrate bile salts sucrose medium

266. Twenty-four hours after returning from a short trip to Asia, a 35-year-old female has a sudden onset of vomiting and massive watery diarrhea that is colorless, odorless, and contains flecks of mucus. Which of the following mediums would most likely be used for isolating *V cholerae*, the suspected organism?

a. Löffler medium
b. Löwenstein-Jensen medium
c. Sheep blood agar
d. Thayer-Martin agar
e. Thiosulfate citrate bile salts sucrose medium

267. A 32-year-old female prostitute is seen at the public health clinic with fever, night sweats, and reports coughing up blood. Her medical history reveals she is HIV positive and has lost 20 lbs over the past month. Acid-fast bacilli are observed in the sputum. After digestion of the sputum, isolation of the suspected organism is best accomplished by using which one of the following media?

a. Löffler medium
b. Löwenstein-Jensen medium
c. Sheep blood agar
d. Thayer-Martin agar
e. Thiosulfate citrate bile salts sucrose medium

268. *Bacillus* and *Clostridium* species are spore-forming bacilli and can survive in the environment for years. Several species cause important disease in humans, although most will respond quickly to appropriate antibiotic therapy. However, which organism listed below would not benefit from such prompt antibiotic treatment?

a. *Bacillus anthracis*
b. *Clostridium botulinum*
c. *Clostridium difficile*
d. *Clostridium perfringens*
e. *Clostridium tetani*

269. A 12-year-old boy has sudden onset of fever, headache, and stiff neck. Two days earlier, he swam in a lake that is believed to have been contaminated with dog excreta. Leptospirosis is suspected. Which of the following laboratory tests is most appropriate to determine whether he has been infected with leptospira?

a. Agglutination test for leptospiral antigen
b. Counterimmunoelectrophoresis of urine sample
c. Gram stain of urine specimen
d. Spinal fluid for dark-field microscopy and culture in Fletcher serum medium
e. Urine culture on EMB and Thayer-Martin agar

270. A 60-year-old female complains of tenderness and pain around a peritoneal catheter. Blood cultures reveal gram-positive, catalase-positive cocci. Which of the following is the most likely organism which is also considered a predominant organism on skin?

a. α-Hemolytic streptococci
b. *Bacteroides fragilis*
c. *Escherichia coli*
d. *Lactobacillus* species
e. *Staphylococcus epidermidis*

271. A healthy 45-year-old female had root canal treatment about 3 weeks ago. She now presents with a new heart murmur, fever, painful skin nodules, abdominal pain, and an abnormal liver function test. Which of the following organisms would mostly likely cause endocarditis and is implicated in dental caries or root canal infections?

a. α-Hemolytic streptococci
b. *Bacteroides fragilis*
c. *Escherichia coli*
d. *Lactobacillus* species
e. *Staphylococcus epidermidis*

272. A 17-year-old man is hospitalized with trauma to the abdomen following a gang-related fight. He develops an intra-abdominal abscess, which is drained and sent to the laboratory. A mixture of gram-negative anaerobes is detected. Which of the following microorganisms is the most likely and is also the most prevalent bacterium in the gut?

a. α-Hemolytic streptococci
b. *Bacteroides fragilis*
c. *Escherichia coli*
d. *Lactobacillus* species
e. *Staphylococcus epidermidis*

273. A 25-year-old female is treated with a course of broad-spectrum antibiotics for severe pelvic inflammatory disease. She now reports a thick milky white pruritic vaginal discharge. Which of the following is the most prevalent microorganism in the vagina and may also be protective?

a. α-Hemolytic streptococci
b. *Bacteroides fragilis*
c. *Escherichia coli*
d. *Lactobacillus* species
e. *Staphylococcus epidermidis*

274. Viridans streptococci (*S mutans, S mitis*) usually have α-hemolysis and are optochin-resistant. They are becoming increasingly important as causes of endocarditis and abscesses (mixed infections). Which of the following best describes *S mutans*?

a. An anaerobic, filamentous bacterium that often causes cervicofacial osteomyelitis
b. A β-hemolytic organism that causes a diffuse, rapidly spreading cellulitis
c. A facultative anaerobe that is highly cariogenic and sticks to teeth by synthesis of a dextran
d. A facultative anaerobe that often inhabits the buccal mucosa early in a neonate's life and can cause bacterial rheumatic fever
e. A facultatively anaerobic, rod-shaped bacterium that sticks to teeth and is cariogenic, commonly involved in problems involving dental procedures, trauma, surgery, or aspiration

275. *Streptococcus salivarius*, a common isolate, which is considered as normal, nonpathogenic flora in the clinical laboratory, is best described by which of the following?

a. An anaerobic, filamentous bacterium that often causes cervicofacial osteomyelitis
b. A β-hemolytic organism that causes a diffuse, rapidly spreading cellulitis
c. A facultative anaerobe that is highly cariogenic and sticks to teeth by synthesis of a dextran
d. A facultative anaerobe that often inhabits the buccal mucosa early in a neonate's life and can cause bacterial rheumatic fever
e. A facultatively anaerobic, rod-shaped bacterium that sticks to teeth and is cariogenic, commonly involved in problems involving dental procedures, trauma, surgery, or aspiration

276. *Actinomyces* species are a large, diverse group of gram-positive bacilli. *Actinomyces israelii* is an organism that causes pyogenic lesions with interconnecting sinus tracts that contain granules of microcolonies embedded in the tissues. It is best described by which of the following?

a. An anaerobic, filamentous bacterium that often causes cervicofacial osteomyelitis
b. A β-hemolytic organism that causes a diffuse, rapidly spreading cellulitis
c. A facultative anaerobe that is highly cariogenic and sticks to teeth by synthesis of a dextran
d. A facultative anaerobe that often inhabits the buccal mucosa early in a neonate's life and can cause bacterial rheumatic fever
e. A facultatively anaerobic, rod-shaped bacterium that sticks to teeth and is cariogenic, commonly involved in problems involving dental procedures, trauma, surgery, or aspiration

277. *Actinomyces viscosus*, a ubiquitous actinomycete, grows under microaerophilic or strict anaerobic conditions and produces a yellow-orange granule in the typical tissue exudates. It is best described by which of the following?

a. An anaerobic, filamentous bacterium that often causes cervicofacial osteomyelitis
b. A β-hemolytic organism that causes a diffuse, rapidly spreading cellulitis
c. A facultative anaerobe that is highly cariogenic and sticks to teeth by synthesis of a dextran
d. A facultative anaerobe that often inhabits the buccal mucosa early in a neonate's life and can cause bacterial rheumatic fever
e. A facultatively anaerobic, rod-shaped bacterium that sticks to teeth and is cariogenic, commonly involved in problems involving dental procedures, trauma to or surgery of the oral cavity, or aspiration

278. A 3-year-old girl from a family that does not believe in immunization presents to the emergency room with a sore throat, fever, malaise, and difficulty breathing. A gray membrane covering the pharynx is observed on physical examination. Which of the following best describes *C diphtheriae*, the etiologic agent?

a. It produces at least one protein toxin consisting of two subunits, A and B, that cause severe spasmodic cough, usually in children.
b. It produces a toxin that blocks protein synthesis in an infected cell and carries a lytic bacteriophage that produces the genetic information for toxin production.
c. It secretes an erythrogenic toxin that causes the characteristic signs of scarlet fever.
d. It secretes an exotoxin that has been called "verotoxin" and "Shiga-like toxin"; infection is mediated by specific attachment to mucosal membranes.
e. It requires cysteine for growth.

279. A 4-year-old boy is taken to see his pediatrician because of a persistent cough that gradually worsened over a 12-day period. On the day of the examination, the cough is so severe that it is frequently followed by vomiting. A blood cell count shows marked leukocytosis with a predominance of lymphocytes. Which of the following best characterizes this microorganism?

a. It produces a toxin that increases cAMP levels, resulting in increased mucus production.
b. It produces a toxin that blocks protein synthesis in an infected cell and carries a lytic bacteriophage that produces the genetic information for toxin production.
c. It secretes an erythrogenic toxin that causes the characteristic signs of scarlet fever.
d. It secretes an exotoxin that has been called "verotoxin" and "Shiga-like toxin"; infection is mediated by specific attachment to mucosal membranes.
e. It requires cysteine for growth.

280. A 48-year-old deer hunter presents to the emergency room with lymphadenopathy and a skin lesion, which started as a painful papule at the site of a tick bite. The papule then ulcerates with a necrotic center and raised border. Aspirate of the ulcer is positive for *F tularensis*. Which one of the following best characterizes this bacterium?

a. It produces at least one protein toxin consisting of two subunits, A and B, that cause severe spasmodic cough, usually in children.
b. It produces a toxin that blocks protein synthesis in an infected cell and carries a lytic bacteriophage that produces the genetic information for toxin production.
c. It secretes an erythrogenic toxin that causes the characteristic signs of scarlet fever.
d. It secretes an exotoxin that has been called "verotoxin" and "Shiga-like toxin"; infection is mediated by specific attachment to mucosal membranes.
e. It requires cysteine for growth.

281. Ten boy scouts are hospitalized with bloody diarrhea and severe hematological abnormalities. An investigation establishes that all of the boys developed symptoms following consumption of hamburgers from the same fast-food restaurant chain. Which of the following best describes *E coli* 0157/H7, the etiologic bacterium responsible for the outbreak?

a. It produces at least one protein toxin consisting of two subunits, A and B, that cause severe spasmodic cough, usually in children.
b. It produces a toxin that blocks protein synthesis in an infected cell and carries a lytic bacteriophage that produces the genetic information for toxin production.
c. It secretes an erythrogenic toxin that causes the characteristic signs of scarlet fever.
d. It secretes an exotoxin that has been called "verotoxin" and "Shiga-like toxin"; infection is mediated by specific attachment to mucosal membranes.
e. It requires cysteine for growth.

282. A 4-year-old girl awakens at midnight complaining of a sore throat and headache, and she has a fever of 101°F. Physical examination reveals an erythematous throat. A rapid strep test is positive. A throat swab is sent to the laboratory for further testing. Which of the following best characterizes *S pyogenes* as the presumed etiologic agent?

a. It produces at least one protein toxin consisting of two subunits, A and B, that cause severe spasmodic cough, usually in children.
b. It produces a toxin that blocks protein synthesis in an infected cell and carries a lytic bacteriophage that produces the genetic information for toxin production.
c. It secretes an erythrogenic toxin that causes the characteristic signs of scarlet fever.
d. It secretes an exotoxin that has been called "verotoxin" and "Shiga-like toxin"; infection is mediated by specific attachment to mucosal membranes.
e. It has capsules of polyglutamic acid, which is toxic when injected into rabbits.

283. A 19-year-old military recruit who lives in the barracks develops a macular papular skin rash, severe headache, photophobia, fever, stiff neck, and blurred vision. He is presumed to have *N meningitidis*. Which of the following is a characteristic physiological trait of this organism?

a. It causes spontaneous abortion and has tropism for placental tissue due to the presence of erythritol in allantoic and amniotic fluid.
b. It has a capsule of polyglutamic acid, which is toxic when injected into rabbits.
c. It possesses N-acetylneuraminic acid capsule and adheres to specific tissues by pili found on the bacterial cell surface.
d. It secretes two toxins, A and B, in the large bowel during antibiotic therapy.
e. It synthesizes protein toxin as a result of colonization of vaginal tampons.

284. A 45-year-old cattle-farm worker goes to the public health clinic after experiencing 6 weeks of undulating fever, chills, sweating, headache, fatigue, muscle pain, and weight loss. History reveals that he enjoys drinking fresh unpasteurized milk with his other coworkers during the mid-morning breaks. A blood sample is sent to the state laboratory for serologic testing because the physician assistant suspects *Brucella* infection. Which of the following best characterizes this organism?

a. It causes spontaneous abortion and has tropism for placental tissue due to the presence of erythritol in allantoic and amniotic fluid.
b. It has a capsule of polyglutamic acid, which is toxic when injected into rabbits.
c. It has 82 polysaccharide capsular types; capsule is antiphagocytic; type 3 capsule (β-d-glucuronic acid polymer) most commonly seen in infected adults.
d. It secretes two toxins, A and B, in the large bowel during antibiotic therapy.
e. It synthesizes protein toxin as a result of colonization of vaginal tampons.

285. An 18-year-old male patient presents to the emergency room with a 3-day history of fever, dry cough, difficulty in breathing, and muscle aches and pains. His chest x-ray shows a diffuse left upper lobe infiltrate. *Mycoplasma pneumoniae* pneumonia (walking pneumonia) may be rapidly identified by which of the following procedures?

a. Cold agglutinin test
b. Culture of respiratory secretions in HeLa cells after centrifugation of the inoculated tubes
c. Culture of respiratory secretions on monkey kidney cells
d. Detection of specific antigen in urine
e. Electron microscopy of sputum

286. A 50-year-old male presents with severe bilateral pulmonary infiltrate, elevated temperature leucocytosis, elevated enzymes, and elevated creatine kinase. He recently visited his favorite restaurant that had a large water fountain, which was misty on the day of his visit. Which of the following procedures would most rapidly diagnose the suspected organism that is the etiologic agent of Legionnaires' disease in this patient?

a. Cold agglutinin test
b. Culture of respiratory secretions on a charcoal-based nutrient agar
c. Detection of antigen in respiratory secretions
d. Detection of specific antigen in urine
e. Electron microscopy of sputum

287. A group of elementary school-age children meet for a birthday party and in the next few days about half of them experience a mild upper respiratory illness, with sore throat and runny nose. One family gets laboratory work done and finds that *Chlamydia pneumoniae* (TWAR) is involved. Which of the following procedures would be best if the laboratory wanted to isolate this bacterium?

a. Cold agglutinin test
b. Culture of respiratory secretions in HeLa cells after centrifugation of the inoculated tubes
c. Culture of respiratory secretions on monkey kidney cells
d. Detection of specific antigen in urine
e. Electron microscopy of sputum

288. A 5-year-old boy is brought to the local public health clinic because of a severe, intractable cough. During the previous 10 days, he had a persistent cold that had worsened. The cough developed the previous day and was so severe that vomiting frequently followed it. The child appears exhausted from the coughing episodes. A blood cell count shows a marked leukocytosis with a predominance of lymphocytes. Which of the following procedures can best detect the etiologic agent?

a. Cold agglutinin test
b. Culture of respiratory secretions in HeLa cells after centrifugation of the inoculated tubes
c. Culture of respiratory secretions on Bordet-Gengou agar
d. Direct microscopy of sputum by Gram stain
e. Fluorescent antibody detection of the organism in sputum

Bacteriology

Answers

180. The answer is d. *(Brooks, pp 275-276. Levinson, pp 146, 496. Murray, pp 328-332. Ryan, pp 381-383. Toy, p 90.)* Helicobacter pylori was first recognized as a possible cause of gastritis and peptic ulcer by Marshall and Warren in 1984. This organism is readily isolated from gastric biopsies but not from stomach contents. It is similar to *Campylobacter* species and grows on chocolate agar at 98.6°F (37°C) in the same microaerophilic environment suitable for *C jejuni* (Campy-Pak or anaerobic jar [Gas Pak] without the catalyst). *Helicobacter pylori*, however, grows more slowly than *C jejuni*, requiring 5 to 7 days' incubation. *Campylobacter jejuni* grows optimally at 107.6°F (42°C), not 98.6°F (37°C), as does *H pylori*.

DIAGNOSTIC TESTS FOR *HELICOBACTER PYLORI*		
	Advantages	**Disadvantages**
Noninvasive		
Serum ELISA[a]	Inexpensive	Not useful for follow-up
Urea breath test	Useful for follow-up	Expensive; may be falsely negative in patients on acid suppression therapy
Stool antigen test	Inexpensive; useful for follow-up	Inconvenient
Whole blood assay	Inexpensive; rapid	Less accurate than serum ELISA
Invasive (endoscopic)		
Histology	Visualization of pathology	May miss low-grade infection
Rapid urease	Rapid	May be falsely positive in bacterial overgrowth
Culture	Antibiotic susceptibility	Not maximally sensitive; not available routinely; requires 4-7 days

[a]Enzyme-linked immunosorbent assay.

(Reprinted, with permission, from Wilson WR, Sande MA. Current Diagnosis and Treatment in Infectious Disease. *New York: McGraw-Hill;2001: 584.)*

181. The answer is a. *(Brooks, pp 280-282. Levinson, pp 152-153. Murray, pp 343-348. Ryan, pp 399-400.)* The major determinant of virulence in *H influenzae* is the presence of a capsule. There is no demonstrable exotoxin, and the role of endotoxin is unclear. While one would expect that IgA protease would inhibit local immunity, the role of this enzyme in pathogenesis is as yet unclear. Flagella production would not be considered a virulence factor. See the table on the following page for a comparison of gram-negative rods associated with the respiratory tract.

182. The answer is e. *(Brooks, pp 270-272. Levinson, pp 45, 143-145. Murray, pp 317-322. Ryan, pp 348, 375. Toy, p 102.)* The toxin of *V cholerae* and LT enterotoxin from *E coli* are similar. The B subunits of the toxins bind to ganglioside GM1 receptors on the host cell. The A subunits catalyze transfer of the ADP-ribose moiety of ADP to a regulatory protein known as G_s. This activated G_s stimulates adenyl cyclase. Cyclic AMP is increased, as is fluid and electrolyte release from the crypt cells into the lumen of the bowel. Watery, profuse diarrhea ensues. *Brucella abortus* disease starts in humans with an acute bacteremic phase followed by a chronic stage that may last for years. They are adapted to an intracellular habitat with complex nutritional requirements. *Brucella abortus* does not produce any product similar to the toxin of V cholerae, *C diphtheriae's* toxin causes an abrupt arrest of protein synthesis that results in the necrotizing and neurotoxic effects. Listeria enters the body through ingestion and infects cells of the CNS. No virulence factor similar to that of *V cholerae* is produced by Listeria organisms. *Pseudomonas* aeruginosa is pathogenic only when introduced into areas where there are no normal defenses. It produces exotoxin A, which causes tissue necrosis and blocks protein synthesis similar to *C diphtheriae*.

183. The answer is d. *(Brooks, pp 317, 751. Levinson, pp 25, 189, 503. Ryan, p 904.)* Microscopic examination can readily demonstrate clue cells (epithelial cells with *Gardnerella* bacteria attached) or pseudohyphae *(Candida)*. A wet mount will be needed to demonstrate motile *Trichomonas* cells. *Candida, Trichomonas,* and bacterial vaginitis are seen most often. *Staphylococcus aureus* is involved much less frequently. While *E coli* may be a common cause of genitourinary infection, clue cells are usually absent. See the table on the following page for a comparison of these bacteria.

GRAM-NEGATIVE RODS ASSOCIATED WITH THE RESPIRATORY TRACT

Species	Major Diseases	Laboratory Diagnosis	Factors X and V Required for Growth	Vaccine Available	Prophylaxis for Contacts
Haemophilus influenzae	Meningitis[a], otitis media, sinusitis, pneumonia, epiglottitis	Culture; capsular polysaccharide in serum or spinal fluid	+	+	Rifampin
Bordetella pertussis	Whooping cough (pertussis)	Fluorescent antibody on secretions; culture	−	+	Erythromycin
Legionella pneumophila	Pneumonia	Serology; urinary antigen; culture	−	−	None

[a]In countries where the *H influenzae* b conjugate vaccine has been deployed, the vaccine has greatly reduced the incidence of meningitis caused by this organism.

(Reprinted, with permission, from Levinson W, Jawetz E. Medical Microbiology and Immunology: 7th ed. New York, NY: McGraw-Hill; 2002.)

CLINICAL FEATURES OF VAGINITIS

	Normal	Vulvovaginal Candidiasis	Trichomoniasis	Bacterial Vaginosis
Symptoms	None	Pruritus Soreness Dyspareunia	Soreness Dyspareunia Often asymptomatic	Often asymptomatic Occasional abdominal pain
Discharge				
Amount	Variable	Scant/moderate	Profuse	Moderate
Color	Clear/white	White	Green-yellow	White/gray
Consistency	Nonhomogenous floccular	Clumped, adherent	Homogenous, frothy	Homogenous adherent
Vaginal Fluid pH	4.0-4.5	4.0-4.5	5.0-6.0	>4.5
Amine test (fish odor)	None	None	Usually positive	Positive
Microscopy				
Saline	PMN:EC[a] ratio < 1 Lactobacilli predominate	PMN:EC < 1 Pseudohyphae (~40%)	PMN:EC > 1 Motile trichomonads PMNs predominate	PMN:EC< 1 Clue cells Coccobacilli
10% KOH	Negative	Pseudohyphae (~70%)	Negative	Negative

[a]PMN—polymorphonuclear leukocytes; EC—epithelial cells.

(Reprinted, with permission, from Wilson WR, Sande MA. Current Diagnosis and Treatment in Infectious Disease. New York: McGraw-Hill;2001: 209.)

184. The answer is d. (*Brooks, pp 224-230. Levinson, pp 106-110, 484. Murray, pp 209-220. Ryan, p 268.*) *Staphylococcus aureus* is a well-known pathogen that is very opportunistic and commonly causes abscess lesions. It routinely may resist phagocytosis by WBCs due to protein A. Osteomyelitis and arthritis, either hematogenous or traumatic, are commonly caused by *S aureus*, especially in children. *Salmonella* are gram-negative. *Staphylococcus saprophyticus* is a common skin flora and is usually not pathogenic. *Streptococcus pneumoniae* is seldom or never involved in osteomyelitis infections, as is true for *L monocytogenes*.

185. The answer is c. (*Brooks, p 293. Levinson, pp 160, 495. Murray, pp 344-350. Ryan, p 490.*) *Pasteurella* (gram-negative coccobacilli) are primarily animal pathogens, but they can cause a wide range of human diseases. They have a bipolar appearance on stained smears. *Pasteurella multocida* occurs worldwide in domestic and wild animals. It is the most common organism in human wounds inflicted by bites of cats and dogs. It is a common cause of hemorrhagic septicemia in a variety of animals. Wounds commonly present with an acute onset (within hours) of redness, swelling, and pain. The other organisms are routinely found in the environment and may be opportunistic pathogens. *Pasteurella multocida* is a gram-negative rod that usually responds to penicillin treatment. *Aeromonas, Campylobacter, Pseudomonas,* and *Yersinia* are also gram-negative rods.

186 to 188. The answers are 186-c, 187-a, 188-a. (*Brooks, pp 344-348. Levinson, pp 8, 67, 171-172. Murray, pp 421-424. Ryan, pp 410-411.*) *Mycoplasma pneumoniae* causes a respiratory infection known as primary atypical pneumonia, or walking pneumonia. Although disease caused by *M pneumoniae* can be contracted year-round, thousands of cases occur during the winter months in all age groups. The disease, if untreated, will persist for 2 weeks or longer. Rare but serious side effects include cardiomyopathies and CNS complications. Infection with *M pneumoniae* may be treated with either erythromycin or tetracycline. The organism lacks a cell wall and so is resistant to the penicillin and the cephalosporin groups of antibiotics.

Until recently, diagnostic tests have been of limited value. Up to 50% of cases may not show cold agglutinins, an insensitive and nonspecific acute-phase reactant. However, if cold agglutinins for group O human RBCs are present, a quick diagnosis can be made if signs and symptoms are characteristic. Complement fixation tests that measure an antibody to a glycolipid antigen of M pneumoniae are useful but not routinely performed in most laboratories. Also, cross-reactions may occur. Culture of M pneumoniae, while not technically difficult, may take up to 2 weeks before visible growth is observed.

A DNA probe is available. It is a 125I probe for the 16S ribosomal RNA of M pneumoniae. Evaluations in a number of laboratories indicate that compared with culture it is highly sensitive and specific. Recently, DNA probes have been applied to the detection of M pneumoniae in clinical specimens. Mycoplasma have no cell walls and do not react to gram stain reagents. Mycoplasma would grow in cell culture medium but would be of little use as a diagnostic tool since the organism cannot be easily seen or identified under a microscope.

189. The answer is a. *(Brooks, pp 320-326. Levinson, pp 161-165. Murray, pp 278-281. Ryan, pp 445-446.)* Most cases of tuberculosis are caused when patients inhale droplet nuclei containing infectious organisms. While the bacilli are deposited on the alveolar spaces, they do not clog up the alveoli but are engulfed by macrophages. Tissue injury is not a result of toxin secretion but of cell-mediated hypersensitivity, that is, "immunologic injury."

(Reproduced, with permission, from Brooks GF, et al. Jawetz's Medical Microbiology. 24th ed. New York: McGraw-Hill; 2007: 322.)

Humoral (antibodies) immunity would not be responsible for tissue damage since CMI is reacting against the organism. Adhesion sites are not implicated as virulence factors and toxins apparently are not made by the organisms.

190. The answer is c. (*Brooks, p 190. Levinson, pp 70, 78-79. Murray, pp 207, 816-817. Ryan, p 33.*) A new class of antibiotics, the quinolones, has one member, nalidixic acid, that has been available for years. The new representatives are much more active biologically and are effective against virtually all gram-negative bacteria and most gram-positive bacteria. They include norfloxacin, ofloxacin, ciprofloxacin, enoxacin, and the fluorinated quinolones such as lomefloxacin. These antibiotics kill bacteria by inhibition of synthesis of nucleic acid, more specifically, DNA gyrase. Resistance to quinolones has been observed and appears to be a class-specific phenomenon. An exception is when an organism is resistant to nalidixic acid, elevated minimal inhibitory concentrations (MICs) will generally apply to other quinolones, although these MICs will still be within the range of susceptibility. PBPs (penicillin-binding proteins) and β-lactamase involve penicillins, not quinolones, as does the glycine cross-linking. Inhibition of reverse transcriptase (RNA-dependent DNA polymerase) would not be involved in this clinical situation since RT inhibition would indicate HIV or HBV involvement.

191. The answer is c. (*Brooks, pp 225, 229. Levinson, pp 106-110. Murray, pp 211-220. Ryan, pp 269-270.*) VISA was first recognized in Japan. Emergence in the United States soon followed. It is likely that the human VISA isolates have resulted from increased use of vancomycin for patients with MRSA or perhaps an increased pool of VISA in the environment selected out by the use of glycopeptides such as avoparcin, a growth promoter used in food-producing animals. In patients with VISA, the Centers for Disease Control and Prevention (CDC) strongly recommend compliance with isolation procedures and other infection control practices geared to control of VISA. Staphylococci are susceptible to vancomycin if the MIC is equal to or less than 2 μg/mL and of intermediate susceptibility if the MIC is 4 to 8 μg/mL. Vancomycin resistance in *S aureus* is of major concern worldwide and surveillance should be maintained. VISA strains are usually nafcillin-resistant.

192. The answer is a. *(Brooks, pp 198, 280. Levinson, pp 62-64. Murray, p 808. Ryan, pp 854-855. Toy, p 90.)* Many sputum specimens are cultured unnecessarily. Sputum is often contaminated with saliva or is almost totally made up of saliva. These specimens rarely reveal the cause of the patient's respiratory problem and may provide laboratory information that is harmful. The sputum in the question appears to be a good specimen because there are few epithelial cells. The pleomorphic, gram-negative rods are suggestive of *Haemophilus*, but culture of the secretions is necessary. Normal flora from a healthy oral cavity consists of gram-positive cocci and rods, with few or no PMNs. Pneumococci are gram-positive diplococci. Vincent disease is an oral infection, which involves oral tissue only. Presence of PMNs indicates an inflammatory response.

193. The answer is b. *(Brooks, pp 306-309. Levinson, pp 150-151, 497. Murray, pp 400-403. Ryan, pp 324-325.)* *Bacteroides fragilis* is a constituent of normal intestinal flora and readily causes wound infections often mixed with aerobic isolates. These anaerobic, gram-negative rods are uniformly resistant to aminoglycosides and usually to penicillin as well. Reliable laboratory identification may require multiple analytical techniques. Generally, wound exudates smell bad owing to production of organic acids by such anaerobes as *B fragilis*. Black exudates or a black pigment (heme) in the isolated colony is usually a characteristic of *Bacteroides (Porphyromonas) melaninogenicus*, not *B fragilis*. Potent neurotoxins are synthesized by the gram-positive anaerobes such as *C tetani* and *C botulinum*.

194. The answer is b. *(Brooks, pp 296-301. Levinson, pp 119-123. Murray, pp 292-298. Ryan, p 336.)* Typical *Neisseria* are gram-negative diplococci. *Neisseria gonorrhoeae* contain pili, hairlike appendages that may be several micrometers long (see figure). They enhance attachment of the organism to mucous membranes, helping to make the organism more resistant to phagocytosis by WBCs. Gonococci isolated from clinical specimens produce small colonies containing piliated bacteria. Capsules appear to be less important in gonococcal infection than *N meningitidis* infections. Flagella, peptidoglycan, LPS, and F pili do not significantly relate to pathogenesis, other than that LPS (endotoxin) release may become significant later in infection.

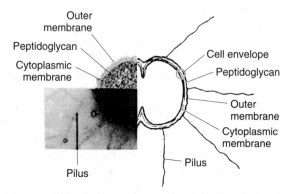

Collage and drawing of *N gonorrhoeae* showing pili and the three layers of the cell envelope. *(Reproduced, with permission, from Brooks GF, et al. Jawetz's Medical Microbiology. 22nd ed. New York: McGraw-Hill;2001: 256.)*

195. The answer is d. *(Brooks, pp 218-219. Levinson, pp 131-132. Murray, pp 255-258. Ryan, pp 302-304. Toy, p 102.)* Listeria multiplies both extracellularly and intracellularly, but under most circumstances a competent immune system eliminates *Listeria*. As expected, listeriosis is seen in the very young and the very old, and in people with compromised immune systems. Reports of *Listeria* food outbreaks have implicated such foods as coleslaw and milk products, especially if not pasteurized. Early-onset-syndrome listeriosis is the result of infection in utero and characterized by sepsis and lesions in multiple organs. None of the other options (*Corynebacterium, Escherichia, streptococci* type B, or *S pneumoniae*) would be likely to cause an in utero infection.

196 to 199. The answers are 196-d, 197-a, 198-c, 199-d. *(Brooks, pp 332-335. Levinson, pp 8, 173, 501. Murray, pp 405-411. Ryan, pp 424-430. Toy, p 164.)* This patient appears to have primary syphilis, as evidenced by a penile chancre that was not tender. One of the differences between syphilis and herpes simplex virus (HSV) is that an HSV lesion is excruciatingly painful. The herpes lesion is vesicular in appearance whereas the classic syphilis chancre has an eroded appearance. Treponemal organisms may be seen microscopically in the lesion if the lesion is scraped. The syphilis lesion will resolve with antibiotic therapy. Acyclovir prescription at this time would be premature. If not treated, the chancre will disappear and the patient will be asymptomatic until he/she exhibits the signs and symptoms of secondary syphilis, which include a disseminated rash and systemic involvement such as meningitis, hepatitis, or nephritis. There are two kinds of tests for the detection of syphilis antibodies: nonspecific tests such as the RPR and VDRL, and specific tests such as the FTA, *T pallidum* hemagglutination test (TPHA), and the microhemagglutination—*T pallidum* (MHTP). The difference is that the nonspecific tests use a cross-reactive antigen known as cardiolipin, while the specific tests use a *T pallidum* antigen. Although the nonspecific tests are sensitive, they lack specificity and often cross-react in patients who have diabetes, hepatitis, or infectious mononucleosis, or who are pregnant. Some patients, especially those with autoimmune diseases, will have both nonspecific (RPR) and specific tests (FTA) positive even if they do not have syphilis. Resolution of such a situation can be done by molecular methods for *T pallidum*, such as PCR, or by

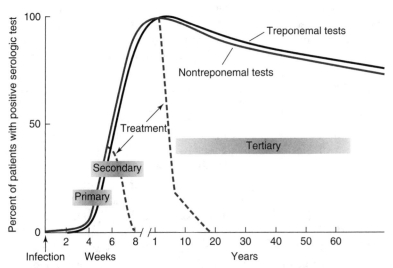

Treponemal and nontreponemal tests in syphilis. The time course of treated and untreated syphilis in relation to serologic tests is shown. The nontreponemal tests (VDRL, RPR) rise during primary syphilis and reach their peak in secondary syphilis. They slowly decline with advancing age. With treatment they revert to normal over a few weeks. The treponemal tests (FTA-Abs, MHTP) follow the same course but remain elevated even following successful treatment. *(Reprinted, with permission, from Ryan KJ, et al. Sherris Medical Microbiology. 4th ed. New York: McGraw-Hill;2001: 429.)*

the immobilization test using live spirochetes and the patient's serum. In the TPI test, the spirochetes will die in the presence of specific antibody (see figure).

200. The answer is c. (*Brooks, pp 313-314. Levinson, pp 35, 155-156. Murray, pp 365, 367-369. Ryan, pp 415-419.*) The symptoms of Legionnaires' disease are similar to those of mycoplasmal pneumonia and influenza. Affected persons are moderately febrile, complain of pleuritic chest pain, and have a dry cough. Unlike *Klebsiella* and *Staphylococcus*, *L pneumophila* exhibits fastidious growth requirements. Charcoal yeast extract agar either with or without antibiotics is the preferred isolation medium.

While sputum may not be the specimen of choice for *Legionella*, the discovery of small, gram-negative rods by direct fluorescent antibody (FA) technique should certainly heighten suspicion of the disease. *Legionella pneumophila* is a facultative intracellular pathogen and enters macrophages without activating their oxidizing capabilities. The organisms bind to macrophage C receptors, which promote engulfment. *Chlamydiae* need cell culture to be isolated and *Mycoplasma* isolation requires a biphasic (agar + broth) medium. Neither of these will grow on the charcoal yeast extract agar.

201. The answer is b. (*Brooks, p 211. Levinson, pp 129, 492-493. Murray, pp 378-387. Ryan, pp 322-324.*) Patients treated with antibiotics develop diarrhea that, in most cases, is self-limiting. However, in some instances, particularly in those patients treated with ampicillin or clindamycin, a severe, life-threatening pseudomembranous enterocolitis develops. This disease has characteristic histopathology, and membranous plaques can be seen in the colon by endoscopy. Pseudomembranous enterocolitis and antibiotic-associated diarrhea are caused by an anaerobic gram-positive rod, *C difficile*. It has been recently shown that *C difficile* produces a protein toxin with a molecular weight of about 250,000. The "toxin" is, in fact, two toxins, toxin A and toxin B. Both toxins are always present in fecal samples, but there is approximately 1000 times more toxin B than toxin A. Toxin A has enterotoxic activity—that is, it elicits a positive fluid response in ligated rabbit ileal loops—whereas toxin B appears to be primarily a cytotoxin. The bacteroides and clostridium organisms are anaerobic and can be found in the intestinal tract. Also, these would be killed by the antibiotics given to the patient. *Staphylococcus aureus* is resistant to many antimicrobials and can cause gastroenteritis if it becomes predominant, but it usually does not cause as serious disease as pseudomembranous enterocolitis. Commercial laboratory tests are available to identify *C difficile* toxin and enterotoxin.

202. The answer is b. (*Brooks, pp 218, 240. Levinson, pp 111-114, 131-132. Murray, pp 233-236, 255-258. Ryan, pp 286-287, 302-305.*) Group B streptococci are normal flora in a sizeable number of women, who show no vaginal adverse disease. *Listeria monocytogenes* also may be present as normal vaginal flora. Streptococci from clinical specimens usually grow in small, pinpoint colonies. *Listeria*, usually growing intracellularly in vivo, also produce small colonies on blood agar. Both also produce β (clear zone) hemolysis. Of the proposed tests, catalase is easy to perform and interpret. Group B streptococci do not produce catalase, while *Listeria* are catalase-positive. Bacitracin sensitivity will determine Group A β-hemolytic streptococci identity. Coagulase is produced by *S aureus*. PCR and sugar fermentation tests are seldom used in gram-positive cocci identification. See the table below for a comparison of medically important streptococci.

STREPTOCOCCI OF MEDICAL IMPORTANCE			
Species	**Lancefield Group**	**Typical Hemolysis**	**Diagnostic Features[a]**
Streptococcus pyogenes	A	β	Bacitracin sensitive
Streptococcus agalactiae	B	β	Bacitracin resistant; hippurate hydrolyzed
Enterococcus faecalis	D	α or β or none	Growth in 6.5% NaCl[b]
Streptococcus bovis[c]	D	α or none	No growth in 6.5% NaCl
Streptococcus pneumoniae	NA[d]	α	Bile-soluble; inhibited by optochin
Viridans group[e]	NA	α	Not bile-soluble; not inhibited by optochin

[a]All streptococci are catalase-negative.
[b]Both *E faecalis* and *S bovis* grow on bile-esculin agar, whereas other streptococci do not. They hydrolyze the esculin, and this results in a characteristic black discoloration of the agar.
[c]*Streptococcus bovis* is a nonenterococcal group D organism.
[d]NA, not applicable.
[e]Viridans group streptococci include several species, such as *Streptococcus anguis, S mutans, S mitis, S gordonii, S salivarius, Streptococcus anginosus, Streptococcus milleri,* and *Staphylococcus intermedius.*

(*Reprinted, with permission, from Levinson W, Jawetz E. Medical Microbiology and Immunology. 7th ed. New York: McGraw-Hill;2002: 95.*)

203. The answer is a. (*Brooks, pp 280-282. Levinson, pp 152-155. Murray, pp 343-349. Ryan, pp 397-401.*) Meningitis caused by *H influenzae* cannot be distinguished on clinical grounds from that caused by pneumococci or meningococci. The symptoms described are typical for all three organisms. *Haemophilus influenzae* is a small, gram-negative rod with a polysaccharide capsule. It is able to grow on laboratory media if two factors are added. Heme (factor X) and NAD (factor V) provide for energy production. Use of the conjugate vaccine (type b polysaccharide) reduces the disease incidence more than 90%. Pneumococci are gram-positive diplococci, and meningococci are gram-negative diplococci, which grow on blood agar and chocolate agar with no X and V factors needed, respectively. Salt-mannitol agar is used to distinguish *S aureus* from other oral flora. Streptococci do not produce catalase while many other organisms do. Coagulase production is another test to identify *S aureus*. Commercial kits are available for immunologic detection of *H influenzae* antigens in spinal fluids, but currently none are available to measure specific antibody in CSF.

204. The answer is a. (*Brooks, p 220. Levinson, pp 169-170, 500-501. Murray, pp 391-393. Ryan, pp 458-459.*) The patient presented with typical symptoms of actinomycosis. *Actinomyces israelii* is normal flora in the mouth. However, it causes a chronic draining infection, often around the maxilla or the mandible, with osteomyelitic changes. Treatment is high-dose penicillin for 4 to 6 weeks. The diagnosis of actinomycosis is often complicated by the failure of *A israelii* to grow from the clinical specimen. It is an obligate anaerobe. Fluorescent antibody (FA) reagents are available for direct staining of *A israelii*. A rapid diagnosis can be made from the pus. FA conjugates are also available for *A viscosus* and *A odontolyticus*, anaerobic actinomycetes that are rarely involved in actinomycotic abscesses. *Corynebacterium diphtheriae* is a gram-positive rod, as is *P acnes*, and *S aureus* would be a large gram-positive cocci.

205. The answer is a. (*Brooks, p 240. Levinson, pp 112-113, 485. Murray, pp 233-236. Ryan, pp 286-287.*) The incidence of GBS disease is 1 to 3 cases per 1000 births. Neonates acquire the disease during birth from mothers who harbor the organism. Risk factors include prematurity, premature rupture of membranes, and group B streptococcal carriage. The Gram stain of

CSF is a rapid test for GBS disease. Although sensitive, the Gram stain requires experience to differentiate these streptococci from other gram-positive cocci. Latex tests for GBS antigen are also available, but sensitivity in CSF is not significantly higher than the Gram stain.

206. The answer is b. *(Brooks, pp 238-240. Levinson, pp 112-113, 485. Murray, pp 233-236. Ryan, pp 286-287.)* GBS can be reduced by intrapartum administration of penicillin. While GBS is relatively more resistant to penicillin than group A streptococci, the great majority of GBS isolates are still penicillin-susceptible. An aminoglycoside such as gentamicin may be added to GBS treatment regimens due to the relative reduced susceptibility of some strains. Experimentally, GBS polysaccharide vaccines have also been used. Screening pregnant females early in pregnancy probably offers little advantage because of the possible acquisition of GBS late in the pregnancy. Identification of possible high-risk births would be part of the physician's care of the pregnant patient and is too general for this question. Screening for GBS at the first office visit is premature since this is a first-time pregnancy with no history of GBS complications. Screening of GBS in the last trimester would probably not be done unless some indication of problems was identified. GBS is part of the normal vaginal flora and would be identified as such on culturing. No polysaccharide vaccine for GBS is currently available.

207. The answer is b. *(Brooks, pp 238-240. Levinson, pp 112-113, 485. Murray, pp 233-236. Ryan, pp 286-287.)* There has been speculation concerning the pathogenesis of GBS. This includes failure to activate complement pathways and immobilization of polymorphonuclear leukocytes due to the inactivation of complement C5a, a potent chemoattractant.

208. The answer is a. *(Brooks, pp 332-335. Levinson, pp 173-175. Murray, pp 405-411. Ryan, pp 424-429.)* In men, the appearance of a hard chancre on the penis characteristically indicates syphilis. Even though the chancre does not appear until the infection is 2 or more weeks old, the VDRL test for syphilis still can be negative despite the presence of a chancre (the VDRL test may not become positive for 2 or 3 weeks after initial infection). However, a lesion suspected of being a primary syphilitic ulcer should be examined by dark-field microscopy, which can reveal motile treponemes. Sending the patient home untreated would never occur, especially in light of the lesion being present. Since syphilis was suspected, the spirochete would not grow on T-M medium, and no pus discharge (suspect gonorrhea) was reported to justify culture for *N gonorrhoeae*.

209. The answer is a. (*Brooks, pp 285-286. Levinson, pp 157, 491-492. Murray, pp 358, 361-363. Ryan, pp 483-484.*) *Brucella* are small, aerobic, gram-negative coccobacilli. Of the four well-characterized species of *Brucella*, only one—*B melitensis*—characteristically infects both goats and humans. Brucellosis may be associated with gastrointestinal and neurologic symptoms, lymphadenopathy, splenomegaly, hepatitis, and osteomyelitis. Susceptibility to dyes (thionin and basic fuchsin) can help in differentiation of the species. None of the remaining options (*C jejuni, S enteritidis, and S marcesens*) are known to routinely be passed from animals to humans. *Francisella tularensis* is known to be so (see chart), but usually in connection with hunting and cleaning game animals. See the table below for a listing of gram-negative rods associated with animal sources.

GRAM-NEGATIVE RODS ASSOCIATED WITH ANIMAL SOURCES				
Species	Disease	Source of Human Infection	Mode of Human Transmission from Animal to Human	Diagnosis
Brucella species	Brucellosis	Pigs, cattle, goats, sheep	Dairy products; contact with animal tissues	Serology or culture
Francisella tularensis	Tularemia	Rabbits, deer, ticks	Contact with animal tissues; ticks	Serology
Yersinia pestis	Plague	Rodents	Flea bite	Immunofluorescence or culture
Pasteurella multocida	Cellulitis	Cats, dogs	Cat or dog bite	Wound culture

(*Reprinted, with permission, from Levinson W, Jawetz E. Medical Microbiology and Immunology. 7th ed. New York: McGraw-Hill; 2002: 139.*)

SPIROCHETES OF MEDICAL IMPORTANCE

Species	Disease	Mode of Transmission	Diagnosis	Morphology	Growth in Bacteriologic Media	Treatment
Treponema pallidum	Syphilis	Intimate (sexual) contact; across the placenta	Microscopy; serologic tests	Thin, tight, spirals, seen by dark-field illumination, silver impregnation, or immunofluorescent stain	–	Penicillin G
Borrelia burgdorferi	Lyme disease	Tick bite	Clinical observations; microscopy	Large, loosely coiled; stain with Giemsa stain	+	Tetracycline or am oxicillin for acute; penicillin G for chronic
Borrelia recurrentis	Relapsing fever	Louse bite	Clinical observations; microscopy	Large, loosely coiled; stain with Giemsa stain	+	Tetracycline
Leptospira interrogans	Leptospirosis	Food or drink contaminated by urine of infected animals (rats, dogs, pigs, cows)	Serologic tests	Thin, tight spirals, seen by dark-field illumination	+	Penicillin G

(Reprinted, with permission, from Levinson W, Jawetz E. Medical Microbiology and Immunology. 7th ed. New York: McGraw-Hill; 2002: 154.)

210. The answer is a. (*Brooks, pp 270-272. Levinson, pp 143-145. Murray, pp 317-320. Ryan, pp 376-377.*) Cholera is a toxicosis. The mode of action of cholera toxin is to stimulate the activity of adenyl cyclase, an enzyme that converts ATP to cyclic AMP. Cyclic AMP stimulates the secretion of chloride ion, and affected patients lose copious amounts of fluid. A drug that inhibits adenyl cyclase thus might block the effect of cholera toxin. Water and electrolyte replacement are primary management mechanisms, while oral tetracycline may help reduce stool output. Many antimicrobial agents are effective against *V chloerae*, notably oral tetracycline. Sensitively test would be needed for choosing the best drug to kill the bacteria. Fluid secretion would be lessened if adenyl cyclase was inhibited. Our patient would not die with the described medical treatment, but be helped to overcome the infection. Reduction of bacterial motility has no association with bacterial virulence.

211. The answer is d. (*Brooks, pp 226-228. Levinson, pp 106-110. Murray, pp 210-223. Ryan, pp 263-264.*) Certain strains of staphylococci elaborate an enterotoxin that is frequently responsible for food poisoning. Typically, the toxin is produced when staphylococci grow on foods rich in carbohydrates and is present in the food when it is consumed. The resulting gastroenteritis is dependent only on the ingestion of toxin and not on bacterial multiplication in the gastrointestinal tract. Characteristic symptoms are nausea, vomiting, abdominal cramps, and explosive diarrhea. The illness rarely lasts more than 24 hours. *Campylobacter perfringens* toxin contributes to a form of food poisoning, but the organism is ingested and grows in the patient, then releasing the toxin. *Campylobacter perfringens* also have toxins that can damage various tissues (gas gangrene). *Staphylococcus aureus* produces coagulase that clots plasma and does not contribute to *S aureus* food poisoning. Penicillinase (β-lactamase) does not contribute to food poisoning symptoms. Leukocidin inactivates WBCs in the laboratory, but clinical significance is uncertain.

212. The answer is e. (*Brooks, pp 224-229. Levinson, pp 106-110. Murray, p 222, Ryan, pp 269-270.*) Staphylococci are gram-positive, non-spore-forming cocci. Clinically, their antibiotic resistance poses major problems. Many strains produce β-lactamase (penicillinase), an enzyme that destroys penicillin by opening the lactam ring. Drug resistance, mediated by plasmids, may be transferred by transduction. No known allergic reactions occur by release of staphylococcal proteins. Even if the penicillin penetrates the *S aureus* membrane, external penicillinase would probably have broken the β-lactam ring, inactivating the drug. *Staphylococcus aureus* most likely contains PBP's (penicillin-binding proteins) but nothing happens if the penicillin is inactivated. Acetyl is CH_3CO. The acetylase would break this bond, but it is uncertain whether this inactivates penicillin like beta-lactamase does.

213. The answer is c. *(Brooks, p 207. Levinson, pp 127-128, 492. Murray, pp 383-386. Ryan, pp 320-322.)* *Campylobacter botulinum* growing in food produces a potent neurotoxin that causes diplopia, dysphagia, respiratory paralysis, and speech difficulties when ingested by humans. The toxin is thought to act by blocking the action of acetylcholine at neuromuscular junctions. Botulism is associated with high mortality; fortunately, *C botulinum* infection in humans is rare. Activation of cyclic AMP is important in cholera disease, not botulism. Clostridia are gram-positive and have no endotoxin. Ingestion of the botulism toxin initiates the disease. The actual organism may or may not be alive when ingested. An enterotoxin, by definition, would affect the intestinal tract.

214. The answer is a. *(Brooks, pp 296-303. Levinson, pp 119-123. Murray, pp 73-78, 291-299. Ryan, p 327.)* Several *Neisseria* species make up part of the normal (nonpathogenic) flora of the human upper respiratory tract. While commensal organisms seldom cause disease, they may occasionally be opportunistic. These organisms are also "foreign" to the immune system and cause immune responses to occur, especially humoral (antibody). The pathogens (*N gonorrhea* and *N meningitidis*) produce factors that ensure successful colonization of tissue in spite of local immune defense mechanisms. *Neisseria* organisms are gram-negative and have endotoxin but not lipoteichoic acid residues. These are part of gram-positive cell walls. Since even nonpathogenic neisseria are foreign to the immune system, any antibody response would be specific to the bacterial strain.

215. The answer is d. *(Brooks, pp 273-275. Levinson, pp 145-146. Murray, pp 325-328. Ryan, pp 379-380.)* Until recently, both erythromycin and ciprofloxacin were the drugs of choice for *C jejuni* enterocolitis. Recently, resistance to the quinolones (ciprofloxacin) has been observed. Ampicillin is ineffective against this gram-negative, curved rod. While Pepto-Bismol may be adequate for a related ulcer-causing bacterium, *Helicobacter*, it is not used for *C jejuni*. While the pathogenesis of *C jejuni* suggests an entero-toxin, an antitoxin is not available.

216. The answer is b. (*Brooks, pp 280-282. Levinson, pp 152-153. Murray, pp 344-348. Ryan, pp 397-401. Toy, p 96.*) *Haemophilus influenzae* is a gram-negative bacillus. In young children, it can cause pneumonitis, sinusitis, otitis, and meningitis. Occasionally, it produces a fulminative laryngotra-cheitis with such severe swelling of the epiglottis that tracheostomy becomes necessary. Clinical infections with this organism after the age of 3 years are less frequent, especially since approval of the type b vaccine. *Haemophilus haemolyticus* is a hemolytic variant of *H influenzae* which only occasionally causes disease. *Klebsiella pneumoniae* is present in about 5% of individuals and causes about 1% of pneumonias. *Treponema pneumoniae* is a prominent cause of pneumonia in persons 5 to 20 years old. *Neisseria meningitidis* can be part of the oral flora but is significant in disease when it enters the blood stream and CNS.

217. The answer is a. (*Brooks, pp 240-243. Levinson, pp 27, 140, 537. Murray, pp 243-246. Ryan, pp 294-295. Toy, p 70.*) Enterococci cause a wide variety of infections ranging from less serious—for example, urinary tract infections—to very serious, such as septicemia. A gram-positive coccus resistant to penicillin must be assumed to be enterococcus until other, more definitive biochemical testing places the isolate in one of the more esoteric groups of gram-positive cocci. Group A streptococci can cause a wide variety of diseases, including rheumatic fever. Certain antigens of the Group A streptococci cross react with human heart antigens, causing dam-age to heart muscles and valves. GBS are part of the normal vaginal flora, are β-hemolytic, and test positive to the cAMP test. Gram-negative *Neisseria* species are seldom involved in heart disease, even as oppor-tunists. *Streptococcus pneumoniae* can cause upper respiratory disease, bac-teremia, and meningitis.

218. The answer is d. (*Brooks, p 243. Levinson, pp 111, 489-490. Murray, pp 243-246. Ryan, pp 294-295.*) *Enterococcus faecalis* causes 85% to 90% of enterococcal infections, while *E faecium* causes 5% to 10%. The enterococci are among the most frequent causes of nosocomial infections, especially in intensive care units. *Streptococcus bovis* is a nonenterococcal Group D streptococcus. *Streptococcus pyogenes* is a Group A streptococcus, responsible for 95% of streptococci infections. *Streptococcus pneumoniae* are sensitive to many antimicrobials. Once isolated, there are a variety of tests to speciate enterococci. However, penicillin-resistant, non-β-lactamase-producing, vancomycin-resistant, gram-positive cocci are most likely *E faecium or E faecalis*.

219. The answer is e. (*Brooks, pp 240-243. Levinson, pp 77, 112. Murray, pp 243-246. Ryan, pp 294-295.*) There are a variety of mechanisms for vancomycin resistance in *E faecium*, and they have been termed Van A, B, or C. These isolates have become one of the most feared nosocomial pathogens in the hospital environment. Unfortunately, no approved antibiotics can successfully treat vancomycin-resistant enterococci (VRE)—only some experimental antibiotics such as Synercid. Enterococci are highly resistant to cephalosporins, β-lactamase resistant penicillins, and monolactams. They have low-level resistance to aminoglycosides and intermediate resistance to fluoroquinolones. They are inhibited by β-lactams (ampicillin) but not killed by them.

220. The answer is c. (*Brooks, pp 224-229. Levinson, pp 107-109, 484. Murray, pp 211-220. Ryan, p 824.*) *Staphylococcus aureus* is implicated in the majority of cases of acute osteomyelitis, which affects children most often. A superficial staphylococcal lesion frequently precedes the development of bone infection. In the preantibiotic era, *Streptococcus pneumoniae* was a common cause of acute osteomyelitis. *M tuberculosis* and gram-negative organisms are implicated less frequently in this infection.

(Reproduced, with permission, from Brooks GF, et al. Jawetz's Medical Microbiology. 24th ed. New York: McGraw-Hill; 2007: 225.)

221. The answer is d. *(Brooks, pp 213-216. Levinson, pp 130-131, 481. Murray, pp 261-265. Ryan, p 170. Toy, p 64.)* All toxigenic strains of *C diphtheriae* are lysogenic for β-phage carrying the *Tox* gene, which codes for the toxin molecule. The expression of this gene is controlled by the metabolism of the host bacteria. The greatest amount of toxin is produced by bacteria grown on media containing very low amounts of iron. Fragment B of the toxin is required for cell entry, while Fragment A stops protein production by inhibiting elongation factor 2 (EF-2). *Corynebacterium diphtheriae* does not possess a capsule, which is normally used to impede phagocytosis by WBCs. Glucose and/or sucrose fermentation is not a virulence factor. Endotoxin comes from gram-negative bacteria while corynebacteria are gram positive.

222 to 224. The answers are 222-c, 223-e, 224-b. *(Brooks, pp 226-228. Levinson, pp 40-44, 107-108. Murray, pp 211-220. Ryan, pp 264-266. Toy, p 156.)* TSS is a febrile illness seen predominantly, but not exclusively, in menstruating women. Clinical criteria for TSS include fever greater than 102°F (38.9°C), rash, hypotension, and abnormalities of the mucous membranes and the gastrointestinal, hepatic, muscular, cardiovascular systems, or CNS. Usually three or more systems are involved. Treatment is supportive, including the aggressive use of antistaphylococcal antibiotics. Certain types of tampons may play a role in TSS by trapping O_2 and depleting magnesium. Most people have protective antibodies to the toxic shock syndrome toxin (TSST-1). Chicken pox (VZV) or varicella presents with a typical vesicular rash. Guillain-Barre syndrome is a demyelinating condition of the peripheral nerves. Scalded skin syndrome is caused by *S aureus* exfoliative toxin that produces epidermal skin layer sloughing. Food poisoning is caused by *S aureus* enterotoxins, which are produced in contaminated food and symptoms appear after ingestion.

TSS is caused by a toxin-producing strain of *S aureus* (TSST-1). In this case no actual organisms would likely be isolated since TSS is caused by an excreted toxin, not the actual organism. Blood culture would also most likely be negative. While there have been reports that *S epidermidis* produces TSS, they have largely been discounted. Vaginal colonization with *S aureus* is a necessary adjunct to the disease. *Staphylococcus aureus* is isolated from the vaginal secretions, conjunctiva, nose, throat, cervix, and feces in 45% to 98% of cases. The organism has infrequently been isolated from the blood. *Clostridium difficile* and *C perfringens* produce pseudomembranous colitis and gas gangrene, respectively. *Gardnerella vaginalis* can be found in the normal vaginal flora and in vaginosis, where inflammatory cells are not present. "Clue cells" are vaginal epithelial cells covered with many gram-variable bacteria, including *G vaginalis*.

Epidemiologic investigations suggest strongly that TSS is related to use of tampons, in particular, use of the highly absorbent ones that can be left in for extended periods of time. An increased growth of intravaginal *S aureus* and enhanced production of TSST-1 have been associated with the prolonged intravaginal use of these hyperabsorbent tampons and with the capacity of the materials used in them to bind magnesium. The most severe cases of TSS have been seen in association with gram-negative infection. TSST-1 may enhance endotoxin activity. Recently, group A streptococci have been reported to cause TSS. Purchased fast-food ingestion, heavy menstrual flow, rubella exposure, and travel to Vermont would have no relevance to this clinical situation.

225 and 226. The answers are 225-c, 226-d. (*http://en.wikipedia.org/wiki/ Bayesian_statistics.*) Bayesian statistics are often used to determine sensitivity, specificity, and predictive values of new diagnostic tests. A square is set up and the experimental numbers inserted: a = true positive, b = false positive, c = false negative, and d = true negative. The formulas for sensitivity, specificity, and predictive values are also given. (See table.)

It is necessary to note that the incidence of the disease in the population affects predictive values but not sensitivity or specificity. At a given level of sensitivity and specificity, as the incidence of the disease in the population increases, the predictive value of a positive (PVP) increases, and the predictive value of a negative (PVN) decreases. For this reason, predictive values are difficult to interpret unless true disease incidence is known.

	Culture	
LA Test	**Positive**	**Negative**
Pos	(a) 25	(b) 5
NEG	(c) 5	(d) 95

$$\text{Sensitivity} = \frac{a}{a+c} = \frac{25}{25+5} = 85\%$$

$$\text{Specificity} = \frac{d}{d+b} = \frac{95}{95+5} = 95\%$$

$$\text{PVP} = \frac{a}{a+b} = \frac{25}{25+5} = 85\%$$

$$\text{PVN} = \frac{d}{d+c} = \frac{95}{95+5} = 95\%$$

227. The answer is d. (*Brooks, pp 263-265. Levinson, pp 149-150. Murray, pp 333-337. Ryan, pp 387-388.*) Pseudomonads occur widely in soil, water, plants, and animals. They are gram-negative, motile, aerobic rods that produce water-soluble pigments (blue and green). They are very opportunistic when abnormal host defenses are encountered. While motile, they do not "swarm" over the surface of an agar plate, as *Proteus* does. Being gram-negative, as many enteric and environmental organisms are, their cell walls contain endotoxin (LPS). Many of the pseudomonads are resistant to a wide range of antimicrobials, enhancing their opportunistic characteristics.

228. The answer is c. (*Brooks, pp 203-211. Levinson, pp 127-129. Murray, pp 377-389, 247-251. Ryan, pp 308, 314-317.*) *Clostridium* and *Bacillus* organisms exist widely in nature. While many *Clostridium* are pathogenic due to exotoxin production (*C tetanis, C botulism*), and anthrax has multiple virulence factors (capsule, LF, EF, and PA), *C perfringens* and *B cereus* are found routinely in gastroenteritis outbreaks. Since both are spore formers, the usual epidemiological investigation finds that heating foods kills vegetative bacteria but not spores. If food is inappropriately stored (>40°F-140°F), spores may germinate into vegetative bacteria and be ingested, causing the disease. Most episodes are self-limited. Both produce enterotoxins that account for similar disease presentations.

229. The answer is e. *(Brooks, pp 224-229. Levinson, pp 48, 107-109. Murray, pp 211-220. Ryan, pp 269-270.)* The incidence of oxacillin and MRSA has been rapidly increasing. MRSA and methicillin-sensitive *S aureus* (MSSA) coexist in heterologous populations. Treatment of a patient harboring this heterologous population may provide a selective environment for the MRSA. Prior to changing therapy, the susceptibility of the isolate should be determined. Vancomycin has often been used effectively for MRSA, but it is expensive and nephrotoxic. There is no evidence that MRSA is any more virulent or invasive than susceptible strains. See the table below for a listing of medically important staphylococci.

STAPHYLOCOCCI OF MEDICAL IMPORTANCE				
Species	Coagulase Production	Typical Hemolysis	Important Features[a]	Typical Disease
Staphylococcus aureus	+	Beta	Protein A on surface	Abscess, food poisoning, toxic shock syndrome
Staphylococcus epidermidis	–	None	Sensitive to novobiocin	Infection of prosthetic heart valves and hips; common member of skin flora
Staphylococcus saprophyticus	–	None	Resistant to novobiocin	Urinary tract infection

[a]All staphylococci are catalase-positive.
(Reprinted, with permission, from Levinson W, Jawetz E. Medical Microbiology and Immunology. *7th ed. New York: McGraw-Hill; 2002: 92.)*

230. The answer is c. *(Brooks, pp 253-255. Levinson, pp 136-140, 492. Murray, pp 303-307. Ryan, pp 355-357. Toy, p 76.)* Food poisoning with *E coli* 0157/H7 causes hemorrhagic colitis; it is often seen in people who have eaten beef hamburgers. The same organism also causes a hemorrhagic uremic syndrome. The toxin, called *Shiga-like toxin*, can be demonstrated in Vero cells, but the cytotoxicity must be neutralized with specific antiserum. With the exception of sorbitol fermentation, there is nothing biochemically distinctive about these organisms.

231. The answer is b. *(Brooks, pp 253-255. Levinson, pp 136-140, 492. Murray, pp 303-307. Ryan, pp 355-357.)* ETEC is an important cause of traveler's diarrhea, producing a heat-labile exotoxin (LT) and a heat-stable enterotoxin (ST). To cause diarrhea, *E coli* must produce not only LT and ST toxins but also adhere to the lining of the small intestine. Fimbrial antigens are involved in adherence. O657/H7 stain is called EHEC, while EPEC is also an important cause of diarrhea in infants. EIEC produces a shigellosis-type disease.

232. The answer is d. *(Brooks, pp 291-292. Levinson, pp 159-160. Murray, pp 311-313. Ryan, pp 484-488.)* Bubonic plague and pneumonic plague differ clinically. Bubonic plague, characterized by swollen lymph nodes and fever, is usually transmitted through a flea bite. Pneumonic plague, which is characterized by sepsis and pneumonia, is transmitted by the droplet route, usually after contact with an infected human or animal. Age of the patient, geographic location and/or health of the animal vector, and season of the year would all be insignificant in considering epidemiological differences between the clinical presentations of the two plagues.

233. The answer is a. *(Brooks, pp 315, 316. Levinson, pp 32, 186-187. Murray, p 372. Ryan, p 479.)* While the essential information (ie, the evidence that the child in question was scratched by a cat) is missing, the clinical presentation points to a number of diseases, including cat scratch disease (CSD). Until recently, the etiologic agent of CSD was unknown. Evidence indicated that it was a pleomorphic, rod-shaped bacterium that had been named *Afipia*. It was best demonstrated in the affected lymph node by a silver impregnation stain. However, it now appears that *Afipia* causes relatively few cases of CSD and that the small, pleomorphic, gram-negative rods present mainly in the walls of capillaries primarily responsible are

Rochalimaea henselae, which has recently been renamed *B henselae*. *Brucella*, *Mycobacterium*, and *Yersinia* species have not been shown to have any association with cat scratch disease.

234. The answer is c. *(Brooks, pp 233-239. Levinson, pp 110-115. Murray, pp 225-233. Ryan, p 273.)* There has been a marked increase in fatal streptococcal infections, including those that are described as "necrotizing fasciitis." The strains of group A streptococci isolated have a pyrogenic exotoxin with properties not unlike those of the toxic shock toxin of *S aureus*. Mortality is high (30%) in spite of aggressive antibiotic therapy.

235. The answer is b. *(Brooks, pp 275-276. Levinson, pp 146-147, 496. Murray, pp 328-332. Ryan, pp 383-384.)* *Helicobacter pylori* antigen tests from a stool sample using an ELISA format and a monoclonal antibody to *H pylori* are as sensitive as culture of the control portion of the stomach. Urea breath tests are also widely used. *Helicobacter pylori* has an active enzyme (urease) that breaks down radioactive urea. The patient releases radioactive CO_2 if *H pylori* are present. *Helicobacter pylori* antibody tests, IgG and IgA, indicate the presence of *H pylori* and usually decline after effective treatment. Culture of stomach contents is insensitive and not appropriate as a diagnostic procedure for *H pylori*. Direct tests, such as antigen or culture of gastric mucosa, are preferred because they are the most sensitive indication of a cure.

236. The answer is e. *(Brooks, pp 337-338, Levinson, pp 24, 176-177. Murray, pp 411-415. Ryan, pp 434-437. Toy, p 40.)* At present, Lyme disease may be diagnosed clinically and serologically. Patients who are from endemic areas such as eastern Pennsylvania and report joint pain and swelling months subsequent to exposure to ticks must be evaluated for Lyme disease and treated if the test is positive. Patients may also report a variety of neurologic problems such as tingling of the extremities, Bell palsy, and headache. IgM antibody appears soon after the tick bite (10 days-3 weeks) and persists for 2 months; IgG appears later in the disease but remains elevated for 1 to 2 years, especially in untreated patients. A significant IgG titer is at least 1:320. Most investigators feel that IgM titers of 1:100 are significant; some investigators say that any IgM titer is significant. Management of this patient would best be done by immediately starting treatment with tetracycline, effective against *B burgdorferi*.

237. The answer is c. (*Brooks, pp 320-327. Levinson, pp 161-168. Murray, pp 282-285, 289. Ryan, p 613.*) There are some interesting characteristics of *M avium* from AIDS patients. According to data from the National Jewish Hospital and Research Center in Denver and the CDC, 75% of the isolates were serovar 4, and 76% produced a deep-yellow pigment. Yellow pigment is not a characteristic of most isolates of *M avium*. The significance of these findings is unknown. Most *M avium* isolates are resistant to isoniazid and streptomycin but susceptible to clofazimine and ansamycin. In vitro susceptibility testing, however, may not be reliable for *M avium*. A blood culture is often the most reliable way to diagnose the disease. Finally, all isolates of *M avium* are acid-fast, by definition.

238. The answer is b. (*Brooks, pp 142, 170, 238. Levinson, pp 115, 470. Murray, pp 231, 233. Ryan, p 279.*) Rheumatic fever (RF) is a disease that causes polyarthritis, carditis, chorea, and erythema marginatum. The mechanism of damage appears to be autoimmune; that is, antibodies are synthesized to a closely related streptococcal antigen such as M-protein, but these same antibodies cross-react with certain cardiac antigens such as myosin. Until recently, RF was very rare in the United States. In 1986, there were at least 135 cases of RF in Utah. Subsequently, scattered cases of RF have occurred in other states. Epidemiologists do not have a reason for this increase in RF. Some evidence suggests that there may be a genetic predisposition to the disease. Intramuscular injection of benzathine penicillin is effective treatment for and prophylaxis against group A streptococcal infection. While it appears that certain strains of streptococci contain cell membrane antigens that are identical to human heart tissue antigens, the strains can infect skin and cause pharyngitis. The first attack of RF (rheumatic fever) usually produces only slight cardiac damage. It is important to protect such patients from recurrent *S pyogenes* infections by prophylactic penicillin use to prevent increased damage from multiple future bacterial attacks. Answer option (e) refers to a staphylococcal antigen as similar, but the correct comparison would be with streptococcal antigen and cardiac antigen.

239. The answer is d. (*Brooks, pp 198, 240. Levinson, pp 27, 112. Murray, pp 73-78. Ryan, pp 293-294.*) In the healthy oral cavity, gram-positive, α-hemolytic streptococci make up the predominant flora. Any dental manipulation causes bleeding, allowing the oral flora to get into the blood (bacteremia). Phagocytic activity by WBCs usually clears this in a few minutes.

However, these same organisms are quite efficient at attaching to and colonizing heart valve defects. *Streptococcus viridians* is a typical member of this α-hemolytic group and is commonly found in subacute bacterial endocarditis (SBE). *Staphylococcus aureus* and *S epidermidis* are present in the oral flora in very small numbers, as is *S pneumoniae*. If *E faecalis* gets into the blood stream from the gastrointestinal tract, it could potentially also cause heart valve problems. The α-hemolytic viridians streptococci are reported as being isolated from SBE most often.

240. The answer is e. *(Brooks, pp 241-242. Levinson, pp 11, 66, 153. Murray, p 241. Ryan, p 291.)* The quellung test determines the presence of bacterial capsules. Specific antibody is mixed with the bacterial suspension or with clinical material. The polysaccharide capsule-antibody complex is visible microscopically. The test is also termed *capsular swelling.* The capsules of *S pneumoniae* as well as *N meningitidis*, *H influenzae*, and *K pneumoniae* play a role in the pathogenicity of the organisms. These surface structures inhibit phagocytosis, perhaps by preventing attachment of the leukocyte pseudopod. *Corynebacterium diphtheriae, Enterobacter,* and *H parainfluenzae* are nonencapsulated.

241. The answer is b. *(Brooks, pp 218, 280. Levinson, pp 112, 114, 136, 139. Murray, pp 255-258. Ryan, pp 302-305. Toy, p 102.)* No vaccine is available for *Listeria*. Except during a meningococcal epidemic, *H influenzae* is the most common cause of bacterial meningitis in children. The organism is occasionally found to be associated with respiratory tract infections or otitis media. *Haemophilus influenzae, N meningitidis, S pneumoniae,* and *Listeria* account for 80% to 90% of all cases of bacterial meningitis. A purified polysaccharide vaccine conjugated to protein for *H influenzae* type B is available. A tetravalent vaccine is available for *N meningitidis* and a 23-serotype vaccine for *S pneumoniae*.

242. The answer is e. *(Brooks, p 149. Levinson, pp 30-37. Murray, pp 73-76.)* Organisms may be transmitted in a number of ways, such as by air, food, hands, sexual contact, and infected needles. However, for each disease or disease category, there is usually a portal of entry not always unique to the organism. The skin is a tough integument and, in fact, is resistant to most infectious organisms except those that may breakdown human skin. Breaches of the skin as by wounds, burns, and the like predispose patients to a variety of infections such as tetanus caused by wound contamination with spores of *C tetani*, or direct infection by *Staphylococcus*, *Streptococcus*, or gram-negative rods (such as *Serratia* or *Pseudomonas*).

243 to 245. The answers are 243-d, 244-a, 245-b. *(Brooks, pp 148-151. Levinson, pp 30-37. Murray, pp 73-76.)* The respiratory tract is a common portal of entry to such airborne organisms as *M tuberculosis*. This is why respiratory precautions must be taken when patients are harboring viable *M tuberculosis*. The gastrointestinal tract is usually infected from ingestion of contaminated food or water (*Shigella, Salmonella, and Campylobacter*) or by an alteration of the normal microbial flora such as with *C difficile* disease. The genital tract may become infected either by sexual contact or by alteration of the genital environment, as often occurs with yeast infections. Several bacteria such as *N gonorrhoeae, Chlamydia,* and *T pallidum* are transmitted by direct sexual contact with infected partners.

246. The answer is d. *(Brooks, pp 268, 296, 303-304. Levinson, pp 190, 504. Murray, pp 334, 338-340. Ryan, pp 390-391.)* While admittedly rare in human medicine, the bacteria referred to should be appreciated for their role in human disease. *Branhamella* is a gram-negative diplococcus. It has recently been renamed *Moraxella catarrhalis*. While it is a member of the normal flora, it may cause severe upper and lower respiratory tract infection, particularly in the immunosuppressed patient. Most isolates produce β-lactamase and are resistant to penicillin. *M catarrhalis* is not a gram-negative rod that causes endocarditis, nor a gram-negative, fusiformed (pointed ends) rod associated with periodontal disease or sepsis. It is not the cause of rat-bite fever or the causative agent of trench fever.

247. The answer is b. *(Brooks, pp 220, 267. Levinson, p 187. Murray, pp 372, 374. Ryan, pp 390-391.)* *Capnocytophaga* grows best in a carbon dioxide atmosphere, as the name implies. It is isolated frequently from patients with periodontal disease but may also cause septicemia in susceptible patients. Rat-bite fever is caused by *Spirillum*, and the agent of CSD is *B henselae*.

248. The answer is b. *(Brooks, pp 350-354. Levinson, pp 183, 503. Murray, pp 436-440. Ryan, pp 477-478.)* *Coxiella burnetii* is a rickettsial organism that causes upper respiratory infections in humans. These can range from subclinical infection to influenza-like disease and pneumonia. Transmission to humans occurs from inhalation of dust contaminated with rickettsiae from placenta, dried feces, urine, or milk, or from aerosols in slaughterhouses. *Campylobacter burnetii* can also be found in ticks, which can transmit the agent to sheep, goats, and cattle. No skin rash occurs in these infections. Treatment includes tetracycline and chloramphenicol. *Coxiella burnetii* is not transmitted by flea or tick vectors. Since Q fever involves the upper respiratory tract, liver, or CNS, there is no transmission by urethral discharge.

249 to 251. The answers are 249-a, 250-d, 251-b. (*Brooks, pp 243, 219-221. Levinson, pp 69-84. Murray, pp 199-208. Ryan, pp 294, 457-459, 870-871.*) These questions demonstrate commonly occurring clinical infectious diseases and microbiologic problems. Enterococci may be resistant to ampicillin and gentamicin. Vancomycin would be the drug of choice. However, laboratory results do not always correlate well with clinical response. The National Committee on Clinical Laboratory Standards recommends testing enterococci only for ampicillin and vancomycin. Some symptomatic patients may have 10 leukocytes per milliliter of urine but relatively few bacteria. The patient is likely infected and the organisms, particularly if in pure culture, should be further processed.

The patient in Question 251 probably has actinomycosis. These laboratory data are not uncommon. There is no reason to work up all the contaminating bacteria. A fluorescent microscopy test for *A israelii* is available. If positive, the FA provides a rapid diagnosis. In any event, it may be impossible to recover *A israelii* from such a specimen. High-dose penicillin has been used to treat actinomycosis. One of the options suggests no further clinical work-up on the patients be done. Clearly, laboratory results may help the clinician make patient management decisions but each of these three cases show that physicians need to have a good understanding that laboratory tests may give conflicting information for the patient being treated. The physician must help the laboratory to understand how to use the data produced to give the patient the best possible medical care. Antibiotic sensitivity tests today are mostly automated and reliable. If a repeat is needed, a new blood sample should be drawn for the new test.

252 to 256. The answers are 252-c, 253-d, 254-b, 255-d, 256-e. (*Brooks, pp 170-172. Levinson, pp 69-84. Murray, pp 199-208. Ryan, p 195. Toy, p 40.*) There are few bacteria for which antimicrobial susceptibility is highly predictable. However, some agents are the drug of choice because of their relative effectiveness. Among the three antibiotics that have been shown to treat legionellosis effectively (erythromycin, rifampin, and minocycline), erythromycin is clearly superior, even though in vitro studies show the organism to be susceptible to other antibiotics.

Penicillin remains the drug of choice for *S pneumoniae* and the group A streptococci, although a few isolates of penicillin-resistant pneumococci have been observed. Resistance among the pneumococci is either chromosomally mediated, in which case the minimal inhibitory concentrations (MICs) are relatively low, or plasmid-mediated, which results in highly resistant bacteria. The same is generally true for *H influenzae*. Until the mid-1970s, virtually all isolates of *H influenzae* were susceptible to ampicillin. There has been a rapidly increasing incidence of ampicillin-resistant isolates—almost 35% to 40% in some areas of the United States. Resistance is ordinarily mediated by β-lactamase, although ampicillin-resistant, β-lactamase-negative isolates have been seen. No resistance to penicillin has been seen in group A streptococci.

Lyme disease, caused by *B burgdorferi*, has been treated with penicillin, erythromycin, and tetracycline. Treatment failures have been observed. Ceftriaxone has become the drug of choice, particularly in the advanced stages of Lyme disease.

The most common infection due to beta-hemolytic *S pyogenes* (GAS) is strep sore throat or pharyngitis. From here, the infection is able to spread to all parts of the body. Significant symptoms, as described, are often experienced, with only 20% of infections being asymptomatic. The organisms grow fairly well in the laboratory and easily identified. All *S pyogenes* strains are susceptible to penicillin G, and most are susceptible to erythromycin. Antimicrobial drugs have no effect on established glomerulonephritis and rheumatic fever. In acute infections, efforts must be made to eradicate streptococci from the patient quickly to eliminate the antigenic stimulus.

Campylobacter difficile causes toxin-mediated pseudomembranous enterocolitis as well as antibiotic-associated diarrhea. Pseudomembranous enterocolitis is normally seen during or after administration of antibiotics. One of the few agents effective against *C difficile* is vancomycin. Alternatively, bacitracin can be used.

257 to 260. The answers are 257-a, 258-d, 259-b, 260-c. (*Brooks, pp 270-276. Levinson, pp 133-146. Murray, pp 325-328. Ryan, pp 373-378.*

Toy, p 172.) Some organisms originally thought to be vibrios, such as *C jejuni*, have been reclassified. *Campylobacter jejuni*, which grows best at 107.6°F (42°C), has its reservoir in birds and mammals and causes gastroenteritis in humans.

Vibrio cholerae causes cholera, which is worldwide in distribution. Vibrios are the most common bacteria in surface waters worldwide. They are curved rods with a polar flagellum. *Vibrio cholerae* subgroups O1 and O139 (older serotype designations: Ogawa [AB], Inaba [AC], Jolpka [ABC]) cause cholera in humans. A person with normal gastric acidity may have to ingest 10^{10} or more *V cholerae* to become infected when the vehicle is water because the organisms are susceptible to acid. When ingested with food, as few as 10^2 to 10^4 may be able to produce disease. The organisms do not reach the bloodstream but remain in the intestinal tract.

Vibrio parahaemolyticus is a halophilic marine vibrio that causes gastroenteritis in humans, primarily from ingestion of cooked seafood. It is lactose-negative and sucrose-negative.

Vibrio vulnificus is also halophilic. It has been suggested that these halophilic vibrios do not belong in the genus *Vibrio* but in the genus *Beneckea*. *Vibrio vulnificus* is lactose-positive and produces heat-labile, extracellular toxin. Organisms that, unlike *V cholerae*, do not agglutinate in 0 to 1 antiserum were once called nonagglutinable (NAG), or noncholera (NC), vibrios. Such a classification can be confusing because *V vulnificus*, which is an NCV, nevertheless causes severe cholera-like disease. In addition, *V vulnificus* can produce wound infections, septicemia, meningitis, pneumonia, and keratitis.

261 to 264. The answers are 261-b, 262-d, 263-a, 264-e. *(Brooks, pp 280-287. Levinson, pp 152-156. Murray, pp 311-313, 358-363. Ryan, pp 401-402, 481-488.)* All the organisms described in the questions are short, ovoid, gram-negative rods. For the most part, they are nutritionally fastidious and require blood or blood products for growth. These and related organisms are unique among bacteria in that, though they have an animal reservoir, they can be transmitted to humans. Humans become infected by a variety of routes, including ingestion of contaminated animal products (*B abortus* in cattle), direct contact with contaminated animal material or with infected animals themselves (*Y enterocolitica* and *B bronchiseptica* in dogs), and animal bites (*P multocida* in many different animals). The laboratory differentiation of these microbes may be difficult and must rely on a number of parameters, including biochemical and serologic reactions, development of specific antibody response in affected persons, and epidemiologic evidence of infection.

Yersinia enterocolitica are motile at 77°C (25°C) and nonmotile at 98.6°F (37°C). They are found in the intestinal tract of animals and cause a variety of clinical syndromes in humans. Transmission to humans probably occurs via animal fecal contamination of food, drink, or fomites.

The brucellae are obligate parasites of animals and humans and are located intracellularly. *Brucella abortus* is typically found in cattle. Brucellosis (undulant fever) has an acute bacteremic phase followed by a chronic stage that may last years and involve many tissues. *Brucella abortus* requires CO_2 for growth and is most often isolated from blood and bone marrow. Species differentiation is due to dye (thionine) sensitivity.

Bordetella bronchiseptica causes diseases in animals (kennel cough in dogs) and occasionally respiratory disease and bacteremia in humans. *Bordetella* requires enriched medium (Bordet-Gengou) and is strongly urease-positive.

Pasteurella multicida occurs worldwide in the respiratory and gastrointestinal tracts of many domestic and wild animals. It is the most common organism in human wounds inflicted by cat and dog bites. It is one of the common causes of hemorrhagic septicemia in rabbits, rats, horses, sheep, fowl, cats, and swine. It can affect many systems in humans, as well as bite wounds.

265 to 267. The answers are 265-d, 266-e, 267-b. *(Brooks, pp 63-71. Levinson, pp 62-68. Murray, pp 189-198. Ryan, pp 339, 373, 449. Toy, p 122.)* The medium of choice for the isolation of pathogenic Neisseriae is Thayer-Martin (TM) agar. TM agar is both a selective and an enriched medium; it contains hemoglobin, the supplement Isovitalex, and the antibiotics vancomycin, colistin, nystatin, and trimethoprim. *Vibrio cholerae* as well as other vibrios, including *V parahaemolyticus* and *V alginolyticus*, are isolated best on thiosulfate citrate bile salts sucrose medium, although media such as mannitol salt agar also support the growth of vibrios. Maximal growth occurs at a pH of 8.5 to 9.5 and at 98.6°F (37°C) incubation. Löwenstein-Jensen slants or plates, which are composed of a nutrient base and egg yolk, are used routinely for the initial isolation of mycobacteria. Small inocula of *M tuberculosis* can also be grown in oleic acid albumin media; large inocula can be cultured on simple synthetic media.

Loeffler medium is an enriched nonselective medium used for the cultivation of corynebacteria, especially *C diphtheriae*. Horse serum and egg coagulate during sterilization and provide nutrients. This medium enhances the production of metachromatic granules (observed with methylene blue stain). Columbia agar with 5% sheep blood is a general-purpose medium for isolation of a variety of organisms, including fastidious organisms. Along with nutrition, blood agar allows the observation of alpha (incomplete) and beta (complete lysis) hemolysis caused by bacteria.

268. The answer is b. *(Brooks, pp 206-207. Levinson, pp 127-128. Murray, pp 383-386. Ryan, pp 320-322.)* Botulism is a disease brought about by ingesting a preformed toxin. Anaerobic bacteria have grown in food, deposited the botulism toxin, and died. The toxin affects the CNS by inhibiting the release of acetylcholine at the neuronal synapse. This results in a flaccid paralysis and death by respiratory failure. At no stage of the disease will any antibiotic be able to modify or arrest the disease. Antitoxins (A, B, and E) must be promptly administered, and ventilation assisted mechanically. In all other choices, antibiotics will provide a mechanism to kill or inhibit the microorganisms, bringing the infection under control.

269. The answer is d. *(Brooks, pp 339-340. Levinson, pp 67, 174-177, 541. Murray, pp 416-418. Ryan, pp 430-431.)* Leptospirosis is a zoonosis of worldwide distribution. Human infection results from ingestion of water or food contaminated with leptospirae. Rats, mice, wild rodents, dogs, swine, and cattle excrete the organisms in urine and feces during active illness and during an asymptomatic carrier state. Drinking, swimming, bathing, or food consumption may lead to human infection. Children acquire the disease from dogs more often than do adults. Treatment can include doxycycline, ampicillin, or amoxicillin. Symptoms in humans range from fever and rash to jaundice through aseptic meningitis.

Leptospirae are tightly coiled, thin, flexible spirochetes 5 to 15 μm long, with one end bent into a hook. It stains best where silver can be impregnated into the organism. The gram stain would not be useful. The organisms derive energy from oxidation of fatty acids, so EMB or Thayer-Martin agar would be inadequate. Agglutination testing and CIE is complicated by the fact that all *Leptospirae* strains exhibit cross-reactivity in serologic tests.

270 to 273. The answers are 270-e, 271-a, 272-b, 273-d. *(Brooks, pp 196-201. Levinson, pp 25-30. Murray, pp 73-78. Ryan, p 143.)* An understanding of normal, or indigenous, microflora is essential in order to appreciate the abnormal. Usually, anatomic sites contiguous to mucous membranes are not sterile and have characteristic normal flora.

The skin flora differs as a function of location. Skin adjacent to mucous membranes may share some of the normal flora of the gastroin-testinal system. Overall, the predominant bacteria on the skin surface are *S epidermidis* and *Propionibacterium*, an anaerobic diphtheroid.

The mouth is part of the gastrointestinal tract, but its indigenous flora shows some distinct differences. While anaerobes are present in large numbers, particularly in the gingival crevice, the eruption of teeth at 6 to 9 months of age leads to colonization by organisms such as *S mutans* and *Streptococcus sanguis*, both α-hemolytic streptococci. An edentulous person loses β-hemolytic streptococci as normal flora.

The gastrointestinal tract is sterile at birth and soon develops charac-teristic flora as a function of diet. In the adult, anaerobes such as *B fragilis* and *Bifidobacterium* may outnumber coliforms and enterococci by a ratio of 1000:1. The colon contains 10^{11} to 10^{12} bacteria per gram of feces.

Soon after birth, the vagina becomes colonized by lactobacilli. As the female matures, lactobacilli may still be predominant, but anaerobic cocci, diphtheroids, and anaerobic, gram-negative rods also are found as part of the indigenous flora. Changes in the chemical or microbiologic ecology of the vagina can have marked effects on normal flora and may promote infec-tion such as vaginitis or vaginosis.

Escherichia coli are among the most common group of gram-negative rods isolated in the laboratory. It is fairly easily identified in the laboratory. It ferments mannitol and is lactose positive. The organism is part of normal body flora, but is a very efficient opportunist. Urinary tract infections are commonly caused with this organism.

274 to 277. The answers are 274-c, 275-d, 276-a, 277-e. (*Brooks, pp 196-201. Levinson, pp 25-30. Murray, pp 73-78. Ryan, pp 274-275, 457-459.*) *Streptococcus salivarius, S mutans, A israelii,* and *A viscosis* are all part of the normal microbiota of the human mouth. Both genera are common causes of bacterial endocarditis. *Streptococcus mutans* is highly cariogenic (ie, capable of producing dental caries), in large part because of its unique ability to synthesize a dextran bioadhesive that sticks to teeth. *Streptococcus salivarius* settles onto the mucosal epithelial surfaces of the human mouth soon after birth and is often found in the saliva. Streptococcus pyogenes (group A streptococcus) is responsible for about 95% of human infections caused by streptococci and is the cause of rheumatic fever. Members of the genus *Actinomyces* that are clinically significant and can be differentiated by specific fluorescent antibody microscopy as well as a battery of physiologic tests, such as those assessing requirements for oxygen. *Actinomyces* organisms are opportunistic members of the normal oral microbiota. Both *A Israelii* and *A viscosis* are pathogenic and can cause osteomyelitis in the cervicofacial region. Of the two species, *A israelii*, which is anaerobic, is the more common causative agent of actinomycosis. *A viscosis*, a facultative anaerobe, appears to be cariogenic. Group A streptococci (GAS) are β-hemolytic and produces cellulitis as a typical lesion. Cellulitis is recognized as a diffuse, rapidly spreading lesion in the body tissues.

278 to 284. The answers are 278-b, 279-a, 280-e, 281-d, 282-c, 283-c, 284-a. *(Brooks, pp 213-216, 283-287, 253-255. Levinson, pp 130-131, 138, 153-155, 158-159. Murray-2009, pp 261-265, 303-307, 351-361. Toy, p 122.)* Diphtheria, a disease caused by *C diphtheriae*, usually begins as pharyngitis associated with pseudomembrane formation and lymphadenopathy. Growing organisms lysogenic for a prophage produce a potent exotoxin that is absorbed in mucous membranes and causes remote damage to the liver, kidneys, and heart; the polypeptide toxin inhibits protein synthesis of the host cell. Although *C diphtheriae* may infect the skin, it rarely invades the bloodstream and never actively invades deep tissue. Diphtheria toxin (DT) kills sensitive cells by blocking protein synthesis. DT is converted to an enzyme that inactivates EF-2, which is responsible for the translocation of polypeptidyl-tRNA from the acceptor to the donor site on the eukaryotic ribosome. The reaction is as follows:

$$NAD + EF\text{-}2 = ADP\text{-}ribosyl - EF\text{-}2 + nicotinamide + H+$$

Bordetella pertussis and *B parapertussis* are similar and may be isolated together from a clinical specimen. However, *B parapertussis* does not produce pertussis toxin. Pertussis toxin, like many bacterial toxins, has two subunits: A and B. Subunit A is an active enzyme, and B promotes binding of the toxin to host cells. Pertussis toxin has ADP-ribosylating activity, with an A/B structure and mechanism of action similar to that of cholera toxin (cAMP).

Francisella tularensis is a short, gram-negative organism that is markedly pleomorphic; it is nonmotile and cannot form spores. It has a rigid growth requirement for cysteine. Human tularemia usually is acquired from direct contact with tissues of infected rabbits but also can be transmitted by the bites of flies and ticks. *Francisella tularensis* causes a variety of clinical syndromes, including ulceroglandular, oculoglandular, pneumonic, and typhoidal forms of tularemia.

The pathogenesis of infection with *E coli* is a complex interrelation of many events and properties. *Escherichia coli* may serve as a model for other members of the Enterobacteriaceae. Some strains of *E coli* are EIEC, some ETEC, some EHEC, and others EPEC. At present, there is little clinical significance in routinely discriminating the various types, with the possible exceptions of the ETEC and the *E coli* 0157/H7 that are hemorrhagic. *Escherichia coli* 0157/H7 secretes a toxin called *verotoxin*. The toxin is very active in a Vero cell line. More correctly, the toxin(s) should be called *Shiga-like*.

Streptococcal infection usually is accompanied by an elevated titer of antibody to some of the enzymes produced by the organism. Among the antigenic substances elaborated by group A β-hemolytic streptococci are erythrogenic toxin, streptodornase (streptococcal DNase), hyaluronidase, and streptolysin O (a hemolysin). Streptolysin S is a nonantigenic hemolysin. Specifically, erythrogenic toxin causes the characteristic rash of scarlet fever.

Many factors play a role in the pathogenesis of *N meningitidis*. A capsule containing N-acetylneuraminic acid is peculiar to *Neisseria* and *E coli* K1. Fresh isolates carry pili on their surfaces, which function in adhesion. *Neisseria* has a variety of membrane proteins, and their role in pathogenesis can only be speculated upon at this time. The lipopolysaccharide (LPS) of *Neisseria*, more correctly called lipooligosaccharide (LOS), is the endotoxic component of the cell.

There are no known toxins, hemolysins, or cell-wall constituents known to play a role in the pathogenesis of disease by *Brucella*. Rather, the ability of the organisms to survive within the host phagocyte and to inhibit neutrophil degranulation is a major disease-causing factor. In infectious abortion of cattle caused by *Brucella*, the tropism for placenta and the chorion is a function of the presence of erythritol in allantoic and amniotic fluid.

285 to 288. The answers are 285-a, 286-c, 287-b, 288-c. *(Ryan, pp 851-855. Toy, pp 90, 96.)* "Atypical pneumonia" is an old classification used for respiratory disease that is not lobar and is not "typical." That is, it does not include pneumonia caused by pneumococcus, *Klebsiella*, *Haemophilus*, or β-hemolytic streptococci that results in a typical lobular infiltrate. In recent years, the atypical pneumonias have become much more frequent than pneumococcal pneumonia. They are characterized by a slower onset with headache, joint pain, fever, and signs of an acute upper respiratory infection. There are usually no signs of acute respiratory distress, but patients report malaise and fatigue. The most common cause of atypical pneumonia is *M pneumoniae*. A quick test for *M pneumoniae* infection is cold agglutinins. The test may lack both sensitivity and specificity, but it is rapid and readily available compared with culture of *M pneumoniae* or specific antibody formation.

In certain age groups (men over 55 years old), Legionnaires' disease must be ruled out. While direct microscopy, culture, and serology are available, the detection of *Legionella* antigen in respiratory secretions is the most sensitive test available.

Campylobacter pneumoniae may also cause respiratory infection particularly in, but not limited to, children. Diagnosis is best made by growing these energy-defective bacteria in tissue culture such as HeLa cells. Serology is usually not helpful.

During the winter months, *Bordetella* infection may be quite prevalent, particularly in those patients whose immunizations are not updated. Adult *Bordetella* infection may not present with typical whooping cough symptoms and must be differentiated from other forms of acute bronchitis by culture on specific media or direct fluorescent microscopy.

Direct microscopy of sputum is an important preliminary test for sputum and other exudate specimens. One needs to be aware that the information obtained is limited in interpretation. No specific identity of a microorganism can be determined by gram staining and even mixtures of bacteria can be inferred. On the other hand, examination of gram stains may provide enough information for the physician to make immediate decisions on treatment and other management that may be modified by future laboratory results. Fluorescent Ab detection of an organism in sputum is more specific than gram staining. Here specific known Abs (single or in a mixture) are used to identify organisms present.

Rickettsiae, Chlamydiae, and Mycoplasmas

Questions

289. Mycoplasmas have been cultivated from human mucus membranes and tissues, especially from the genital, urinary, and respiratory tracts. Chlamydia can be isolated from many of these sources as well. Both cause respiratory and genital tract infections. Adults may present with asymptomatic respiratory infection to serious pneumonitis, and identification of the etiologic agent usually determines the best antimicrobial treatment. Which of the following best describes the difference between mycoplasmas and chlamydiae?

a. Able to cause disease in humans
b. Able to cause urinary tract infection
c. Able to grow on artificial cell-free media
d. Being Able to stain well with Gram stain
e. Susceptible to penicillin

290. A 39-year-old man presents with sudden, influenza-like symptoms. He states that he works in a slaughterhouse, and several of his coworkers have similar symptoms. Early stages of pneumonia are detected. Which of the following is the most likely etiologic organism?

a. *Coxiella burnetii*
b. *Rickettsia rickettsiae*
c. *Taenia solium*
d. *Taenia saginata*

291. Many survivors of military or natural disasters are at risk of infection due to loss of public health services. Rickettsial infections—except Q fever and the ehrlichiosis—typically are manifested by fever, rashes, and vasculitis. Which of the following best characterizes rickettsiae, which include the spotted fevers, Q fever, typhus, and scrub typhus?

a. Easily stained (gram-negative) with a Gram stain
b. Maintained in nature, with humans as the mammalian reservoir
c. Obligate intracellular parasites
d. Stable outside the host cell
e. The cause of infections in which a rash is always present

292. A man with chills, fever, and headache is thought to have "atypical" pneumonia. History reveals that he raises chickens, and that approximately 2 weeks ago he lost a large number of them to an undiagnosed disease. Which of the following is the most likely diagnosis of this man's condition?

a. Anthrax
b. Leptospirosis
c. Ornithosis
d. Relapsing fever
e. Q fever

293. An ill patient denies being bitten by insects. However, he spent some time in a milking barn and indicates that it was dusty. Of the following rickettsial diseases, which one has he most likely contracted?

a. Brill-Zinsser disease
b. Q fever
c. Rickettsial pox
d. Rocky Mountain spotted fever (RMSF)
e. Scrub typhus

294. A 23-year-old college senior presents to the student health clinic with symptoms of a suspected sexually transmitted disease (STD). Neisseria and chlamydia agents are ruled out. Which of the following organisms is the most likely cause of his nongonococcal urethritis (NGU)?

a. *Mycoplasma fermentans*
b. *Mycoplasma hominis*
c. *Mycoplasma mycoides*
d. *Mycoplasma pneumoniae*
e. *Ureaplasma urealyticum*

295. A young man, home on leave from the military, went camping in the woods to detect deer movement for future hunting. Ten days later, he developed fever, malaise, and myalgia. Leukopenia and thrombocytopenia were observed, as well as several tick bites. Which of the following statements best describes human monocytic ehrlichiosis (HME)?

a. Clinical diagnosis is based on the presence of erythema migrans (EM).
b. Diagnosis is usually made serologically but morulae may be seen in the cytoplasm of monocytes.
c. It is a fatal disease transmitted by the bite of a dog.
d. Symptoms include vomiting and paralysis.
e. The human monocytic ehrlichiosis agent grows on artificial media.

296. A couple, who did not know each other very well, dated and had sexual contact. Several weeks later, the man noticed a small, painless vesicle on his penis, which ruptured and then healed. Soon, his inguinal lymph nodes enlarged and discharged pus through multiple sinus tracts. Lymphogranuloma venereum (LGV) is a venereal disease caused by serotype L1, L2, or L3 of *Chlamydia trachomatis*. The differential diagnosis should include which of the following?

a. Babesiosis
b. Chancroid
c. Mononucleosis
d. Psittacosis
e. Shingles

297. A forest worker experiences a sudden onset of fever, headache, myalgias, and prostration. A macular rash develops several days later, with it appearing first on the hands and feet before moving onto his trunk. Which of the following treatments is most appropriate?

a. Amphotericin B
b. Cephalosporin
c. Erythromycin
d. Sulfonamides
e. Tetracycline

298. Both *C trachomatis* and *C psittaci* can be isolated in McCoy tissue culture, although *C psittaci* is much more dangerous to work with in the laboratory. The species of *Chlamydia* that infect humans exhibit similar morphologic features, share a common group antigen, and multiply in the cytoplasm of their host cells by a distinctive developmental cycle. Which of the following criteria can be used to distinguish these organisms from each other?

a. *Chlamydia psittaci* forms inclusions that contain glycogen.
b. *Chlamydia psittaci* is an obligate prokaryotic parasite.
c. *Chlamydia trachomatis* can be stained with Giemsa.
d. *Chlamydia trachomatis* has a different lipopolysaccharide antigen.
e. *Chlamydia trachomatis* is sensitive to sulfonamides.

299. Chlamydiae are true bacteria with an unusual three-stage cycle of development. These characteristics are important to understand to be able to distinguish them from other bacteria and viruses that can cause similar disease presentations and choice of treatments. For the growth of *Chlamydia*, which of the following is the correct sequence of these events?

a. Development of an initial body, synthesis of elementary body progeny, penetration of the host cell
b. Penetration of the host cell, development of an initial body, synthesis of elementary body progeny
c. Penetration of the host cell, synthesis of elementary body progeny, development of an initial body
d. Synthesis of elementary body progeny, development of an initial body, penetration of the host cell
e. Synthesis of elementary body progeny, penetration of the host cell, development of an initial body

300. Young children in a small Egyptian village have eye infections that presents with lacrimation, discharge, and conjunctival hyperemia. Scarring of the conjunctiva and noticeable loss of vision occurs in some. Which of the following statements best describes the etiologic agent that caused these infections and relative treatment?

a. The organisms are gram-positive and treatable with penicillin.
b. The organisms have no cell wall and will only respond to tetracycline.
c. The organisms are gram-negative, and prophylactic use of tetracyclines can prevent infections.
d. Gram stains of conjunctival scrapings are useful diagnostic tests to justify treatment with sulfonamides.
e. The organisms are isolated on blood agar plates and respond to cell wall–inhibiting antibiotics.

301. The ehrlichia group organisms are obligate intracellular bacteria that are taxonomically grouped with the rickettsiae and have tick vectors. Human granulocytic ehrlichiosis (HGE) is a disease transmitted to humans by the bite of a tick, *Ixodes scapularis*. Three ehrlichia species are present in different parts of the United States and produce inclusions in circulating WBCs. Which of the following statements about HGE is correct?

a. Clinical diagnosis is based on the presence of erythema migrans.
b. Human granulocytic ehrlichiosis is caused by *Ehrlichia chaffeensis*.
c. Human granulocytic ehrlichiosis is a self-limiting disease.
d. Human granulocytic ehrlichiosis is characterized by an acute onset of fever, severe headache, and influenza-like symptoms.
e. The causative organism can be grown on ordinary laboratory media.

302. The "spotted fever" group of rickettsial diseases is caused by a variety of rickettsial species. While not critical for treatment of disease, the speciation of these organisms is essential for epidemiologic studies. Which of the following rickettsiae is found in the United States and is a member of the spotted fever group?

a. *Rickettsia akari*
b. *Rickettsia australis*
c. *Rickettsia conorii*
d. *Rickettsia prowazekii*
e. *Rickettsia sibirica*

303. A 36-year-old man presents to his primary care physician's office complaining of fever and headache. On examination, he has leucopenia, increased liver enzymes, and inclusion bodies are seen in his monocytes. History reveals that he is outdoorsman and that he remembers removing a tick from his leg. Which of the following is the most likely diagnosis?

a. Ehrlichiosis
b. Lyme disease
c. Q fever
d. Rocky Mountain spotted fever
e. Tularemia

304. Rickettsial organisms infect humans worldwide, although geographic locations may be limited for some species and possibly produce some challenges in medical diagnosis. All are obligate intracellular parasites, except *C burnetii,* and transmitted by an insect vector. Typhus, spotted fever, and scrub typhus share which of the following manifestations of disease?

a. Arthritis
b. Common vector
c. Fever and rash
d. Short incubation period (<48 hours)
e. Similar geographic distribution

305. Humans are the natural hosts for *C trachomatis,* which is widespread in the population and a well-known cause of sexually transmitted disease. The organism is a well-documented cause of nongonococcal urethritis in men and urethritis, cervicitis, and pelvic inflammatory disease in women. This organism is also implicated in which of the following?

a. Blindness
b. Middle ear infection in young children
c. Perinatal retinitis
d. Sexually transmitted cardiac disease in adults
e. Urinary tract infection in children

306. A homosexual male presents to his physician with bilateral inguinal buboes (lymph nodes), one of which seems ready to rupture. He recalls having two small, painless genital lesions that healed rapidly. The etiologic agent is isolated using McCoy cells. Which of the following statements best characterizes Lymphogranuloma venereum?

a. It is most common in temperate regions.
b. In the United States, it is more common among women.
c. The causative agent is *C trachomatis*.
d. Lymphogranuloma venereum does not become chronic.
e. Penicillin is effective in early treatment.

307. Dozens of political refugees fleeing from active warfare and living in a dense forest environment with crowded, unsanitary conditions experienced nonspecific symptoms, followed by high fever, severe headache, chills, myalgia, and arthralgia. All had body lice. Improved living conditions in a refugee camp and treatment with tetracycline brought resolution to most individuals. Which of the following statements describes the etiological agent responsible for their infection?

a. The disease was caused by an organism with no cell walls.
b. The disease was caused by a viral agent.
c. The disease was derived from rodents living in the forest area.
d. Reoccurrence of milder disease may occur in later years.
e. The disease was caused by a tick vector.

308. The three *Chlamydia* species that infect humans are small, gram-negative rods once thought to be viruses. Chlamydiae and viruses are obligate intracellular parasites but which of the following best characterizes chlamydiae from viruses?

a. Cannot visualize with light microscope
b. Independent synthesis of proteins
c. Intracellular reproduction
d. Susceptibility to antimicrobial agents (penicillins)
e. Synthesis of adenosine triphosphate (ATP)

309. Several members of a high school study club develop pharyngitis that progresses to an atypical pneumonia. *Mycoplasma* infection is considered but specimens were submitted to the clinical laboratory to determine the correct agent and antimicrobial therapy. *Chlamydia pneumoniae* (TWAR) is diagnosed and is the most recent *Chlamydia* species to be associated with human disease. Which one of the following statements best describes *C pneumoniae* and human disease today?

a. *Chlamydia pneumoniae* has been associated with atherosclerotic coronary artery disease.
b. *Chlamydia pneumoniae* infections are generally severe.
c. *Chlamydia pneumoniae* infections are uncommon—up to 10% of adults may show specific antibody.
d. Infections with *C pneumoniae* usually arise from bacterial overgrowth in the colon.
e. Nonpsittacine birds are reservoirs of *C pneumoniae*.

310. An 18-year-old student develops symptoms consistent with primary atypical pneumonia (PAP). This is generally a mild disease, ranging from subclinical infection to serious pneumonitis; the latter characterized by onset of fever, headache, sore throat, and cough but requires laboratory tests to determine which organism is involved and a basis for antimicrobial choices. Which of the following organisms causes this disease in humans?

a. *Mycoplasma fermentans*
b. *Mycoplasma hominis*
c. *Mycoplasma pneumoniae*
d. *Mycoplasma orale*
e. *Ureaplasma urealyticum*

311. Nongonococcal urethritis (NGU) is the most common sexually transmitted disease in men. Within 2 weeks, the symptoms usually include painful urination and a urethral discharge. Because of the similarity of NGU symptoms with *Neisseria gonococcus* infection, diagnosis depends on culture of the discharge. While the majority of NGU are caused by *C trachomatis,* which of the following organisms is very significant in causing additional cases in humans?

a. *Mycoplasma fermentans*
b. *Mycoplasma hominis*
c. *Mycoplasma pneumoniae*
d. *Mycoplasma orale*
e. *Ureaplasma urealyticum*

312. A healthy oral cavity has a microbial population consisting of gram-positive streptococci and diphtheroids. Anaerobic rods and spirochetes are present in low numbers and may be opportunistic for disease. Which of the following organisms also normally inhabits the healthy human oral cavity?

a. *Mycoplasma fermentans*
b. *Mycoplasma hominis*
c. *Mycoplasma pneumoniae*
d. *Mycoplasma orale*
e. *Ureaplasma urealyticum*

313. At least 15 species of *Mycoplasma* are of human origin, and five are of primary importance. Which of the following organisms normally inhabits the female genital tract and is strongly associated with salpingitis and ovarian abscesses?

a. *Mycoplasma fermentans*
b. *Mycoplasma hominis*
c. *Mycoplasma pneumoniae*
d. *Mycoplasma orale*
e. *Ureaplasma urealyticum*

314. Suppurative inguinal adenitis usually starts by the appearance of small, painless lesions on the external genitalia that heal spontaneously. Then regional lymph nodes enlarge and become painful and often discharge pus through multiple sinus tracts. Which organism listed below is responsible for this sexually transmitted disease?

a. *Bartonella (Rochalimaea) henselae*
b. *Chlamydia trachomatis*
c. *Coxiella burnetii*
d. *Ehrlichia chaffeensis*
e. *Rickettsia rickettsii*

315. Which of the following is transmitted by the bite of a hard *Ixodes* tick, where circulating leukocytes are infected and morulae (clusters of microorganisms) form, which can be treated with tetracyclines and rifamycins?

a. *Bartonella (Rochalimaea) henselae*
b. *Chlamydia trachomatis*
c. *Coxiella burnetii*
d. *Ehrlichia chaffeensis*
e. *Rickettsia rickettsii*

316. Cat scratch disease is usually a benign, self-limited illness manifested by fever and lymphadenopathy that develops about 2 weeks after contact with a cat. Which of the following microorganisms is the causative agent of this infection?

a. *Bartonella (Rochalimaea) henselae*
b. *Chlamydia trachomatis*
c. *Coxiella burnetii*
d. *Ehrlichia chaffeensis*
e. *Rickettsia rickettsii*

317. Six laboratory technicians at the state health laboratory were working on a study using rabbits. The experiments involved an outbreak of acute febrile illnesses in workers from a slaughterhouse. The organism of interest was a gram-negative bacteria with tropism for mononuclear cells. A dysfunction of the animal cage air safety system allowed contaminated air to escape into the animal care facility and research laboratories. Four of the six technicians now suffer from a flu-like illness and pneumonitis. Which organism listed below is most likely the cause of this outbreak?

a. *Bartonella (Rochalimaea) henselae*
b. *Chlamydia trachomatis*
c. *Coxiella burnetii*
d. *Ehrlichia chaffeensis*
e. *Rickettsia rickettsii*

318. The patient shown below in the photo presented with petechial and hemorrhagic lesions. He had experienced a fever and demonstrated evidence of a tick bite. Which of the following is the etiologic agent of a disease found in the western hemisphere and may exhibit a wide range of systemic manifestations?

(Photo contributor: Daniel Noltkamper, MD. Reproduced, with permission, from Knoop KJ, Stack LB, Storrow AB, et al. The Atlas of Emergency Medicine. 3rd ed. New York: McGraw-Hill; 2009:372.)

a. *Bartonella (Rochalimaea) henselae*
b. *Chlamydia trachomatis*
c. *Coxiella burnetii*
d. *Ehrlichia chaffeensis*
e. *Rickettsia rickettsii*

Rickettsiae, Chlamydiae, and Mycoplasmas

Answers

289. The answer is c. *(Brooks, pp 344-345. Levinson, pp 171-172. Murray, pp 421-426. Ryan, pp 409, 463. Toy, p 116.)* Unlike chlamydiae, mycoplasmas can replicate in cell-free media. They lack a rigid cell wall and are bound by a triple-layer unit membrane. For this reason, they are completely resistant to the action of penicillins.

290. The answer is a. *(Brooks, pp 353-354. Levinson, pp 182-184. Murray, pp 438-439. Ryan, p 477.)* Q fever is an acute, flu-like illness caused by *C burnetii*. It is one rickettsial disease not transmitted by the bite of a tick. *Chlamydia burnetii* is found in high concentrations in the urine, feces, and placental tissue/amniotic fluid of cattle, goats, and sheep. Transmission to humans is by aerosol inhalation of those specimens. *Rickettsia* is present in the United States and South America, but is transmitted by ticks that feed on rodents or dogs. The parasitic *Taenia* species are transmitted by ingestion of undercooked meat.

291. The answer is c. *(Brooks, pp 350-354. Levinson, pp 182-184. Murray, pp 427-436. Ryan, pp 472-473.)* Rickettsiae are obligate intracellular parasites that depend on host cells for their phosphorylated energy compounds. The significant rickettsial diseases in North America include RMSF (*R rickettsii*), Q fever (*C burnetii*), and typhus (*R prowazekii, R typhi*). Laboratory diagnosis of rickettsial disease is based on serologic analysis rather than isolation of the organism.

292. The answer is c. *(Brooks, pp 364-365. Levinson, pp 179-181. Murray, pp 441-450. Ryan, p 469.)* Ornithosis (psittacosis) is caused by *C psittaci*. Humans usually contract the disease from infected birds kept as pets or from infected poultry, including poultry in dressing plants. Although ornithosis may be asymptomatic in humans, severe pneumonia can develop. Fortunately, the disease is cured easily with tetracycline. *Bacillus anthracis* is a spore-forming, gram-positive bacillus that has a protective capsule made of glutamic acid (amino acid) residues. Humans are infected accidentally by contact with infected animals or their products. Skin lesions, seen most often, is known as woolsorter's disease. *Leptospira* organisms are tightly coiled spirochetes. Human contact is often in water, where the organism enters breaks in the skin. They produce hemorrhage and necrosis in the liver and kidneys and often present as aseptic meningitis. Relapsing fever is caused by *Borrelia recurrentis* and is transmitted by the body louse or *Ornithodoros* ticks. An unusual feature of this disease is the selection of new antigenic forms of the organism after host antibody formation. Q fever is caused by a rickettsial organism, *C burnetii*.

293. The answer is b. (*Brooks, pp 350-354. Levinson, pp 182-184. Murray, pp 427-436. Ryan, p 477.*) Most rickettsial diseases are transmitted to humans by way of arthropod vectors. The only exception is Q fever, which is caused by *C burnetii*. This organism is transmitted by inhalation of contaminated dust and aerosols or by ingestion of contaminated milk. Brill-Zinsser disease is a recurrence of epidemic typhus (louse borne). Rickettsial pox is transmitted by a mite from the mouse reservoir. RMSF is caused by *R rickettsii* and is transmitted by ticks from the rodent or dog reservoirs. Scrub typhus is an Asian/Pacific area disease with a mite transferring the organism from a rodent reservoir.

294. The answer is e. (*Brooks, p 347. Levinson, pp 171-172. Murray, pp 421-426. Ryan, p 413.*) *Ureaplasma urealyticum* has been associated with NGU as well as infertility. *Mycoplasma pneumoniae* is the etiologic agent of PAP. *Mycoplasma hominis*, although isolated from up to 30% of patients with NGU, has yet to be implicated as a cause of that disease. *Mycoplasma fermentans* has on rare occasions been isolated from the oropharynx and genital tract. *Mycoplasma mycoides* causes bovine pleuropneumonia.

295. The answer is b. (*Brooks, p 355. Levinson, pp 182-184. Murray, pp 435-437. Ryan, p 478.*) HME, caused by the bite of the tick *Amblyomma americanum* infected with *E chaffeensis*, causes an illness not unlike RMSF, except a rash usually does not occur. Diagnosis is usually made serologically, and treatment of choice is tetracycline. Symptoms include high fever, severe headache, and myalgias. Erythema migrans is the characteristic skin lesion seen in Lyme disease. HME is transmitted by a tick vector, as mentioned previously, and not by a dog bite. Vomiting and paralysis are not usual symptoms seen in HME cases. Cultures can be isolated using tissue culture cell lines, but not artificial media (agar, broth, etc).

296. The answer is b. *(Brooks, p 362. Levinson, pp 179-181. Murray, pp 441-450. Ryan, pp 466-467.)* The differential diagnosis of LGV includes syphilis, genital herpes, and chancroid. Several clinical tests can be used to rule out syphilis and genital herpes. These include a negative (negative to rule out; positive to rule in) dark-field examination as well as positive serologic findings for syphilis and the demonstration of herpes simplex virus by cytology or culture. *Haemophilus ducreyi* can usually be isolated from the ulcer in chancroid. Babesiosis is an RBC-infecting tick-borne disease, usually derived from dogs or Texas cattle. Most cases are asymptomatic, but clindamycin or azithromycin are effective treatments. Mononucleosis is seen most often in infectious mononucleosis caused by EBV. Psittacosis is caused by inhaling aerosols or direct contact with birds infected with *C psittaci* and is usually a mild upper respiratory illness. Shingles would be evidenced by masses of painful herpetic lesions caused by reactivation of VZV (chicken pox).

297. The answer is e. *(Brooks, pp 350-354. Levinson, pp 182-184. Murray, pp 427-436. Ryan, p 475.)* Tetracyclines and chloramphenicol are effective, provided treatment is started early for rickettsial diseases, including RMSF, as in this case. Those should be given orally daily and continued for several days after the rash subsides. Intravenous dosage can be used in severely ill patients. Sulfonamides enhance the disease and are contraindicated. The other antibiotics are ineffective. Antibiotics only suppress the bacteria's growth, and the patient's immune system must eradicate them.

298. The answer is e. *(Brooks, pp 359-364. Levinson, pp 179-181. Murray, pp 441-450. Ryan, p 463.)* The chlamydiae are obligate prokaryotic parasites of eukaryotic cells. For many years, they were considered to be viruses but are now considered to be bacteria. The two species, *C trachomatis* and *C psittaci,* can be distinguished by two criteria: the susceptibility of *C trachomatis* to sulfonamides and its ability to form inclusions containing glycogen. Chlamydiae are obligate intracellular bacteria and are seen using Giemsa staining. Differences in LPS antigens have not been reported to be useful in distinguishing one species from another.

299. The answer is b. *(Brooks, p 359. Levinson, pp 179-181. Murray, pp 441-450, Ryan, p 465. Toy, p 52.)* The developmental cycle of *Chlamydia* begins with the elementary body attaching to and then penetrating the host cell. The elementary body, now in a vacuole bounded by host-cell membrane, becomes an initial body. Within about 12 hours, the initial body has divided to form many small elementary particles encased within an inclusion body in the cytoplasm; these progeny are liberated by host-cell rupture.

300. The answer is c. *(Brooks, pp 360-361. Levinson, pp 179-181. Murray, pp 441-450. Ryan, pp 464-466.)* *Chlamydia trachomatis* serovars A, B, Ba, and C are responsible for endemic trachoma. While diagnosis is usually dependent upon observation of intracellular inclusions with a glycogen matrix in which elementary bodies are embedded, Gram stain preparations are not useful diagnostic tools. The cell wall most closely resembles a high lipid content and may stain gram-negative or variable. A single monthly dose of doxycycline can result in significant clinical improvement and be preventative. Cell wall inhibitors (penicillins, cephalosporins) result in cell-wall defective forms but are not effective in clinical diseases treatment. Inhibitors of protein synthesis (tetracyclines, erythromycin) are effective in most clinical infections.

301. The answer is d. *(Brooks, p 355. Levinson, pp 182-184. Murray, pp 435-437. Ryan, p 478.)* HGE is caused by the bite of *I scapularis* infected with either *E phagocytophila* or *E ewingii* or *Ehrlichia equi*. A rash rarely occurs and EM does not occur, but the symptoms (fever, chills, headache, myalgia, nausea, vomiting, anorexia, and weight loss) are similar to those seen in RMSF. Serological tests show that subclinical ehrlichiosis occurs frequently. Ehrlichia chaffeensis causes human monocyte ehrlichiosis and may cause severe or fatal illness. Seroprevalence studies suggest that subclinical ehrlichiosis occurs frequently. The organisms can be isolated using cell culture procedures.

302. The answer is a. *(Brooks, pp 350-354. Levinson, pp 182-184. Murray, pp 427-436. Ryan, p 473.)* The primary cause of RMSF is *R rickettsii*, although rickettsial pox is caused by *R akari*, the only other member of the spotted fever group that resides in the United States. *Rickettsia sibirica* is responsible for tick typhus in China; *R australis* causes typhus in Australia, as the name signifies; and *R conorii* causes European and African rickettsioses.

Rickettsia prowazekii is not a member of the spotted fever group; it causes epidemic typhus.

303. The answer is a. *(Brooks, p 355. Levinson, pp 182-184. Murray, pp 435-437. Ryan, p 478.)* All the listed diseases except Q fever are tick-borne. Two human forms of ehrlichiosis can occur: HME, caused by *E chaffeensis*, and HGE, caused by *E ewingii*. Ehrlichiosis was previously recognized only as a veterinary pathogen. HME infection is transmitted by the brown dog tick and *A americanum*. HGE infection is transmitted by *I scapularis*, the same tick that transmits Lyme disease. Both infections cause fever and leukopenia. A rash rarely occurs. *Ehrlichia chaffeensis* infects monocytes, and HGE infects granulocytes; both organisms produce inclusion bodies called *morulae*. *Francisella tularensis* is a small, gram-negative, nonmotile coccobacillus. Humans most commonly acquire the organism after contact with the tissues or body fluid of an infected mammal or the bite of an infected tick. The Rickettsia *C burnetii* causes Q fever, and humans are usually infected by aerosol of a sporelike form shed in milk, urine, feces, or placenta of infected sheep, cattle, or goats. Lyme disease is caused by a spirochete, *B burgdorferi*, and produces the characteristic lesion erythema chronicum migrans (ECM). The etiologic agent of RMSF is *R rickettsii*. It usually produces a rash that begins in the extremities and then involves the trunk.

304. The answer is c. *(Brooks, pp 350-354. Levinson, pp 182-184. Murray, pp 427-436. Ryan, pp 473-475.)* Typhus, spotted fever, and scrub typhus are all caused by rickettsiae (*R prowazekii*, *R rickettsii*, and *R tsutsugamushi*, respectively). Clinically, the diseases have several similarities. Each has an incubation period of 1 to 2 weeks, followed by a febrile period, which usually includes a rash. During the febrile period, rickettsiae can be found in the patient's blood, and there is disseminated focal vasculitis of small blood vessels. The geographic area associated with these diseases is usually different. Scrub typhus is usually found in Japan, Southeast Asia, and the Pacific, while spotted fever is usually found in the Western hemisphere. Typhus has a worldwide incidence. (Typhus is caused by lice and fleas, spotted fever is caused by ticks and mites, and scrub are caused by mites.)

305. The answer is a. *(Brooks, p 360. Levinson, pp 179-181. Murray, pp 441-450. Ryan, p 464. Toy, p 52.)* Trachoma has been the greatest single cause of blindness in the world. *Chlamydia trachomatis* is the most common cause of STD in the United States and is also responsible for the majority of cases of infant conjunctivitis and infant pneumonia. Middle ear infection in children is most often caused by bacteria normally found in the oral cavity or upper respiratory system. Gram-positive cocci, *Pseudomonas* species, and a host of other normal flora can be involved. Trachoma involves the keratoconjunctiva area of the eye, not the retina. Sexually transmitted cardiac in adults and children's urinary tract infections are not reported to be caused by *C trachomatis*.

306. The answer is c. *(Brooks, p 362. Levinson, p 179. Murray, pp 441-450. Ryan, pp 466-468.)* LGV is an STD caused by *C trachomatis* of immunotypes L1, L2, and L3. It is more commonly found in tropical climates. In the United States, the sex ratio is reported to be 3.4 males to 1 female. Tetracycline has been successful in treating this disease in the early stages; however, late stages usually require surgery. Unless effective antimicrobial drug treatment is given promptly, chronic inflammatory processes can lead to fibrosis, lymphatic obstruction, and rectal strictures.

307. The answer is d. *(Brooks, pp 350-354. Levinson, pp 182-184. Murray, pp 427-436. Ryan, pp 475-476.)* The disease described is epidemic typhus or louse-borne typhus. It is caused by *R prowazekii* and is spread by the human body louse, *Pediculus humanus*. Lice obviously occur most readily in unsanitary conditions brought on by war or natural disasters, where normal healthy living conditions are unavailable. Rickettsial diseases respond to tetracycline treatment and vector control. The organisms replicate in endothelial cells, resulting in vasculitis. Recrudescent disease (recurrence in later years) has been demonstrated in people exposed to epidemic typhus during World War II. This form of disease is generally milder, and convalescence is shorter. Rickettsiae are pleomorphic coccobacilli with cell walls that do not stain well in Gram stain procedures. No viruses were involved in this problem because tetracycline was able to kill the infecting organisms. Humans are the main reservoir of the causative agent.

308. The answer is b. *(Brooks, p 359. Levinson, pp 179-181. Murray, pp 441-450. Ryan, pp 463-464.)* Although both chlamydiae and viruses are obligate, intracellular parasites and depend on the host cell for ATP and phosphorylated intermediates, they differ in many respects. Unlike viruses, chlamydiae synthesize proteins and reproduce by fission. Chlamydiae are readily seen under the light microscope and possess bacteria-like cell walls.

309. The answer is a. *(Brooks, p 363. Levinson, pp 179-181. Murray, pp 441-450. Ryan, p 470.)* A distinct group of chlamydia, first designated "TWAR," has been given the name *Chlamydia pneumoniae*. The strain was first isolated in Taiwan and usually causes mild acute respiratory disease. *Chlamydia psittaci* causes a respiratory syndrome and is associated with avian contact. *Chlamydia pneumoniae* has no avian vector. Recent evidence suggests that *C pneumoniae* may be involved in cardiac disease, possibly as part of an autoimmune phenomenon. This organism has recently had a genus name change to *Chlamydophila*. Most infections with *C pneumoniae* are asymptomatic or associated with mild illness. Five to 20% of community-acquired pneumonia in young persons is thought to be caused by *C pneumoniae*. *Chlamydia pneumoniae* may cause upper and lower airway disease, but is not associated with colon infections. Humans are the only hosts.

310 to 313. The answers are 310-c, 311-e, 312-d, 313-b. *(Brooks, pp 344-347. Levinson, pp 171-172. Murray, pp 421-426. Ryan, pp 409-412. Toy, p 116.)* Members of the mycoplasma group that are pathogenic for humans include *M pneumoniae* and *U urealyticum*. *Mycoplasma pneumoniae* is best known as the causative agent of PAP, which may be confused clinically with influenza or legionellosis. It also is associated with arthritis, pericarditis, aseptic meningitis, and the Guillain-Barré syndrome. *Mycoplasma pneumoniae* can be cultivated on special media and identified by immunofluorescence staining and "fried egg" colonies on agar.

Ureaplasma urealyticum (once called *tiny*, or *T strain*) has been implicated in cases of NGU. As the name implies, this organism is able to split urea, a fact of diagnostic significance. *Ureaplasma urealyticum* is part of the normal flora of the genitourinary tract, particularly in women.

Both *M orale* and *M salivarium* are inhabitants of the normal human oral cavity. These species are commensals and do not play a role in disease.

The only other species of *Mycoplasma* associated with human disease is *M hominis*. A normal inhabitant of the genital tract of women, this organism has been demonstrated to produce an acute respiratory illness that is associated with sore throat and tonsillar exudate, but not with fever. *Mycoplasma hominis* can cause disease outside the urinary tract in immunosuppressed patients or immunocompetent patients after trauma of the genitourinary tract. Other opportunistic infections known to be caused by *M hominis* includes wound infections, osteomyelitis, brain abscess, pneumonia, and peritonitis. It has been associated with neonatal pneumonia and sepsis. *Mycoplasma fermentans* is an animal isolate.

314. The answer is b. *(Brooks, pp 360-361. Levinson, pp 179-181. Murray, pp 441-450. Ryan, pp 463-470, 471-479. Toy, p 52.)* Chlamydiae are gram-negative bacteria that are obligate, intracellular parasites. They are divided into three species: *C trachomatis, C pneumoniae,* and *C psittaci.* Chlamydiae have a unique developmental cycle. The infectious particle is the elementary body. Once inside the cell, the elementary body undergoes reorganization to form a reticulate body. After several replications, the reticulate bodies differentiate into elementary bodies, are released from the host cell, and become available to infect other cells. Three of the 15 serovars of *C trachomatis* (L1, L2, and L3) are known to cause LGV, an STD. *Chlamydia trachomatis* is a leading cause of STD in the United States. It is insidious because so many early infections are asymptomatic, particularly in women. The painless papule or vesicle develops on any part of the external genitalia, anus, rectum, or elsewhere. This lesion may ulcerate and heal without notice. Lymph nodes enlarge and discharge pus through sinuses. Unless effective antibiotics (tetracycline, erythromycin) are given promptly, a chronic inflammatory process may lead to fibrosis and lymphatic obstruction.

315. The answer is d. *(Brooks, p 355. Levinson, pp 182-184. Murray, pp 435-437. Ryan, pp 463-470, 471-479.)* Ehrlichia is an obligate, intracellular parasite that resembles *Rickettsia. Ehrlichia chaffeensis* has been linked to human ehrlichiosis, although this infection is primarily seen in animals. The majority of patients with this disease report exposure to ticks. It is thought that *I scapularis* carries *Ehrlichia,* although the Lone Star tick, *A americanum,* may also transmit the disease. These gram-negative bacteria infect circulating leukocytes where they multiply within phagocytic vacuoles, forming clusters with inclusion-like appearance. These clusters of ehrlichiae are called morulae (mulberry-like). Diagnosis is confirmed by observing these morulae in white blood cells.

316. The answer is a. *(Brooks, pp 315-317. Levinson, pp 186-187. Murray, pp 371-373. Ryan, pp 463-470, 471-479.)* Bartonella henselae is a fastidious, gram-negative rod that causes bacillary angiomatosis, a disease that forms dermal or subcutaneous nodules. The role of *B henselae* in cat scratch disease has recently been recognized. Molecular taxonomic studies have indicated that the causative organism is more closely related to *Bartonella* than to *Rochalimaea,* hence the change in name. Cat scratch disease is usually a benign, self-limited illness with fever and lymphadenopathy that develops about 2 weeks after contact with a cat (bite or scratch). Lymph nodes may discharge pus. Treatment is mostly supportive, although tetracycline or erythromycin may be helpful.

317. The answer is c. *(Brooks, pp 350-351. Levinson, pp 182-184. Murray, pp 438-439. Ryan, pp 463-470, 471-479.)* *Coxiella* is transmitted through the respiratory tract rather than through the skin, and *B henselae* from animal scratches. *Coxiella* may cause chronic endocarditis that is not very responsive to either antimicrobial therapy or valve replacement. About 50% of Q-fever cases in humans are asymptomatic. Symptomatic cases usually present with an acute febrile illness (flu-like disease, fever, pneumonitis, possibly hepatitis). Diagnosis depends on a history with contact with newborn or infected adult animals (sheep, cattle, cats, rabbits, dogs). About 2% to 10% of Q-fever patients progress to a chronic infection with endocarditis, which occurs in about 60% to 70% of those cases. No vaccine exists and doxycycline is effective when symptoms appear.

318. The answer is e. *(Brooks, pp 350-354. Levinson, pp 182-184. Murray, pp 427-436. Ryan, pp 463-470, 471-479.)* Rickettsiae are small bacteria that are obligate, intracellular parasites. Most but not all rickettsiae are transmitted to humans by arthropods. RMSF is a spotted fever caused by *R rickettsii* and is characterized by acute onset of fever, severe headache, and myalgias. The rash occurs 2 to 6 days later, first in the hands and feet, and then moves to the trunk. Diagnosis must be made on clinical presentations, and therapy instituted immediately. Laboratory diagnosis is made on a rising antibody titer (delayed). Untreated disease can be fatal.

Mycology

Questions

319. A leukemic patient complains of respiratory symptoms including frequent coughs. An examination of the left lung reveals the presence of a coin-sized lesion characterized by the presence of an air space surrounding the cavity. The patient's sputum shows the presence of a thick, uniformly septate hyphae. The culture yields hairy colonies firmly adhering to the medium's surface. The patient is tuberculin test negative. Which of the following is the most likely cause of the respiratory problem in this patient?

a. Aspergillosis
b. Candidiasis
c. Histoplasmosis
d. Mucormycosis
e. Tuberculosis

320. A 62-year-old white male is admitted to the hospital complaining of shortness of breath. His medical history indicates he has smoked one pack of cigarettes per day for the past 40 years. Recently, he has been on immunosuppressive therapy for severe arthritis. A biopsy specimen of the lung is obtained, and septate hyphae that form V-shaped branches are observed. Culture on agar shows conidia with spores in radiating columns (see the figure). Which of the following is consistent with these diagnostic findings?

x1000

(Reproduced, with permission, from Brooks GF et al. Jawetz's Medical Microbiology. 22nd ed. New York: McGraw-Hill;2001: 534.)

a. Aspergillosis
b. Emphysema
c. Lung cancer
d. *Pneumocystis jiroveci* pneumonia
e. Viral pneumonia
f. Zygomycosis

321. An AIDS patient complains of headache and neck stiffness and appears disoriented. Brain tumor and abscess are ruled out, and chronic meningitis is diagnosed. Pathological studies discover the object designated by the arrow in the following photomicrograph. This object designated by the arrow is which of the following?

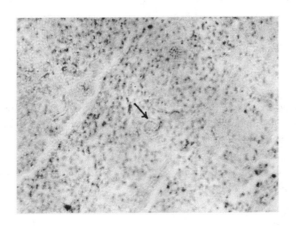

a. An encapsulated yeast
b. A hyphal strand
c. A macroconidium
d. A spherule
e. A thick-walled spore

322. A 6-year-old girl presents to the clinic with scaly patches on the scalp. Primary smears and culture of the skin and hair are negative. A few weeks later, she returns and is found to have inflammatory lesions. The hair fluoresces under Wood light, and primary smears of skin and hair contain septate hyphae. On speaking with the parents, it is discovered that there are several pets in the household. Which of the following is the most likely infecting agent?

a. *Epidermophyton floccosum*
b. *Microsporum audouinii*
c. *Microsporum canis*
d. *Trichophyton rubrum*
e. *Trichophyton tonsurans*

323. A patient with AIDS has a persistent cough and has shown progressive behavioral changes in the past few weeks after eating an under-cooked hamburger. A cerebrospinal fluid (CSF) sample is collected and an encapsulated, yeastlike organism is observed. Based only on these observations, which of the following is the most likely organism?

a. *Candida*
b. *Cryptococcus*
c. *Cryptosporidium*
d. *Pneumocystis*
e. *Toxoplasma*

324. A chronically ill, young, white male is unable to work due to his frequent illnesses. He spends most of his time raising and training pigeons. He develops a mild pulmonary infection and eventually presents to his primary care physician with headache, mental status changes, and fever. A clinical diagnosis of meningitis is confirmed with a latex agglutination test on CSF for the capsular polysaccharide of the organism. Which of the following is the most likely causative agent?

a. *Aspergillus fumigatus*
b. *Candida albicans*
c. *Cryptococcus neoformans*
d. *Histoplasma capsulatum*
e. *Paracoccidioides brasiliensis*

325. A section of tissue from the foot of a person assumed to have eumycotic mycetoma shows a white, lobulated granule composed of fungal hyphae. In the United States, the most common etiologic agent of this condition is a species of which of the following?

a. *Acremonium*
b. *Actinomyces*
c. *Madurella*
d. *Nocardia*
e. *Pseudallescheria*

326. A healthy middle-aged construction worker who engaged in a demolition task 10 days earlier complains of respiratory symptoms similar to those of pneumonia. No causative agent has been isolated from his sputa. The patient does not respond to any antibacterial antibiotics and dies before a definitive diagnosis is established. Microscopic examination of specimens taken of granulomatous and suppurative lesions of the lung obtained during necropsy reveal the presence of large budding yeast cells. The bud is attached to the parent cell by a broad base. Based on this information, which of the following is the most likely diagnosis?

a. Blastomycosis
b. Coccidioidomycosis
c. Cryptococcosis
d. Histoplasmosis
e. Sporotrichosis

327. A 40-year-old woman working in her rose garden trips and falls into a mature rose bush. Her right arm and hand receive deep punctures from several large thorns. Several days later, raised, erythematosus lesions develop at several of the puncture sites. Lines of secondary lesions spread from the initial wound sites. Based on this information, which of the following is the most likely cause of these lesions?

a. *Blastomyces* species
b. *Coccidioides* species
c. *Cryptococcus* species
d. *Histoplasma* species
e. *Sporothrix* species

328. Several young men from the local high school's football team complain of a sudden onset of athlete's foot (tinea pedia). They all experience itching between the toes, vesicle rupture with a thin fluid release, and peeling skin. There are three genera of dermatophytes. Which of the following characterizes the infections caused by these organisms?

(Courtesy of MG Rinaldi, San Antonio, TX)

a. Characterized by aflatoxin-induced hallucinations
b. Confined to keratinized tissues
c. Easily treatable with penicillin
d. Marked by alveolar irritation
e. Rarely associated with chronic lesions

329. A 57-year-old obese, white female is referred to your clinic due to a sore throat characterized by a white pseudomembranous lesion of epithelial cells and organisms. The patient's history reveals type 1 diabetes mellitus and recent penicillin use for a severe bacterial infection in her right foot. Which of the following will most likely be present on microscopic examination?

a. Abundance of septate rhizoids
b. Asci containing 2 to 8 ascospores
c. Metachromatic granules
d. Spherules containing endospores
e. Yeasts and pseudohyphae

330. Superficial (cutaneous or mucosal) candidiasis is established by an increase in local numbers of *Candida* and damage to the skin or epithelium that permits local invasion. Systemic infection occurs when *Candida* enters the blood stream and the host's immune system is inadequate. The mechanism of mucosal invasion by *C albicans* is at least partially understood. Which of the following modifications in the structure or function of this yeast is most likely to affect its invasive ability?

a. Loss of ability to produce ethanol from glucose
b. Loss of ability to produce germ tubes or hyphae
c. Loss of ability to produce a polysaccharide capsule
d. Reduced ability to grow at 37°C
e. Replacement of mannans in the cell wall with glucan

331. You have been designated as coordinator of construction of a bone marrow transplant unit (BMTU). There will be extensive removal of walls and floors in order to install the laminar flow rooms required for a BMTU. From the standpoint of frequency and lethality, which of the following fungi should be your biggest concern?

a. *Aspergillus* species
b. *Blastomyces* species
c. *Candida* species
d. *Cryptococcus* species
e. *Wangiella* species

332. A middle-aged man, employed for several years in a commercial farm that supplies eggs and chickens to industry develops a flu-like syndrome with fever, chills, myalgias, headaches, and a nonproductive cough. *Histoplasma capsulatum* is isolated and identified. Which of the following best describes the presence of the organism in tissue biopsies?

a. Arthrospores
b. Oval budding yeasts inside macrophages
c. Single-cell yeasts with pseudohyphae
d. Spherules containing endospores
e. Yeasts with broad-based bud

333. A 65-year-old female patient is admitted to an intensive care unit because of sudden swelling on the right side of the face and an episode of bleeding from the right nostril. According to her daughter, these signs were not apparent a few days ago. She has a long history of diabetes, high blood pressure, and recently developed clinical signs of ketoacidosis and renal insufficiency. Her blood sugar level at the time of admission is 700 mg/dL. The facial lesion becomes partially necrotic and shows slight protrusion of the right eye and facial paralysis. The patient dies on the second day. Histopathologic examination of the lesions reveals occlusion of the small vessels and the presence of nonseptate hyphae. This is most likely caused by which of the following?

a. Candadiasis
b. Erysipelis
c. Gas gangrene
d. Mucormycosis
e. Nocardiosis

334. A healthy young man in Arizona develops fever, malaise, cough, and headache. Radiographs show a pulmonary infiltrate, and the patient also has a skin rash. Inhalation of fungal spores can cause primary lung infections. Which of the following organisms is associated with this mode of transmission?

a. *Candida albicans*
b. *Candida tropicalis*
c. *Coccidioides immitis*
d. *Sporothrix schenckii*
e. *Toxoplasma tonsurans*

335. An immunocompromised patient is suspected of having an infection with *A fumigatus*. Which of the following clinical conditions is most likely to occur?

a. Invasive infection causing thrombosis and infarction
b. Superficial rash
c. Thrush
d. Urinary tract infection
e. Wound infection

336. A 25-year-old pregnant woman, living in the San Joaquin Valley (California), experiences an influenza-like illness with fever and cough. She is diagnosed with *Coccidioides* infection that disseminated from her lungs to other organs while in the third trimester of pregnancy. Patients who have disseminated coccidioidomycosis usually demonstrate which of the following?

a. Absence of complement-fixing (CF) antibodies
b. A negative coccidioidin skin test and a rising CF titer
c. A negative coccidioidin skin test and a stable CF titer
d. A positive skin test and a mildly elevated CF titer
e. Lack of immunity to reinfection

337. A young adult being treated for AIDS develops thrush. His tongue, lips, and gums are affected, and *C albicans* (see figure) is isolated and identified. Which of the following best describes this organism?

(Reproduced, with permission, from Brooks GF et al. Jawetz's Medical Microbiology. 23rd ed. New York: McGraw-Hill;2004: 646.)

a. Round, black sporangia filled with endospores; sporangia unbranched, rising from a runner called a stolon
b. Single-tipped sporangiophores; no rhizoids or stolons; nonseptate hyphae, which show branching
c. Widespread in environment; conidia may be inhaled; microscopic appearance in specimen reveals dichotomous branching and septate hyphae
d. Yeast forms with budding blastoconidia often showing pseudohyphae; positive germ tube test; chlamydospores present

338. A patient with lymphocytic leukemia is handling the care and treatment of her disease until she develops an acute pneumonic infection. *Aspergillus* organisms are isolated and identified. *Aspergillus* is best described by which of the following?

a. Round, black sporangia filled with endospores; sporangia unbranched, rising from a runner called a stolon
b. Single-tipped sporangiophores; no rhizoids or stolons; nonseptate hyphae, which show branching
c. Widespread in environment; conidia may be inhaled; microscopic appearance in specimen reveals dichotomous branching and septate hyphae
d. Yeast forms with budding blastoconidia often showing pseudohyphae; positive germ tube test; chlamydospores present

339. A diabetic patient develops acidosis and inhales conidia. He develops a mild pulmonary infection, but the organism also causes a rhinocerebral complication. Mucormycosis is an opportunistic mycosis in which the major clinical form is rhinocerebral infection, where sporangiospores germinate in the nasal passages and hyphae invade into the blood vessels. The genus *Mucor* is best described by which of the following?

a. Round, black sporangia filled with endospores; sporangia unbranched, rising from a runner called a stolon
b. Single-tipped sporangiophores; no rhizoids or stolons; nonseptate hyphae, which show branching
c. Widespread in environment; conidia may be inhaled; microscopic appearance in specimen reveals dichotomous branching and septate hyphae
d. Yeast forms with budding blastoconidia often showing pseudohyphae; positive germ tube test; chlamydospores present

340. Zygomycetes (including *Rhizopus* species) have been reported as pathogens in transplant patients, while the acidotic state associated with diabetic ketoacidosis is a risk factor for zygomycosis. Such opportunistic Zygomycetes can be associated with rhinocerebral, pulmonary, GI, cutaneous, and disseminated infections. *Rhizopus* is best described by which of the following?

a. Round, black sporangia filled with endospores; sporangia unbranched, rising from a runner called a stolon
b. Single-tipped sporangiophores; no rhizoids or stolons; nonseptate hyphae, which show branching
c. Widespread in environment; conidia may be inhaled; microscopic appearance in specimen reveals dichotomous branching and septate hyphae
d. Yeast forms with budding blastoconidia often showing pseudohyphae; positive germ tube test; chlamydospores present

341. A 37-year-old Asian male is admitted to the hospital complaining of shortness of breath. He denies use of cigarettes, although he admits a previous history of intravenous drug abuse. His chest films show a diffuse ground-glass pattern. A specimen is obtained by bronchoalveolar lavage, and distinctive thin-walled trophozoites and thick-walled spherical cysts containing 4 to 8 nuclei are observed using methenamine-silver stain. Which of the following is the most likely diagnosis?

a. AIDS-related lymphoma
b. Aspergillosis infection
c. Blastomycosis infection
d. Histoplasmosis infection
e. *Pneumocystis jiroveci* pneumonia

342. An 18-year-old white male high-school student visits the school nurses' office complaining of a diffuse, painful rash extending from his midthigh to his navel region. He indicates that one of his football team-mates gave him topical hydrocortisone to initially treat a minor groin rash. A KOH scraping of the lesion reveals the organisms shown in the figure. Which of the following is the most likely diagnosis?

(Reproduced, with permission, from Brooks GF et al. Jawetz's Medical Microbiology. 22nd ed. New York: McGraw-Hill;2001: 536.)

a. Coccidioidomycosis
b. Herpes simplex infection
c. Herpes zoster infection
d. Secondary syphilis
e. Tinea corporis (incognito)

343. A thorn pierces the glove of a medical student's left hand, when serving as a missionary in Africa, while assisting with the construction of a water project. Several days after the inflammation from the initial wound subsides, necrotizing lesions begin to form that spread toward the elbow. Which of the following is the most likely etiological agent?

a. *Coccidioides immitis*
b. *Malassezia furfur*
c. *Microsporum canis*
d. *Sporothrix schenckii*
e. *Stachybotrys chartarum*

344. A 30-year-old patient is generally healthy until his impacted wisdom tooth is removed by an oral surgeon. The area where the tooth had been is sore, but the appearance of eruptions through the skin beneath the area of the jaw where the tooth had been is more alarming. The exudate draining through the skin eruptions is cultured aerobically, but the results were negative. Which of the following is the most likely etiologic agent responsible for the patient's condition?

a. *Actinomyces bovis*
b. *Actinomyces israelii*
c. *Candida albicans*
d. *Histoplasma capsulatum*
e. *Nocardia asteroides*

345. Several laboratory tests are researched for their usefulness in evaluating suspected histoplasmosis in patients who reside in an area where the disease is endemic. If the prevalence of histoplasmosis is 25%, which of the following sensitivity and specificity combinations would be the most useful confirmatory test for diagnosing the disease?

a. Sensitivity of 50%, specificity of 98%
b. Sensitivity of 90%, specificity of 80%
c. Sensitivity of 92%, specificity of 70%
d. Sensitivity of 99%, specificity of 90%

346. A man living near the Ohio river develops a mild fever and cough. His physician finds a pulmonary infiltrate evidenced on a radiograph. *Histoplasma capsulatum* is a dimorphic soil saprophyte that causes histoplasmosis, the most prevalent pulmonary mycotic infection in humans and animals. As such, laboratories must be familiar with identification characteristics of this organism. Which of the following is associated with *H capsulatum?*

a. Arthroconidia
b. Sclerotic bodies
c. Spherules
d. Tuberculate macroconidia

347. A middle-aged man, living in an area where water contamination is believed to be responsible for gastrointestinal and septic illness, is taking tetracycline as treatment for a sepsis. As a result of taking this broad-spectrum antibiotic, he develops oral candidiasis. Which of the following best describes what has happened in this situation?

a. The antibiotic enhances the growth of *C albicans*.
b. Tetracycline is known to inhibit ergosterol synthesis.
c. Broad-spectrum antibiotics upset the balance of normal microbial flora.
d. The antibiotic damages the host oral epithelium.
e. Tetracycline drastically increases DNA synthesis by *C albicans*.

348. An old man living in a desert community develops a dry cough and joints pain that he had not experienced before. Valley fever or desert rheumatism is asymptomatic in 60% of individuals, while 40% present with a self-limited influenza-like illness with fever, malaise, cough, arthralgia, and headache. Less than 1% develop life-threatening CNS complications. The highly infectious asexual conidia of the etiologic agent are called which of the following?

a. Arthroconidia
b. Blastoconidia
c. Chlamydospores
d. Sporangiospores

349. Two children, who play with the family pets daily, develop tinea corporis infections as evidenced by annular lesions of ringworm, with a clearing, scaly center surrounded by a red advancing border that may be dry or vesicular. This condition is caused by which of the following?

a. *Epidermophyton floccosum*
b. *Exophiala werneckii*
c. *Malassezia furfur*
d. *Microsporum canis*
e. *Trichosporon beigelii*

350. A young man routinely goes to the gym and always takes a shower before heading home, notices itching between his toes. Peeling skin is also present. Tinea pedis is caused by which of the following?

a. *Epidermophyton floccosum*
b. *Exophiala werneckii*
c. *Malassezia furfur*
d. *Microsporum canis*
e. *Trichosporon beigelii*

351. Young students in an inner city school class develop tinea capitis, which is ringworm of the scalp and hair. Lesions begin with hyphal invasion of the skin and spread to the hair follicle, just above the hair root. This results in gray circular patches with scaling and itching. This condition is caused by which of the following?

a. *Epidermophyton floccosum*
b. *Exophiala werneckii*
c. *Malassezia furfur*
d. *Microsporum canis*
e. *Trichosporon beigelii*

352. Pityriasis versicolor (tinea versicolor) invades cornified skin, resulting in discrete, serpentine, hyper- or hypopigmented maculae. The chronic lesions usually occur on the chest, upper back, arms, or abdomen. This is caused by which of the following organisms?

a. *Epidermophyton floccosum*
b. *Exophiala werneckii*
c. *Malassezia furfur*
d. *Microsporum canis*
e. *Trichosporon beigelii*

353. A young man in his mid twenties presents with mucosal lesions in his mouth. Based on his CD4 cell count and other signs during the past few months, he is diagnosed as having AIDS. Which of the following is the most likely etiology of the oral lesions?

a. *Aspergillus* species
b. *Candida* species
c. *Cryptococcus* species
d. *Mucor* species
e. *Rhizopus* species

354. It is difficult to determine whether isolation from one body site or body fluid is suggestive of colonization or infection. Which of the following fungi is often isolated from blood, urine, and sputum in invasive disease?

a. *Aspergillus fumigatus*
b. *Basidiobolus ranarum*
c. *Candida albicans*
d. *Conidiobolus coronata*
e. *Rhizopus arrhizus*

355. A middle-aged woman is diagnosed with diabetes. She fails to follow her physician's advice and plans, in general, and suffers from a series of opportunistic infections. Which of the fungi listed below is the cause of her rhinocerebral zygomycosis (or mucor mycosis)?

a. *Aspergillus fumigatus*
b. *Basidiobolus ranarum*
c. *Candida albicans*
d. *Conidiobolus coronata*
e. *Rhizopus arrhizus*

356. Three weeks after traveling to California to study desert flowers, an AIDS patient develops fever, chest pain, and muscle soreness. Two months later, red, tender nodules appear on the shins, and he has pain and tenderness in the right ankle. An x-ray film of the chest shows a left pleural effusion. Which of the following is the most likely diagnosis?

a. Blastomycosis
b. Coccidioidomycosis
c. Histoplasmosis
d. *Mycobacterium marinum* infection
e. *Mycoplasma pneumoniae* infection

357. Mary is a superb gardener and especially loves roses. She does not think much of thorn sticks until one especially traumatic inoculation progressed to a neurotic lesion and the local draining lymphatics became thickened. Which of the following fungi caused this disease?

a. *Aspergillus fumigatus*
b. *Coccidioides immitis*
c. *Cryptococcus neoformans*
d. *Histoplasma capsulatum*
e. *Sporothrix schenckii*

358. An 18-year-old high school student in rural north Mississippi develops fever, cough, and chest pain. The cough, associated with weight loss, persists. Because of poor performance at football practice, he is advised to see a physician. Lymph node biopsies stained with hematoxylin and eosin (H and E) studies reveal granulomatous inflammation and macrophages engorged with oval structures measuring 2 to 4 μm. Cultures incubated at room temperature grow powdery white colonies, which on microscopic study have tuberculate spores. The high school student most likely acquired his infection from which of the following?

a. Another human via respiratory secretions
b. Bird excrement
c. Cat feces
d. Contaminated drinking water
e. Desert sand

Mycology

Answers

319. The answer is a. (*Brooks, pp 646-647. Levinson, pp 351-352. Murray, pp 763-767. Ryan, pp 655-656, 660-664, 670-672. Toy, p 278.*) Aspergillus is widespread in nature and produces small conidia that are easily aerosolized. Atopic individuals often develop severe allergic reactions to the conidial antigens. In immunocompromised patients, the conidia may germinate to produce hyphae that invade the lungs and other tissues. Both clinical symptoms and cultural characteristics of the causative agent suggest the diagnosis of this patient as aspergillosis, a common infection seen in immunocompromised hosts. Tuberculosis is unlikely because the patient is tuberculin test negative. The causative fungus for mucormycosis (phycomycosis) produces nonseptate hyphae in culture. *Histoplasma capsulatum*, which causes histoplasmosis in humans, grows in yeast form in the infected person. *Candida*, causative agent for candidiasis, does not produce hairy colonies on an agar surface.

320. The answer is a. (*Brooks, pp 646-647. Levinson, pp 351-352. Murray, pp 760-762. Ryan, pp 665-667. Toy, p 278.*) *Aspergillus* species cause infections of the skin, eyes, and ears, and "fungus ball" in the lungs. *Aspergillus* species occur only as molds (not dimorphic). They have septate hyphae that form V-shaped branches, whose walls are parallel. Septate, branching hyphae invading tissue are typically seen in biopsy. On culture, colonies with radiating chains of conidia (see figure in Question 321) are typical. These molds are widely spread in nature, and transmission is by airborne conidia. The organism is very opportunistic in immunocompromised individuals, and antifungal treatment may be difficult. Emphysema is a chronic pulmonary disease marked by an abnormal increase in the size of air spaces distal to the terminal bronchi. Patients often have a barrel chest and wheezing during inspiration. Cancer may appear in the trachea, air sacs, and other lung tubes. It may appear as an ulcer, as a nodule or flattened lump, or on the surface blocking air tubes. *Pneumocystis jiroveci* is an extracellular pathogen, and growth is limited to the surfactant layer above alveolar epithelium. *Pneumocystis jiroveci* exists as thin-walled trophozoites and thick-walled cysts. Viral pneumonia usually presents with cough and shortness of breath with chest films showing diffuse bilateral pulmonary infiltrates.

321. The answer is e. *(Brooks, pp 622-624. Levinson, pp 350-351. Murray, pp 760-762. Ryan, pp 674-678, 680-683. Toy, pp 284, 296.)* Thick-walled spores are characteristic of many fungal infections, including blastomycosis, coccidioidomycosis, and histoplasmosis. Observation of these structures in sputum or in tissue should alert the microbiologist to a diagnosis of systemic fungal infection. The presence of encapsulated yeast in clinical specimens may suggest the presence of *Cryptococcus*. Hyphal strands would be linear filaments and recognized as part of a mold mycelium. *Conidia* are asexual reproductive structures of molds. They may be large (macroconidium) or small (microconidium). Microscopic structures are usually recognized as such and help in identifying the species involved. Spherules usually refer to structures present in tissues infected with *C immitis*. The spherules contain hundreds of endospores.

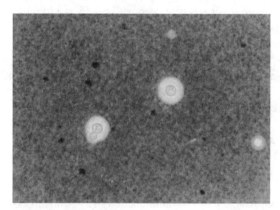

(Reproduced, with permission, from Brooks GF et al. Jawetz's Medical Microbiology. 24th ed. New York: McGraw-Hill; 2007: 645.)

322. The answer is c. *(Brooks, pp 626-629. Levinson, pp 342-343. Murray, pp 718-724. Ryan, pp 649-650.)* Wood light is a device that produces ultraviolet light rays. Hairs infected with both *M canis* and *M audouini* fluoresce with a yellow-green color under Wood light, while *T rubrum*, *T tonsurans*, and *E floccosum* do not. But *M audouini* is an anthropophilic agent of tinea capitis, whereas *M canis* is zoophilic. *Microsporum canis* is seen primarily in children and is associated with infected cats or dogs.

323. The answer is b. *(Brooks, p 645. Levinson, pp 350-351. Murray, pp 760-762. Ryan, pp 669-672. Toy, p 296.)* Patients with paralysis of their cellular immune system, such as in AIDS, are susceptible to a wide variety of diseases, including infection with *Cryptococcus*. A brain abscess caused by *C neoformans* is not unusual in patients with AIDS. Initial laboratory suspicion is usually aroused by the presence of encapsulated yeast in the CSF. There also could be other microorganisms as well as noninfectious artifacts that superficially resemble yeast. While *C neoformans* can be readily cultured, a rapid diagnosis can be made by detecting cryptococcal capsular polysaccharide in CSF or blood. Care must be taken to strictly control the test because rheumatoid factor may cross-react. Once the yeast is isolated, then specific stains as well as panels of assimilatory carbohydrates are available to definitively identify this organism as *C neoformans*. The patient may also be infected with *P jiroveci*, but not in the central nervous system. *Pneumocystis jiroveci* has recently been reclassified as a fungus. It, however, does not have a capsule on either the thin-walled trophozoites or thick-walled cysts. *Pneumocystis carinii* is only found in rats. *Candida* species would be recognized by their large, typical structure which also has no capsule. *Cryptosporidium* typically infects intestines of immunocompromised hosts, while *Toxoplasma* is a coccidian protozoan most often seen when nonimmune mothers are infected during pregnancy.

324. The answer is c. *(Brooks, p 645. Levinson, pp 350-354. Murray, pp 760-762. Ryan, pp 669-672.)* *Cryptococcus neoformans* occurs widely in nature, particularly in soil contaminated with bird droppings. Human infection occurs when inhalation of the organism occurs. Lung infection is often asymptomatic but can result in pneumonia. Meningitis occurs through dissemination, particularly in immunosuppressed patients. India ink preparations of CSF reveal a budding yeast with a wide, unstained capsule in infected persons. *Aspergillus, Candida, Histoplasma,* and *Paracoccidioides* all do not have capsules. *Paracoccidioides brasiliensis* does have large, multiple budding from the parent fungal body.

325. The answer is e. *(Brooks, p 633. Levinson, pp 169-170. Murray, pp 271, 729-730.)* Eumycotic mycetoma is a slowly progressing disease of the subcutaneous tissues that is caused by a variety of fungi. The term *Madura foot* has been used to describe the foot lesion. Although several fungi have been isolated in the United States from persons who have mycetoma,

Pseudallescheria boydii appears to be one of the most common. Other foot infections that may resemble Madura foot are actinomycotic (bacterial) in nature. These are caused by *Nocardia brasiliensis* and *Actinomadura*. *Acremonium falciforme* is another fungal agent that has been suggested to be able to cause mycetoma, but has not been reported to be able to do so in significant number of reports.

326. The answer is a. *(Brooks, p 640. Levinson, p 347. Murray, pp 735-738. Ryan, pp 672-683. Toy, p 284.)* The key diagnostic finding is the morphology of the yeast isolated from the granulomatous, suppurative lesions of the lung. *Blastomyces dermatidis*, which causes blastomycosis, grows in the yeast form in infected tissues. The bud of growing yeast is attached to the parent cell by a broad base. Although the fungi that cause all other diseases listed (coccidioidomycosis, cryptococcosis, histoplasmosis, and sporotrichosis) in the question grow in yeast form in infected tissues, most buds are attached to the parent cell by a narrow base.

327. The answer is e. *(Brooks, p 630-631. Levinson, pp 342-343. Murray, pp 725-727. Ryan, pp 654-656.)* Cutaneous sporotrichosis, caused by *S schenckii*, begins at the site of inoculation, usually on an extremity or the face. The organism often is found on thorns of rose bushes. Ulceration is common, and new lesions appear along paths of lymphatic channels. Extracutaneous sporotrichosis is seen primarily in bones and joints. There is no evidence to suggest that any portal of entry besides skin is important. *Blastomyces, Coccidioides, Histoplasma, and Cryptococcus* species are endemic mycoses, geographically restricted to areas of endemicity. They cause systemic or deep mycoses in infected persons.

328. The answer is b. *(Brooks, p 626. Levinson, pp 342-343. Murray, pp 718-724.)* The dermatophytes (see figure presented in the question) are a group of fungi that infect only superficial keratinized tissue (skin, hair, nails). Dermatophytes are probably restricted to nonviable skin because most are unable to grow at 37°C or in the presence of serum. Such lesions are among the most prevalent in the world. They are not life-threatening, but can be persistent and troublesome. They form hyphae and arthroconidia on the skin; in culture, they develop colonies and conidia. Tinea pedis, or athlete's foot, is the most common dermatophytosis. Several topical antifungal agents, such as undecylenic acid, salicylic acid, and ammoniated

SOME CLINICAL FEATURES OF DERMATOPHYTE INFECTION

Skin Disease	Location of Lesions	Clinical Features	Fungi Most Frequently Responsible
Tinea corporis (ringworm)	Nonhairy, smooth skin	Circular patches with advancing red, vesiculated border and central scaling; pruritic	T rubrum, E floccosum
Tinea pedis[a] (athlete's foot)	Interdigital spaces on feet of persons wearing shoes	Acute: itching, red vesicular Chronic: itching, scaling, fissures	T rubrum, T mentagrophytes, E floccosum
Tinea cruris (jock itch)	Groin	Erythematous scaling lesion in intertriginous area; pruritic	T rubrum, T mentagrophytes, E floccosum
Tinea capitis	Scalp hair; endothrix: fungus inside hair shaft; ectothrix: fungus on surface of hair	Circular bald patches with short hair stubs or broken hair within hair follicles; kerion rare; microsporum-infected hairs fluoresce	T mentagrophytes, M canis
Tinea barbae	Beard hair	Edematous, erythematous lesion	T mentagrophytes
Tinea unguium (onychomycosis)	Nails	Nails thickened or crumbling distally, discolored, lusterless; usually associated with tinea pedis	T rubrum, T mentagrophytes, E floccosum
Dermatophytid (id reaction)	Usually sides and flexor aspects of fingers, palm; any site on body	Pruritic vesicular to bullous lesions; most commonly associated with tinea pedis	No fungi present in lesion; may become secondarily infected with bacteria

[a]May be associated with lesions of hands and nails (onychomycosis)

(Reproduced, with permission, from Brooks GF et al. Jawetz's Medical Microbiology. 24th ed. New York: McGraw-Hill;2007: 629.)

mercury, may be useful in treatment. For serious infection, systemic use of griseofulvin is effective. Since none of the three genera (*Microsporum, Tricophyton, and Epidermophyton*) produce aflatoxin, no hallucinations would have been experienced. Penicillin is not able to inhibit fungal growth either in human infection or on artificial medium. Since these fungi infect only superficial skin, no lung infections would occur. Immunocompromised individuals would probably be the only ones that might develop a chronic infection if such case was not treated with an appropriate medication.

Epidermophyton floccosum

Microsporum gypseum

Microsporum canis

(Reproduced, with permission, from Brooks GF et al. Jawetz's Medical Microbiology. 24th ed. New York: McGraw-Hill; 2007: 627.)

329. The answer is e. *(Brooks, pp 642-644. Levinson, pp 349-350. Murray, pp 754-756. Ryan, pp 660-664. Toy, p 290.)* *Candida albicans* is the most important species of *Candida* and causes thrush, vaginitis, skin and nail infections, and other infections. It is part of the normal flora of skin, mouth, GI tract, and vagina. It appears in tissues as an oval, budding yeast or elongated pseudohyphae. It grows well on laboratory media and is identified by germ-tube formation. A vaccine is not available and serologic and skin tests have little value. *Candida* infection can be treated with topical nystatin or oral ketoconazole. Rhizoids (irregular rootlike system of growth) are not seen in *Candida* growth. Asci are saclike spore cases in which ascospores are formed. Ascomycetes, not *Candida*, produce these. Metachromatic granules would be seen in *Corynebacterium*, a gram-positive bacillus, but not in *Candida*. Spherules containing endospores are found in *C immitis*, not *Candida*.

330. The answer is b. *(Brooks, pp 642-644. Levinson, pp 349-350. Murray, pp 754-756. Ryan, pp 660-664. Toy, p 290.)* *Candida albicans* is part of the normal flora of the gastrointestinal tract, mouth, and genital surfaces. Notwithstanding, *C albicans* causes severe disease, particularly in patients with compromised immunity. It is generally thought that when *C albicans* is unable to adhere to mucosa it is nonpathogenic and that production of germ tubes or hyphae plays a major role in colonization and infection of the mucosal epithelial cells by allowing direct penetration of these cells with specific hydrolytic enzymes. While other mutations such as temperature intolerance, metabolic alterations, and structural substitutions may affect the ability of *Candida* to survive, these changes would not affect adherence.

331. The answer is a. *(Brooks, pp 646-647. Levinson, pp 351-352. Murray, pp 763-767. Ryan, pp 665-667. Toy, p 278.)* While all fungi such as *Candida* and *Cryptococcus* are potentially serious in a bone marrow transplant unit (BMTU), the most frequent cause of fungal infection and death is *Aspergillus*. Aspergilli are ubiquitous in the environment. There are instances of multiple infections in new units that have not been monitored prior to opening or in units adjacent to construction projects. Strict precautions should be taken to exclude dust and debris from the BMTU area during construction, but in any event, the environment should be monitored for airborne microorganisms, especially *Aspergillus*, prior to opening the unit. *Blastomyces* and *Cryptococcus* may be inhaled and cause lung infections, but they are not as prevalent in the atmosphere and ubiquitous as *Aspergillus*. *Candida* is part of the normal human flora and is opportunistic when immune defenses are not working properly. *Wangiella dermatitidis* causes phaeohyphomycosis, darkly pigmented septate hyphae in tissue.

332. The answer is b. *(Brooks, pp 637-639. Levinson, pp 345-346. Murray, pp 743-747. Ryan, pp 672-676.)* *Histoplasma capsulatum* is a dimorphic fungus that forms two types of spores: tuberculate macroconidia and microconidia. Inhalation of the microconidia transmits infection. Inhaled spores (microconidia) are engulfed by macrophages and develop into yeast forms. Most infections remain asymptomatic; small granulomatous foci heal by calcification. However, pneumonia can occur. In tissue, the yeasts are typically seen within macrophages since the organism is a facultative intracellular parasite. Arthrospores (arthroconidia) result from the fragmentation of hyphal cells (eg, *C immitis*). Single-cell yeasts with pseudohyphae would be *C albicans*. Spherules with endospores are made by *C immitis* also. Yeasts with a broad-based bud would be *B dermatidis*.

333. The answer is d. *(Brooks, p 709. Levinson, p 352. Ryan, pp 678-680.)* This description is a typical picture of mucormycosis occurring in a diabetic patient. The organism is a member of *Phycomycetes*, which forms uniseptate hyphae. In candidiasis, septate hyphae and budding yeast are seen in infected tissues. Nocardiosis, erysipelas, and gas gangrene are not mycotic infections. They are caused by bacteria (*Nocardia asteroides, Streptococcus pyogenes, and Clostridium perfringens* respectively).

334. The answer is c. *(Brooks, pp 642-644. Levinson, pp 349-350. Murray, pp 754-756. Ryan, pp 678-680.)* *Candida albicans* and *C tropicalis* are opportunistic fungi, and as part of the normal flora are not transmitted by inhalation. *Coccidioides immitis* is a dimorphic fungus, and inhalation of the spores transmits the infection. *Sporothrix* is also a dimorphic fungus, but its portal of entry is cutaneous. *Trychophyton* is a dermatophyte and one of the causes of athlete's foot.

335. The answer is a. *(Brooks, pp 646-647. Levinson, pp 351-352. Murray, pp 736-737, 791-793. Ryan, pp 665-667. Toy, p 278.)* *Aspergillus* is an opportunistic pathogen that can invade wounds, burns, abraded skin, the cornea, and the outer ear. However, in immunocompromised patients, infection of the wound site is not common. *Aspergillus* does not cause urinary tract infection. In immunocompromised persons, invasive disease occurs. Blood vessel invasion can result in thrombosis and infarction. In pulmonary cavities (due to tuberculosis), "fungus ball" formation can occur, which can be seen on x-ray. Infection of the bronchi can result in allergic bronchopulmonary aspergillosis, characterized by asthmatic symptoms. Thrush is caused by *C albicans*. Rashes are not usually seen with *Aspergillus* infection.

336. The answer is b. *(Brooks, pp 634-636. Levinson, pp 344-345. Murray, pp 738-741. Ryan, pp 680-683.)* In patients with coccidioidomycosis, a positive skin test to coccidioidin appears 2 to 21 days after the appearance of disease symptoms and may persist for 20 years without reexposure to

SUMMARY OF ENDEMIC MYCOSES[a]

	Coccidioidomycosis	Histoplasmosis	Blastomycosis	Paracoccidioidomycosis
Etiology	*C immitis*, *C posadasii*	*H capsulatum*	*Blastomyces dermatidis*	*Paracoccidioides brasiliensis*
Ecology	Soil	Bat and avian habitats (guano); alkaline soil	Unknown (riverbanks?)	Unknown (soil?)
Geographic distribution	Semiarid regions of southwestern United States, Mexico, Central and South America	Global: endemic in Ohio, Missouri, and Mississippi River valleys; central Africa (var *duboisii*)	Endemic along Mississippi, Ohio, and St. Lawrence River valleys and in southeastern United States	Central and South America
Conidia (< [95°F] 35°C)	Hyaline septate hyphae and arthroconidia, 3×6 μm	Hyaline septate hyphae, tuberculate macroconidia, 8-16 μm, and small oval microconidia, 3-5 μm	Hyaline septate hyphae and short conidiophores bearing single globose to piriform conidia, 2-10 μm	Hyaline, septate hyphae, and rare globose conidia and chlamydospores
Tissue form	Spherules, 10-80 μm or larger, containing endospores, 2-4 μm	Oval yeasts, 2×4 μm, intracellular in macrophages	Thick-walled yeasts with broad-based, usually single buds, 8-15 μm	Multiple budding yeasts, 15-30 μm or larger

[a]All four systemic mycoses are caused by dimorphic fungi and are acquired by inhalation of conidia. With the exception of blastomycosis, the evidence is strong that there is a high rate of infection within the endemic areas. Ninety percent or more of infections occur in immunocompetent individuals, and most are asymptomatic and self-limited. Up to 90% of cases of symptomatic disease occur in males. Coccidioidomycosis and histoplasmosis are common among AIDS patients in the endemic areas.

(Reproduced, with permission from, Brooks GF et al. Jawetz's Medical Microbiology. 24th ed. New York: McGraw-Hill; 2007:635.)

the fungus. A decrease in intensity of the skin response often occurs in clinically healthy people who move away from endemic areas. If patients with disseminated disease become anergic (inability to react with antigens administered through skin testing), the skin test will be negative. CF immunoglobulin G (IgG) antibodies, which may not appear at all in mild disease, rise to a high titer in disseminated disease, a poor prognostic sign. For this reason, a persistent or rising CF titer combined with clinical symptoms indicates present or imminent dissemination. Rarely is the CF titer negative. Most persons once infected with *C immitis* are immune to reinfection.

(Reproduced, with permission, from Brooks GF et al. Jawetz's Medical Microbiology. 24th ed. New York: McGraw-Hill; 2007: 635.)

337 to 340. The answers are 337-d, 338-c, 339-b, 340-a. *(Brooks, pp 622-630, 642,646. Levinson, pp 349-352. Murray, pp 730-732, 754-756, 763-767. Ryan, pp 660-668. Toy, p 278.)* Fungi that cause opportunistic infections are diverse, and most of them are represented in this group of questions. Infection occurs primarily in the compromised host with underlying diseases such as lymphoma, leukemia, and diabetes. Unfortunately, most of the opportunistic fungi that cause infection are commonly seen in the laboratory as contaminants.

Candidiasis is the most frequent opportunistic infection. While *C albicans* is most commonly isolated, other species such as *C tropicalis* and *Torulopsis glabrata* are also seen. The yeasts may be identified biochemically, but *C albicans* is distinctive in that it produces germ tubes and chlamydospores.

Aspergillosis, caused by a number of species of *Aspergillus*, is characterized in direct smear by septate hyphae, dichotomously branched.

Aspergillus flavus and *A fumigatus* are often seen as saprophytes in the laboratory but also account for the major species isolated from patients with aspergillosis. Differentiation of species, as with the zygomycetes, is dependent upon isolation of the fungus and precise morphological examination.

Zygomycosis, a term referring to infection by members of the class Zygomycetes, is caused primarily by *Rhizopus, Mucor*, and *Absidia*. Other zygomycetes such as *Basidiobolus* and *Cunninghamella* are rarely encountered. The lack of septate hyphae on a direct smear may be the initial hint of zygomycosis. However, not uncommonly, the occasional hypha of *Mucor* will have a septum. The genera cannot be differentiated on a direct patient specimen. The organism must be isolated and slide cultures performed to observe the characteristic morphology of these filamentous fungi.

Rhizopus species have sporangia that arise from a stolon, while *Mucor* species do not. *Mucor* species have collarettes; *Rhizopus* species do not.

341. The answer is e. *(Brooks, p 648. Levinson, p 352. Murray, pp 638, 772-773, Ryan, pp 685-689.)* *Pneumocystis jiroveci* causes pneumonia in immunocompromised patients. Once considered a protozoan, it is not classified as a fungus. Effective chemoprophylactic regimens have resulted in a dramatic decrease in pneumonia deaths in AIDS patients. *Pneumocystis jiroveci* has the morphologically distinct forms (trophozoite and cyst) described in the question. Cysts stain well with silver stain. In clinical specimens, trophozoites and cysts are present in a tight mass. *Pneumocystis jiroveci* cannot be cultured. The organism is widespread in nature and does not cause disease without immunosuppression. It may represent a member of normal flora. The more familiar *P carinii* is found only in rats. AIDS-related lymphoma would not present the results observed in the chest films. *Aspergillus* hyphae invade the lumens and walls of blood vessels as well as existing cavities where abundant hyphae could fill the spaces. The most common presentation of *Blastomyces* is a pulmonary infiltrate indistinguishable from other lower respiratory infections, which may become chronic. *Histoplasma* invades macrophages and causes granulomatous nodules in the lungs which often heal with calcification.

342. The answer is e. *(Brooks, pp 626-629. Levinson, pp 337, 342-343. Murray, pp 718-724. Ryan, p 653.)* Of the available answer choices, only tinea corporis dermatophyte infection will show numerous, smooth-walled macroconidia, with microconidia being absent. *Epidermophyton* species would be a common cause of this kind of rash. Jock itch (tinia cruruis—groin) can involve particularly bad lesions if inappropriate use of topical steroids is involved. This is also called tinea incognito. Tinea or ringworm designations were used because of the dermatophyte infections. Treatment usually consists of thorough removal of infected and dead epithelial structure and application of a topical antifungal medication. HSV and VZV produce vesicular rashes, not maculopapular ones. Syphilis' secondary lesions consist of a red maculopapular rash anywhere on the body, along with moist, pale papules (condylomas) in the anogenital region. *Coccidioides* (valley fever) may present with a hypersensitivity rash and also involves the pulmonary system.

343. The answer is d. (*Brooks, pp 630-631. Levinson, pp 342-343. Murray, pp 725-727. Ryan, pp 654-656.*) *Sporothrix schenckii* is a dimorphic fungus that lives on vegetation. A mold with branching septate hyphae and conidia at ambient temperature, it grows as a small budding yeast at 37°C. Following traumatic introduction into the skin, a chronic granulomatous infection occurs with secondary spread to local lymph nodes. For systemic treatment, Amphoteracin B is given. *Malassezia* and *Microsporum* produce superficial infections. *Coccidioides* would be transmitted by airborne mechanisms. *Stachybotrys chartarum* is the toxic house mold that is so prevalent in current news reports.

344. The answer is b. (*Brooks, pp 217-221. Levinson, pp 169-170. Murray, pp 391-393.*) Actinomycosis is a chronic suppurative and granulomatous infection that produces pyogenic lesions with interconnecting sinus tracts that contain granules composed of microcolonies of bacteria embedded in tissue components. The etiologic agents are closely related to normal oral flora with most cases being due to *A israelii*, a facultative anaerobe. The three most common forms are cervicofacial, thoracic, and abdominal, with trauma being the mechanism that introduces these organisms into the mucosa tissues. The bacteria bridge the mucosal surfaces of the mouth, respiratory tract, and lower GI tract. Infection is associated with dental caries, gingivitis, surgical complication, or trauma, as mentioned above. Aspiration may lead to pulmonary infection. Cervicofacial disease presents as a swollen, erythematous process in the jaw area, producing draining fistulas. *Actinomyces bovis* seldom causes human disease. Nocardia infection is usually caused by inhalation of the organism and relate to pulmonary infections. *Histoplasma capsulatum* could be identified by microscopic examination of exudate, showing large, spherical thick-walled macroconidia with peripheral projections of cell wall materials.

345. The answer is a. (*http://en.wikipedia.org/wiki/Bayesian_statistics.*) Sensitivity, in medical diagnosis, is the probability of the test finding disease among those who have the disease or the proportion of people with disease who have a positive test result. Sensitivity = true positives/(true positives + false negatives). Specificity is the probability of the test finding *no* disease among those who do *not* have the disease or the proportion of people free of a disease who have a negative test. Specificity = true negatives/(true negatives + false positives). Positive predictive value (PPV) is the percentage of people with a positive test result who actually have the disease. Negative predictive value (NPV) would be the percentage of people who do *not* have the disease. When a diagnostic test or sign has a high sensitivity, a *negative* result rules out the diagnosis. When a diagnostic sign or test has a high specificity, a *positive* result rules in the diagnosis. In our test question, 25% prevalence (total number of cases of a disease in a given population at a given time) is relatively high. Incidence, for comparison, is the number of cases (especially new cases) in a given population over a period of time. In our example, in order to maximize the chances of finding the true number of disease cases, we would want the highest degree of specificity (98%).

346. The answer is c. (*Brooks, pp 637-639. Levinson, pp 345-346. Murray, pp 743-746.*) In *H capsulatum* infection, conidia develop into yeast cells which are engulfed by alveolar macrophages. These may give rise to inflammatory reactions that become granulomatous. In culture at 25°C, *H capsulatum* develops hyphae with microconidia and large, spherical macroconidia with peripheral projections of cell wall materials. The macroconida are also called tuberculate macroconidia. Arthroconidia (arthrospores) result from the fragmentation of hyphal cells of *C immitis*. Spherules result when arthroconidia are inhaled and enlarge into larger bodies that contain endospores. Spherules can be produced in the laboratory using a complex medium. Sclerotic bodies are found in chromoblastomycosis infections. The fungi reside in soil and vegetation and cause skin infections. In tissue, the fungi appear as spherical brown cells termed muniform or sclerotic bodies that divide by transverse separation. Separation in different planes may give rise to a cluster of 4 to 8 cells.

347. The answer is c. (*Brooks, pp 642-644. Levinson, pp 348-350. Murray, pp 679-687. Toy, p 290.*) It has long been recognized that fungi may be part of the normal (usual) microbial flora of humans, but their numbers are kept quite low by the competition for food, and the like, by the faster growing bacteria. If some mechanism (broad-spectrum antibiotics) alter the usual flora, these fungi, especially *Candida*, may become efficient opportunists and cause a disease situation. Removal of the antibiotic will allow reestablishment of normal bacterial flora and control *Candida* numbers again.

348. The answer is a. (*Brooks, pp 634-636. Levinson, pp 344-345. Murray, pp 739-741, 777.*) Valley fever is caused by *C immitis*. It is grown on Sabouraud agar, and the infection is endemic in the semiarid regions of the southwestern United States, as well as Central and South America. Hyphae form chains of arthroconidia (arthrospores) which often develop in alternate cells of a hypha. Individual arthroconidia are released from chains, become airborne, and are resistant to harsh environmental conditions. Following inhalation, arthroconidia become spherical, enlarge forming spherules that contain endospores. Such spherules have a thick, refractive cell wall and are diagnostic of *C immitis*. Blastospores represent conidial formation through a budding process, as seen in yeast or chains of *Cladosporium*. Chlamydospores are large, thick-walled spherical conidia produced from terminal hyphal cells (*C albicans*). Sporangiospores are sexual structures characteristic of zygomycetes (mitotic spores produced within an enclosed sporangium), often supported by one sporangiophore (*Rhizopus, Mucor*).

349 to 352. The answers are 349-d, 350-a, 351-d, 352-c. (*Brooks, pp 626-629. Levinson, pp 342-343. Murray, pp 718-724. Ryan, pp 649-650, 654.*) Dermatomycoses are cutaneous mycoses caused by three genera of fungi: *Microsporum, Trichophyton*, and *Epidermophyton*. These infections are called *tinea* or *ringworm*, a misnomer that has persisted from the days when they were thought to be caused by worms or lice. Tinea capitis (ringworm of the scalp) is due to an infection with *M canis* or *T tonsurans*. It usually occurs during childhood and heals spontaneously at puberty. Circular areas on the scalp, with broken or no hair, are characteristic of this disorder. Tinea corporis (ringworm of the body) is caused by *M canis* and *T mentagrophytes*. This disorder affects smooth skin and produces circular pruritic areas of redness and scaling. Both tinea cruris (ringworm of the groin, "jock itch") and tinea pedis (ringworm of the feet, athlete's foot) are caused by *T rubrum*, *T mentagrophytes*, or *E floccosum*. These common conditions are pruritic and can cause scaling. Tinea versicolor (pityriasis versicolor) is not a dermatomycotic condition but, rather, a superficial mycosis now thought to be caused by *M furfur*. The disorder is characterized by chronic but asymptomatic scaling on the trunk, arms, or other parts of the body. *Hortaea (Exophiala) werneckii* causes tinea nigra, a chronic and asymptomatic infection of the stratum cornea, resulting in a dark discoloration of the skin. This will respond to azole antifungal drugs. *Trichosporon* species cause white piedra, a hair shaft infection with large, soft and yellowish nodules on the hair.

353. The answer is b. *(Brooks, pp 642-644. Levinson, pp 349-350. Murray, pp 751-759. Ryan, pp 660-664. Toy, p 290.)* *Candida* species are normal flora of the skin, mucous membranes, and gastrointestinal tract. The risk of endogenous infection is ever present. Candidiasis is the most common systemic mycosis. Oral thrush develops in most patients with AIDS. Other risk factors include antibiotic use and cellular immunodeficiency. *Mucor* and *Rhizopus* are primarily dermatophytes, while *Aspergillus* is usually derived from an environmental source. While *Aspergillus* is a significant opportunist, the numbers of cases are much lower than those observed to be caused by *Candida*. *Cryptococcus* is usually acquired by inhalation.

354 and 355. The answers are 354-c, 355-e. *(Brooks, pp 642-644. Levinson, pp 349-352. Murray, pp 751-759. Toy, p 290.)* Candidiasis, cryptococcosis, zygomycosis, and aspergillosis are among the most common opportunistic fungal infections. These fungi are commonly observed in the environment and are innocuous to people with intact host defenses. However, when host defenses are compromised by immunosuppression (AIDS), cytotoxic drugs, diabetes, or devices that breach the normal host defenses, these usually harmless fungi become potent pathogenic microorganisms.

Candida albicans is a member of the normal human microflora. This yeast causes such relatively mild infections as "jock itch" and diaper rash. Suppression of cellular immunity often results in more serious yeast infections. Oral candidiasis is one of the earliest and most frequent of the opportunistic infections in patients with AIDS. Diagnosis of invasive candidiasis is difficult, especially when patients are symptomatic and *Candida* is not recovered from blood specimens. Candidal antibody tests, antigen detection, and metabolite detection have not been successful in differentiating between invasive disease and colonization. The figure presented in Question 337 illustrates *C albicans* from a skin smear.

Zygomycosis (sometimes called *mucormycosis*) is caused by a variety of fungi called zygomycetes. These fungi include *Conidiobolus*, *Rhizopus*, and *Basidiobolus*, which can be differentiated mycologically, but all are characterized by large (6-25 mm), irregularly branched, usually nonseptate hyphae. The differentiation of these fungi clinically is a function of the location of the lesion: limbs and trunk, nose, or brain. *Basidiobolus* lesions are most commonly seen on the arms and legs. *Conidiobolus* is usually found in the nasal mucosa and nasal sinuses. *Rhizopus* infection may start in the nasal tissue but spreads rapidly to the eyes and brain. *Aspergillus funigatus* is the most common human pathogen of this worldwide group. Inhalation of *Aspergillus* conidia by atopic persons leads to severe allergic reactions, and in immunocompromised patients, the conidia may germinate into hyphae that invade the lungs and other tissues.

356. The answer is b. *(Brooks, pp 634-636. Levinson, pp 344-345. Murray, pp 739-741, 777. Ryan, pp 678-683. Toy, p 284.)* Endemic areas for *C immitis* are semiarid regions, particularly the central valleys of California and southern Arizona. The infection rate is highest during the dry months of summer and autumn, when dust is prevalent. Inhalation of arthroconidia can lead to an asymptomatic infection in 60% of individuals. The other 40% may develop a self-limited influenza-like illness. Individuals with cell-mediated immunosuppression may lead to dissemination of endospores by the blood. The most frequent sites involved are skin, bones and joints, and the meninges. Histoplasmosis is usually associated with the central river valleys of the United States, while blastomycocis is endemic primarily in the eastern United States. *Mycobacterium marinum* is usually associated with fish and water, while *Mycoplasma pneumoniae* transmission is from person to person.

357. The answer is e. *(Brooks, p 630. Levinson, p 343. Murray, pp 725-727. Ryan, pp 654-656. Toy, p 308.)* *Sporothrix* is a dimorphic fungus that lives on vegetation. While a mold forms at ambient temperatures and produces septate hyphae and conidia, the infection almost always follows traumatic introduction into the skin. A chronic granulomatus infection is typical, with local lymph nodes being involved. Multiple lesions (abscesses) may occur along the lymphatics. *Histoplasma, Coccidioides, Cryptococcus*, and *Aspergillus* are usually acquired by inhalation.

358. The answer is b. *(Brooks, pp 637-639. Levinson, pp 345-346. Murray, pp 743-745. Ryan, pp 672-676. Toy, p 284.)* *Histoplasma capsulatum* infection is highest in the United States, especially in the Ohio and Mississippi river valleys. Numerous outbreaks have resulted from exposure of many persons to inocula of conidia. These occur when the organism is disturbed from its natural habitat, soil mixed with bird feces, or bat guano. Feces provide an excellent culture for fungal growth to occur. Some 80% to 90% of residents in certain endemic areas may have positive skin tests. Histoplasmosis is not transmissible from person to person. It is also not transmissible from cat feces, contaminated drinking water, or desert sands.

Parasitology

Questions

359. Babesiosis (see figure) is a tick-borne disease, resulting in affecting persons with malaise, nausea, fever, sweats, myalgia, and arthralgia and could be confused with *Plasmodium falciparum* ring form in red cells. Infection with Babesia has been most commonly observed in which of the following?

(*Reproduced, with permission, from Wilson WR, Sande MA. Current Diagnosis and Treatment in Infectious Disease. New York, NY: McGraw-Hill; 2001:805.*)

a. AIDS patients
b. Foresters
c. Patients without a spleen
d. Transfusion recipients
e. Transplant recipients

360. An AIDS patient presents to his primary care physician with a 2-week history of watery, nonbloody diarrhea. This stool reveals the organism seen in the figure below. Which of the following is the most likely diagnosis?

(Reproduced, with permission, from Wilson WR, Sande MA. Current Diagnosis and Treatment in Infectious Disease. New York, NY: McGraw-Hill; 2001:827.)

a. Acid-fast bacilli
b. *Enterocytozoon*
c. *Cryptosporidium*
d. *Cyclospora*
e. Yeast

361. A healthy 30-year-old woman consumed half a box of imported raspberries 10 days ago. She experiences a self-limited but prolonged, relapsing watery diarrhea, along with fatigue and low-grade fever. Stool examination reveals oocysts with autofluorescent inclusions which were acid-fast. Which of the following is the most likely cause of her infection?

a. *Escherichia coli* 0157:H7
b. *Cyclospora*
c. *Cryptosporidium*
d. *Isospora*
e. *Vibrio*

362. *Toxoplasma* organisms are normally ingested by humans and produce either congenital or postnatal toxoplasmosis. While most human infections are asymptomatic, fatal infections can occur in patients with AIDS. For control of infection, which of the following steps in the *Toxoplasma* life cycle would be most practical to interrupt?

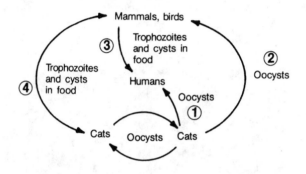

a. Step 1
b. Step 2
c. Step 3
d. Step 4
e. Steps 3 and 4

363. A 30-year-old female stores her contact lenses in tap water. She notices deterioration of vision and visits an ophthalmologist, who diagnoses her with severe retinitis. Culture of the water as well as vitreous fluid would most likely reveal which of the following?

a. *Acanthamoeba*
b. *Babesia*
c. *Entamoeba coli*
d. *Naegleria*
e. *Pneumocystis*

364. A young nurse in a South American city located in the tropics develops classical symptoms of malaria. An accurate diagnosis of the *Plasmodium* species is necessary to provide the best treatment to insure recovery and prevent relapse. Sporozoites from a mosquito bite rapidly enter live cells where asexual merozoites enter the blood stream and RBCs are invaded. This erythrocytic stage provides a basis for laboratory diagnosis. Which of the diagnostic characteristics of *P falciparum* (see figure) is best described by the following?

(Reproduced, with permission, from Lichtman MA, Beutler E, Kipps TJ, et al. Williams Hematology. 7th ed. New York, NY: McGraw-Hill; 2006:Plate I-12.)

a. An important diagnostic feature is the irregular appearance of the edges of the infected red blood cell.
b. A period of 72 hours is required for the development of the mature schizont, which resembles a rosette with only 8 to 10 oval merozoites.
c. Except in infections with very high parasitemia, only ring forms of early trophozoites and the gametocytes are seen in the peripheral blood.
d. Schüffner dot stippling is routinely seen in red blood cells that harbor parasites.
e. The signet-ring-shaped trophozoite is irregular in shape with ameboid extensions of the cytoplasm.

365. After returning from a wilderness camping outing, several children report watery, greasy, and foul-smelling stools. Deer, cattle, and horses were known to be in the vicinity. The life cycle of the parasite responsible for this outbreak consists of two stages: the cyst and the trophozoite, as shown in the figure below. Which of the following is the most likely identification of this organism?

A: "Face" and B: "profile" of vegetative forms; C and D: cysts (binucleate [D] and quadrinucleate stages). 2000×.
(Reproduced, with permission, from Brooks GF et al. Jawetz's Medical Microbiology. 24th ed. New York, NY: McGraw-Hill; 2007:660.)

a. *Clonorchis*
b. *Entamoeba*
c. *Giardia*
d. *Pneumocystis*
e. *Trichomonas*

366. A divorced working mother takes her 4-year-old child to a day-care center. She has noticed that the child's frequent stools are nonbloody with mucus and are foul smelling. The child has no fever, but does complain of "tummy hurting." The increase of fat in the stool directs the pediatrician's concern toward a diagnosis of malabsorption syndrome associated with which of the following?

a. Amebiasis
b. Ascariasis
c. Balantidiasis
d. Enterobiasis
e. Giardiasis

367. A family from a rural area of Central America migrates to the United States. Several members of the family present to a physician with headache, vertigo, and vomiting. Calcified cysts are observed in computed tomography scans, indicating possible cysticercosis. Which of the following statements best describes the basis for the patients' infection and symptoms?

a. Acute intestinal stoppage is less common in beef tapeworm infection.
b. Beef tapeworm eggs cause less irritation of the mucosa of the digestive tract.
c. Larval invasion does not occur in beef tapeworm infection.
d. The adult beef tapeworms are smaller.
e. Toxic by-products are not given off by the adult beef tapeworm.

368. A man coughs up a long (4-6 cm), white worm, and his chief complaint is abdominal tenderness. He reports that he goes to sushi bars at least once a week. The following parasites have been observed in people who eat raw fish: *Anisakis, Pseudoterranova, Eustrongylides,* and *Angiostrongylus.* Which of the following would best differentiate the specific parasitic agent?

a. Antigen detection in tissues
b. Characteristic signs and symptoms
c. Identification of specific species of fish involved
d. Specific antibody tests
e. Study of distinctive morphology of the parasite

369. Several diagnostic tests for antibodies to *Toxoplasma* are directly compared for sensitivity and specificity against the sera of 100 healthy adults. While differences are apparent in the accuracy of the tests, it is able to conclude that 80% of those tested have IgG antibodies against *Toxoplasma.* Which of the following is most compatible in helping to explain this finding?

a. A variety of parasitic infections induce the formation of *Toxoplasma* antibody.
b. The IgM test is more reliable than the IgG test for determination of past infections; retesting for IgM would show that most people do not have *Toxoplasma* antibody.
c. The potential for *Toxoplasma* infection is widespread, and the disease is mild and self-limiting.
d. The test for *Toxoplasma* antibodies is highly nonspecific.
e. Toxoplasmosis is caused by eating meat; therefore, all meat eaters have had toxoplasmosis.

370. A 32-year-old gay man presents to his physician with nonbloody, foul-smelling, greasy stools 3 weeks after traveling to Mexico. While certain enteric protozoan and helminthic infections have been long related to contaminated food or water, sexual transmission of these diseases has produced a "hyperendemic" infection rate among gay males. Which of the following organisms is the most likely etiologic cause of this patient's diarrhea?

a. Amebiasis
b. Ascariasis
c. Enterobiasis
d. Giardiasis
e. Trichuriasis

371. Analysis of a patient's stool reveals small structures resembling rice grains; microscopic examination shows these to be proglottids. Which of the following is the most likely organism in this patient's stool?

a. *Ascaris lumbricoides*
b. *Enterobius vermicularis*
c. *Necator americanus*
d. *Taenia saginata*
e. *Trichuris trichiura*

372. An AIDS patient complains of headaches and disorientation. A clinical diagnosis of *Toxoplasma* encephalitis is made, and *Toxoplasma* cysts are observed in a brain section (see figure below). Which of the following antibody results would be most likely in this patient?

a. IgM nonreactive, IgG nonreactive
b. IgM nonreactive, IgG reactive (low titer)
c. IgM reactive (low titer), IgG reactive (high titer)
d. IgM reactive (high titer), IgG reactive (high titer)
e. IgM reactive (high titer), IgG nonreactive

373. A young boy from an impoverished area in Argentina presents to a public health clinic with Romana sign and a chagoma lesion. Several reduviid insects from the home are shown to the health care workers. In the chronic stage of this disease, where are the main lesions usually observed?

a. Digestive tract and respiratory tract
b. Heart and digestive tract
c. Heart and liver
d. Liver and spleen
e. Spleen and pancreas

374. A woman who recently returned from Africa complains of having paroxysmal attacks of chills, fever, and sweating. These attacks last a day or two at a time and recur every 36 to 48 hours. Examination of a stained blood specimen reveals ringlike and crescent-like forms within red blood cells. Which of the following is the most likely infecting organism?

a. *Plasmodium falciparum*
b. *Plasmodium vivax*
c. *Schistosoma mansoni*
d. *Trypanosoma gambiense*
e. *Wuchereria bancrofti*

Questions 375 and 376

375. A young man, who recently returned to the United States from Vietnam, has severe liver disease. Symptoms include jaundice, anemia, and weakness. Which of the following is the most likely etiologic agent shown in the photomicrographs?

a. *Clonorchis sinensis*
b. *Diphyllobothrium latum*
c. *Plasmodium falciparum*
d. *Taenia saginata*
e. *Taenia solium*

376. An intermediate form of the organism shown in the photomicrographs lives in which of the following?

a. Cows
b. Mosquitoes
c. Pigs
d. Snails
e. Ticks

377. A woman who recently traveled through Central Africa now complains of severe chills and fever, abdominal tenderness, and darkening urine. Her febrile periods last for 28 hours and recur regularly. Which of the following blood smears would most likely be associated with the symptoms described?

a. A
b. B
c. C
d. D
e. E

378. A physician, diagnosed with an HIV infection, is being treated with HAART medications; however, he also develops pneumocystosis. *Pneumocystis jiroveci* pneumonia is a treatable disease; therefore, rapid diagnosis is essential. Which of the following is the method of choice for detection of *P jiroveci* in respiratory specimens?

a. Culture in rat lung cells
b. Direct fluorescent antibody (DFA) microscopy
c. Indirect fluorescent antibody (IFA) microscopy
d. Methenamine-silver stain
e. Toluidine blue stain

379. A young woman reports to her physician with possible urinary tract infection. The doctor finds the vagina and cervix tender, inflamed, and covered with a frothy yellow discharge. Which of the following protozoa described in this case is known to exist only in the trophozoite stage?

a. *Balantidium coli*
b. *Entamoeba histolytica*
c. *Giardia lamblia*
d. *Toxoplasma gondii*
e. *Trichomonas vaginalis*

380. An international photographer returns to the United States from a global picture assignment. He is seen by his physician, giving his major complaint as diarrhea. Which of the following can be ruled out?

a. *Echinococcus granulosus*
b. *Dientamoeba fragilis*
c. *Diphyllobothrium latum*
d. *Giardia lamblia*
e. *Leishmania donovani*

381. A "parasite" that most clearly resembles a fungus when examined by molecular techniques is the initial clinical manifestation in up to 60% to 90% of patients with AIDS and is considered a gold standard in diagnosis for these individuals. Which of the following is this organism?

a. Blastocystis
b. Blastomyces
c. Cryptosporidium
d. Microsporidium
e. Pneumocystis

382. A medical technologist visits Scandinavia and consumes raw fish daily for 2 weeks. Six months after her return home, she has a routine physical and is found to be anemic. Her vitamin B_{12} levels were below normal. Which of the following is the most likely cause of her vitamin B_{12} deficiency anemia?

a. Cysticercosis
b. Excessive consumption of ice-cold vodka
c. Infection with *Diphyllobothrium latum*
d. Infection with Parvovirus B19
e. Infection with *Yersinia*

383. A renal transplant patient is admitted for graft rejection and pneumonia. A routine evaluation of his stool shows rhabditiform larvae. Subsequent follow-up reveals similar worms in his sputum. He has no eosinophils in his peripheral circulation. Which of the following is the most likely organism?

a. *Ascaris lumbricoides*
b. *Hymenolepis nana*
c. *Loa loa*
d. *Necator americanus*
e. *Strongyloides stercoralis*

384. A 56-year-old male immigrant from Bolivia complains of abdominal pain and cramping. He comments that 2 months previous to his current problems, he had numerous bloody stools every day. Physical findings include right upper quadrant pain over the liver with hepatomegaly, and a liver biopsy is performed. Which of the following parasites would most likely be identified in the liver biopsy?

a. *Acanthamoeba castellanii*
b. *Ascaris lumbricoides*
c. *Balantidium coli*
d. *Entamoeba histolytica*
e. *Taenia solium*

385. Human malarial infections start with the bite of a mosquito, and patients may experience the periodic paroxysms of this infection due to events that occur in the bloodstream. Up to one million deaths worldwide have been estimated annually. Which of the following control methods for this disease is currently most effective?

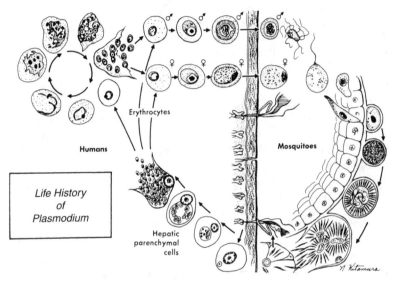

a. Antibiotics
b. A vaccine
c. Chemoprophylaxis
d. Tick repellents
e. White clothing

386. An African local clinic reports seeing increased cases of central nervous system involvement in patients. Genetically induced changes in the glycoprotein coat of which one of the following organisms enhances its escape from the host's immune antibody response by having genes that encode multiple, variant surface glycoproteins?

a. *Trichinella spiralis*
b. *Trichmonas vaginalis*
c. *Toxoplasma gondii*
d. *Trypanosoma gambiense*
e. *Leishmania donovani*

387. Human parasitic amoebas are usually ingested for transmission. In less acute disease, patients may experience abdominal tenderness, abdominal cramps, nausea, vomiting, and diarrhea. Which of the following best describes these intestinal amebas?

a. Infection with *E histolytica* is limited to the intestinal tract.
b. They are usually nonpathogenic.
c. They are usually transmitted as trophozoites.
d. They can cause peritonitis and liver abscesses.
e. They occur most abundantly in the duodenum.

388. *Schistosoma haematobium* is identified in an Egyptian farmer's infection, which has caused dermatitis, fever, and chronic filero-obstructive disease. These symptoms are the result of granulomatous reactions to the ova or to products of the parasite at the place of oviposition. Which of the following clinical manifestations can be routinely observed in these infections?

a. Arthropathies
b. Bladder wall hyperplasia
c. Cardiac abnormalities
d. Pulmonary embolism
e. Hemorrhagic cystitis

389. A boy scout troop goes camping in a New England forest area in the late spring. Two weeks later, several of the boys present with erythema migrans lesions but no other clinical manifestations. *Borrelia burgdorferi*, the causative agent of Lyme disease, has been isolated from a variety of ticks such as *I scapularis, Amblyomma, Dermacentor,* and *I pacificus*. Which of the following statements most accurately describes Lyme disease?

a. *Dermacentor* and *Amblyomma* are significant vectors of *B burgdorferi* to humans.
b. Dogs and cats are naturally immune to Lyme disease.
c. *Ixodes scapularis* and *I dammini* are different types of ticks.
d. Only a small percentage of people who get bitten by a tick develop Lyme disease.
e. White-tailed deer, an important reservoir for *I scapularis*, are dying because of Lyme disease.

390. A male patient in a tropical environment has eosinophilia during acute inflammatory episodes of his illness, but this is not considered to be the definitive diagnostic feature to determine what is causing his disease. Transmission of human parasites may occur via ingestion of contaminated food, water, snails, a variety of insects, and possibly even through pets or rat ectoparasites. Which of the following requires a mosquito for transmission?

a. Babesiosis
b. Bancroftian filariasis
c. Dog tapeworm
d. Guinea worm
e. Leishmaniasis

391. A Brazilian farmer presents to his medical clinic with hepatosplenomegaly with ascetic fluid in the peritoneal cavity. His liver is studded with white granulomas. He is treated with praziquantel. Which of the following organisms is endemic in Africa and South/Central America and is transmitted by skin penetration (by eggs with a large lateral spine), resulting in a dermatitis and katayama fever (serum sickness-like syndrome with fever, lymphadenopathy, and hematosplenomegaly)?

a. *Clonorchis sinensis*
b. *Paragonimus westermanni*
c. *Schistosoma haematobium*
d. *Schistosoma japonicum*
e. *Schistosoma mansoni*

392. The adults in a village in southern China suffer from fever, chills, mild jaundice, eosinophilia, and liver enlargement. Which of the following organisms may be ingested with raw fish, often resulting in an asymptomatic infection but, with a heavy infection, may cause biliary and bile duct obstruction and has an operculated egg?

a. *Clonorchis sinensis*
b. *Paragonimus westermanni*
c. *Schistosoma haematobium*
d. *Schistosoma japonicum*
e. *Schistosoma mansoni*

393. Which of the following organisms is endemic in Asia, and has a small lateral egg spine, and in chronic disease may result in hepatosplenic disease, portal hypertension, and liver granulomas?

a. *Clonorchis sinensis*
b. *Paragonimus westermanni*
c. *Schistosoma haematobium*
d. *Schistosoma japonicum*
e. *Schistosoma mansoni*

394. An African rice farmer, who depends on irrigation water from a regional lake, develops hematuria and dysuria severe enough to have concern for renal failure. Which of the following organisms has large terminal egg spines, may cause a chronic granulomatous bladder disease with urethral obstruction, chronic renal failure, and may be detected via eggs in the urine?

a. *Clonorchis sinensis*
b. *Paragonimus westermanni*
c. *Schistosoma haematobium*
d. *Schistosoma japonicum*
e. *Schistosoma mansoni*

395. Campers in a European forest area drink unfiltered stream water and later experience abdominal cramps with foul-smelling and greasy stools. *Giardia lamblia* infection can occur by ingesting as few as 10 eggs, resulting in asymptomatic cyst passage, self-limited diarrhea, or chronic diarrhea with associated malabsorption and weight loss. Since antimicrobial treatment is available, this infection is best diagnosed by which of the following?

a. Baermann technique
b. Dilution followed by egg count
c. Enzyme immunoassay (EIA)
d. Examination of a cellophane tape swab
e. Sigmoidoscopy and aspiration of mucosal lesions

396. Patients with *E histolytica* have an asymptomatic carrier rate greater than 90%. Chronic disease (intermittent bloody diarrhea and abdominal pain from months to years) is often difficult to distinguish from inflammatory bowel disease. *Entamoeba histolytica* infection is best diagnosed by which of the following?

a. Baermann technique
b. Dilution followed by egg count
c. Enzyme immunoassay (EIA)
d. Examination of a cellophane tape swab
e. Sigmoidoscopy and aspiration of mucosal lesions

397. Many patients with *Strongyloides* low worm burden are asymptomatic. Initial infection occurs by skin penetration and a pulmonary migration occurs. Patients demonstrate dry cough, wheezing, low-grade fever, dyspnea, and hemoptysis. Treatment is available for parasite eradication. Which is the best method listed below for detecting *Strongyloides* larvae?

a. Baermann technique
b. Dilution followed by egg count
c. Enzyme immunoassay (EIA)
d. Examination of a cellophane tape swab
e. Sigmoidoscopy and aspiration of mucosal lesions

398. *Ascaris lumbricoides* are large worms that have a complex life cycle in human hosts involving the digestive system, bloodstream, heart and liver, pulmonary circulation, and back to the small intestine. Serious medical complications may occur in any of these sites making diagnosis critical. *Ascaris* is best observed in human specimens by which one of the following?

a. Baermann technique
b. Dilution followed by egg count
c. Enzyme immunoassay (EIA)
d. Examination of a cellophane tape swab
e. Sigmoidoscopy and aspiration of mucosal lesions

399. A butcher develops a questionable habit of eating various kinds of raw, ground meat over several years. He eventually starts suffering from fatigue and lymphadenopathy. In his extensive physical examination, intensely white focal retinal lesions with vitritis are observed. Chorioretinitis is diagnosed, even though an older laboratory test, the Sabin-Feldman dye test, is found positive. This patient is found to be infected with which of the following?

a. Giardiasis
b. Schistosomiasis
c. Toxoplasmosis
d. Trichinosis
e. Visceral larva migrans

400. One week after eating bear meat, a fur trapper develops diarrhea, nausea, and vomiting. The next week, he experiences systemic symptoms of fever, myalgias, and malaise. His doctor notes periorbital edema and swollen eyelids, and laboratory tests report an eosinophilia. He is diagnosed with which of the following?

a. Giardiasis
b. Schistosomiasis
c. Toxoplasmosis
d. Trichinosis
e. Visceral larva migrans

401. A newspaper correspondent is sent to St Petersburg, Russia, to cover political events occurring there. She drinks only bottled water except on a side trip to the countryside to visit an old monastery. Two weeks later and at home, she develops a chronic diarrhea where the stools are watery, greasy, and foul smelling. Which of the following is the most likely diagnosis?

a. Giardiasis
b. Schistosomiasis
c. Toxoplasmosis
d. Trichinosis
e. Visceral larva migrans

402. A retired air force colonel has had abdominal pain for 2 years; he makes yearly freshwater fishing trips to Puerto Rico and often wades with bare feet into streams. Which of the following should be included in the differential diagnosis?

a. Giardiasis
b. Schistosomiasis
c. Toxoplasmosis
d. Trichinosis
e. Visceral larva migrans

403. A teenager who works in a dog kennel after school for 2 years has had a skin rash, eosinophilia, and an enlarged liver and spleen. Which of the following is the most likely cause of this infection?

a. Giardiasis
b. Schistosomiasis
c. Toxoplasmosis
d. Trichinosis
e. Visceral larva migrans

404. A young woman goes to her doctor with a variety of medical complaints. Her mucosal surfaces are tender, inflamed, eroded, and covered with a yellow discharge. For one problem, the laboratory reports the isolation of a pear-shaped protozoan with a jerky motility. This organism is observed in which of the following?

a. Biopsied muscle
b. Blood
c. Duodenal contents
d. Sputum
e. Vaginal secretions

405. A hunter, successful in his first black bear hunt, takes the meat home to eat. After consuming meals including bear meat over several weeks, two family members develop a flu-like syndrome and mild diarrhea. Several weeks later, two others have fever, GI distress, eosinophilia, muscle pain, and periorbital edema. Which of the specimens listed below would most easily detect the organism responsible for the clinical presentations described?

a. Biopsied muscle
b. Blood
c. Duodenal contents
d. Sputum
e. Vaginal secretions

406. A family of four goes on a vacation for 3 weeks to Central and South America. They consume the usual diets in all the areas they visit, including raw and pickled crustacean. Weeks later, two members produce brown sputum when coughing, hemoptysis, and eosinophilia, while the others are asymptomatic. A tissue-dwelling trematode causing this may be found in feces and which of the following?

a. Biopsied muscle
b. Blood
c. Duodenal contents
d. Sputum
e. Vaginal secretions

407. A forest ranger who routinely drinks untreated stream water and develops minor, intermittent diarrhea, which becomes chronic. Laboratory examination of several stools fail to determine any specific organism. Her physician decides to use the Entero-Test to try to discover the agent causing the symptoms. Cysts of a protozoan adhere to a piece of nylon yarn coiled in a gelatin capsule, which is swallowed. These cysts are usually found in which of the following?

a. Biopsied muscle
b. Blood
c. Duodenal contents
d. Sputum
e. Vaginal secretions

408. A person from Nantucket Island, Massachusetts, develops fever, fatigue, sweats, and arthralgia after hiking with friends in a forest. His physician finds evidence of tick bites that had not been noticed. A parasite resembling malaria that infects both animals and humans and is carried by the same tick that transmits *B burgdorferi* (the bacterium that causes Lyme disease) would most likely be observed in which of the following?

a. Biopsied muscle
b. Blood
c. Duodenal contents
d. Sputum
e. Vaginal secretions

409. A patient with AIDS returns from Haiti with acute diarrhea. The stool reveals an oval organism (8-9 μm in diameter) that is acid-fast and fluoresces blue under ultraviolet light. The most likely identification of this organism is which of the following?

a. *Cryptosporidium hominis*
b. *Cyclospora cayetanensis*
c. *Enterocytozoon bieneusi*
d. *Giardia lamblia*
e. *Prototheca wickerhamii*

410. A 64-year-old sheepherder from the farming region of central California is rushed to the emergency room in anaphylactic shock. The history, as told by the ambulance medic, is that the man was hit in the abdomen during a barroom brawl. Ultrasound reveals a large cyst mass in the liver. A cautious needle aspiration of the liver mass reveals "hydatid sand." Which of the following is the most likely agent involved?

a. *Ascaris lumbricoides*
b. *Clonorchis sinensis*
c. *Echinococcus granulosus*
d. *Fasciolopsis hepatica*
e. *Schistosoma mansoni*

Parasitology

Answers

359. The answer is c. *(Brooks, p 680. Levinson, pp 355, 371. Murray-2009, pp 840-841.)* Babesia is a tick-borne organism transmitted by *I scapularis*, the same tick that transmits Lyme disease. *Babesia* is often mistaken for *Plasmodia* (causative organism of malaria) on a blood smear. Patients become anemic and develop hepatosplenomegaly, but patients who are asplenic are at a much greater risk. Transfusion recipients, foresters, and immunosuppressed patients may be at risk of acquiring disease but not to the same extent as those patients who have been splenectomized.

360. The answer is c. *(Brooks, p 681. Levinson, pp 358-359. Murray-2009, pp 829-830. Ryan, p 702.)* The figure presented in the question shows a *Cryptosporidium* oocyst stained with a fluorescent-labeled specific antibody. *Cryptosporidium* may also be stained with a modified acid-fast stain but are not acid-fast bacilli. Microsporum (phylum Microspora) are a group of intracellular parasites characterized by a unicellular spore containing a coiled springlike polar filament through which the sporoplasm is discharged into a host cell. All vertebrates (especially fish) and many insect groups are infected. Human infection is by ingestion of spores in food or water. Many infections were shown to occur in AIDS patients. *Enterocytozoon* is one example. Few of the sporozoans are acid-fast nor related to yeasts in any way. They are smaller than *Cyclospora*, which are yeast size, but larger than *Enterocytozoon*, one of the microsporidia.

361. The answer is b. *(Brooks, p 680. Levinson, pp 371-372. Murray-2009, pp 830-832.)* Cyclosporiasis is a newly recognized food- and waterborne infectious disease associated with eating contaminated berries imported from some Central American countries. *Cyclospora* are moderately acid-fast but twice the size of *Cryptosporidium*. Patients usually have frequent diarrhea for up to 3 weeks and usually suffer only malaise and fatigue. The disease is self-limiting, but relapses can occur. *Isospora* infection in the United States occurs primarily in patients with AIDS. *Isospora* cysts also autofluoresce and stain acid-fast but are at least twice the size of *Cyclospora* oocysts. *Escherichia coli* and *Vibrio* species are true bacteria and are not considered parasites, per se. They are capable of causing a similar disease presentation and would be one of the potential agents to be considered at the beginning of medical treatment.

362. The answer is a. *(Brooks, pp 682-683. Levinson, pp 365-366. Murray-2009, pp 841-844. Ryan, pp 722-727.)* *Toxoplasma gondii* is a coccidian protozoan of worldwide distribution that infects a wide range of animals and birds, and the infections are mostly asymptomatic. The final normal host appears to be cats, the only host in which the oocysts-producing sexual stage of *Toxoplasma* can develop. *Toxoplasma gondii* may be acquired by inhalation of oocysts in cat feces. It is difficult to control the habits of cats unless they are housed and not let out. Pregnant human females should avoid changing cat litter boxes. While ingestion of oocysts in raw meat may also lead to toxoplasmosis, inhalation of oocysts is the primary cause, particularly among pregnant women in the United States. In the host's duodenum, eight sporozoites are released. They invade other cells, especially macrophages, where trophozoites break out and spread the infection to lymph nodes and other organs. The organism in humans produces either congenital or postnatal toxoplasmosis. Treatment is pyrimethamine and sulfadiazine.

363. The answer is a. *(Brooks, pp 672, 674. Levinson, pp 355, 371. Murray-2009, pp 803, 844-845. Ryan, p 733.)* *Acanthamoeba* is a free-living ameba, as is *Naegleria*. *Naegleria* usually causes severe, often fatal, meningoencephalitis, while *Acanthamoeba* is uncommonly isolated from contact lens fluid and patients with retinitis who do not store their lenses under sterile conditions. *Acanthamoeba* can be grown on nonnutrient agar plates using *E coli* as a food source. They are identified microscopically with use of a nonspecific fluorescent stain. Entry of *Acanthamoeba* into the CNS can occur from skin ulcers or traumatic penetration. Diagnosis is by examination of the CNS, which contains trophozoites and RBCs but no bacteria. *Naegleria*, also a free-living amoeba, produces an explosive, rapid brain infection. *Babesia* are widespread animal parasites, transmitted by ticks. *Entamoeba coli* is ingested and invade the intestinal epithelium. *Pneumocystis jiroveci* (not *P carinii*) causes pneumonia in immunocompromised patients. This agent may be an obligate member of the normal flora.

364. The answer is c. *(Brooks, pp 674-679. Levinson, pp 361-365. Murray-2009, pp 838-839. Ryan, p 712.)* *Plasmodium falciparum* infection is distinguished by the appearance of ring forms of early trophozoites and gametocytes, both of which can be found in the peripheral blood. The size of the RBC is usually normal. Double dots in the rings are common. Irregular edges of the infected RBC do not appear to be a reliable or important diagnostic feature. There are usually more that 12 merozoites (8-32) in *P falciparum*-infected RBCs, and these are rare in peripheral blood. Schüffner dots are found in *P vivax* and *P ovale* infections. *Plasmodium falciparum* peripheral smears show small, delicate-appearing ring trophozoites. *Plasmodium vivax* and *P ovale* produce thicker and larger ring trophozoites.

Synopsis of Malaria			
Infective Stage of Etiologic Agent	Location of Pathogenic Stage	Laboratory Diagnosis Based on Identification of:	Drugs Used in Treatment
Sporozoite (injected by mosquito) of: P vivax P malariae P falciparum P ovale	Liver (primary schizogony) Erythrocytes (schizogonic cycle)	 Blood smears (stages in erythrocytes)	*Prophylaxis* mefloquine *Acute* chloroquine *Chloroquine –resistant* quinine or pyrimethamine +sulfadoxine *Antirelapse* primaquine

(Reproduced, with permission, from Toy EC, DeBord C, Wanger A, et al. Case Files: Microbiology. 2nd ed. New York, NY: McGraw-Hill; 2008:342.)

365. The answer is c. *(Brooks, p 660. Levinson, pp 355-358. Murray-2009, pp 824-826. Ryan, pp 745-748.) Giardia* exists in both trophozoite and cyst form. The "trophs" are fragile and not commonly seen in stools. The cysts are infectious. *Giardia* is the most common parasitic disease in the United States. It is commonly contracted from drinking cyst-contaminated water. Chlorine does not kill *Giardia* cysts, but contaminated water can be made cyst-free by filtration. *Clonorchis* is a trematode and has a soft-bodied syncytial shape (flatworms) and are called flukes. *Clonorchis sinensis* is a fish fluke with a snail host in its life cycle. *Entamoeba* are common parasites of the human large intestine and have no flagella on the active amoeba. *Pneumosystis* was thought to be a protozoan but molecular biology studies have proved it to be a fungus. *Trichomonas* are flagellar protozoa with 3 to 5 anterior flagella and an undulating membrane.

366. The answer is e. *(Brooks, p 660. Levinson, pp 357-358. Murray-2009, pp 824-826. Ryan, pp 745-748.)* *Giardia lamblia* is the only common protozoan found in the duodenum and jejunum. Trophozoites are commonly found in the duodenum and do not penetrate the tissues. Four nuclei cysts (infective stage) can remain viable for up to 4 months. Excystation is via digestive enzymes. The mechanical irritation to tissues leads to diarrhea, with increased fat and mucus in the foul-smelling stool. Malabsorption syndrome (vitamin A and fats) leads to weight loss, anorexia, electrolyte imbalance, and abdominal cramps. Children and immunocompromised individuals are most significantly affected. Giardiasis should be considered in the differential diagnosis of any "traveler's diarrhea." *Entamoeba* species are common parasites of the human large intestines. Mucosal surfaces have discrete ulcers. Trophozoites and RBCs are found in liquid stools and can be identified by microscopy. *Ascaris lumbricoides* use a common round-worm found in the small intestine with larvae in the lungs. *Balantidium coli* is the largest intestinal protozoan found in humans. It is a ciliated, oval organism 60×45 μm or larger. Cysts are passed in human stools and infections occur in areas of poor sanitation and crowding. *Enterobius vermicularis* is the common pinworm, with an anal-oral transmission (self-contamination occurs regularly).

367. The answer is c. *(Brooks, pp 689, 694. Levinson, pp 373-376. Murray-2009, pp 881-884. Ryan, pp 793-797.)* Both beef tapeworm (*T saginata*) and pork tapeworm (*T solium*) can, in the adult form, cause disturbances of intestinal function. Intestinal disorder is due not only to direct irritation but also to the action of metabolic toxic wastes. In addition, *T saginata*, because of its large size, may produce acute intestinal blockage. Unlike

T saginata, T solium produces cysticercosis, which results in serious lesions in humans. In *T saginata*, the cysticercus—encysted larvae stage—develops only in cattle. The eggs of both *Taenia* species are identical, indicating similar reactions on intestinal mucosa. Death of the beef tapeworm larvae releases antigenic material that stimulates a marked inflammatory reaction (fever, muscle pain, and eosinophilia).

368. The answer is e. (*Brooks, pp 686-689t. Levinson, pp 393-394.*) The consumption of raw fish products in Asian restaurants, especially the growing popularity of sushi and sashimi, has led to a variety of infections, most of which are characterized by symptoms consistent with intestinal blockage or meningitis. The parasites are tissue nematodes and parasites of marine mammals. Fish, squid, and other edible marine life are often secondary hosts. The most reliable way to differentiate the specific helminth is by examination of the whole worm or by histologic examination of the parasites in tissue sections. There does not appear to be a great deal of reliable information on nematode antigen differentiation products or procedures, differences in signs and symptoms (S/S), relationship of fish species versus nematode species, or specific antibody tests that could reliably detect and identify the various nematode parasites listed in the question.

369. The answer is c. (*Brooks, pp 682-683. Levinson, pp 365-366, 518. Murray-2009, pp 841-844. Ryan, pp 722-727.*) Serologic tests, such as the Sabin-Feldman dye test and indirect immunofluorescence, have shown that a high percentage of the world's population has been infected with *T gondii*. In adults, clinical toxoplasmosis usually presents as a benign syndrome resembling infectious mononucleosis. However, fetal infections are often severe and associated with hydrocephalus, chorioretinitis, convulsions, and death. Acute toxoplasmosis is best diagnosed by an IgM capture assay. In most patients, specific IgM antibody disappears within 3 to 6 months. Obviously, *Toxoplasma* infection is widespread in animal and bird hosts but does not appear to cause disease in them. Congenital infection occurs only when the nonimmune mothers are infected during pregnancy. Most human infections are asymptomatic. Fatal infections may develop in AIDS patients. *Toxoplasma* antigens do not appear to cross-react with many of the other parasites' antigens. IgM and IgG antibodies can be detected with equal reliability. IgM levels drop eventually while IgG antibodies may be measured for years. The diagnostic test for *Toxoplasma*, in order to be approved for use, must be highly specific and sensitive. There is no evidence that *Toxoplasma* is spread by water.

370. The answer is d. *(Brooks, p 660. Levinson, pp 357-358. Murray-2009, pp 824-826. Ryan, pp 745-748. Toy, p 314.)* The infection rate with *G lamblia* in male homosexuals has been reported to be from 21% to 40%. These high-prevalence rates are probably related to three factors: the endemic rate, the sexual behavior that facilitates transmission (the usual barriers to spread have been interrupted), and the frequency of exposure to an infected person. Amebiasis is infection with amoebas and asymptomatic cyst carriers exist, forming part of a pool that potentially could contribute to this problem. However, the foul-smelling greasy stools point to *Giardia*. *Ascaris* is a nematode worm that also inhabits the intestine of vertebrates. This life cycle includes swallowing eggs (from contaminated water), hatching of eggs in the intestine, migration of nematode to the lungs, and finally reaching the duodenum. Diarrhea episodes do not appear to be routinely reported in this infection. *Enterobius vermicularis* infections are noted for perirectal irritation and pruritis, not diarrhea episodes. Trichuriasis (whipworm) transmission is via fecally contaminated soil, not person to person.

371. The answer is d. *(Brooks, pp 686, 690. Levinson, pp 373-376. Murray-2009, pp 881-884. Ryan, pp 793-795. Toy, pp 314, 332.)* *Enterobius* (pinworm), *Ascaris* (roundworm), *Necator* (hookworm), and *Trichuris* (whipworm) are roundworms, or nematodes. *Taenia saginata* (tapeworm), a segmented flatworm, affects the small intestine of humans. Tapeworm segments, called *proglottids*, appear in the stool of infected persons. The *Taenia* group of tapeworms are considered to be the large (3-10 m in length) ones that infect humans. "Measly pork" contain bladderlike larvae (cysticerci) which are the size of rice grains. These develop into giant tapeworms in the intestine and egg-filled terminal proglottids break off and are eliminated in the feces. *Ascaris lumbricoides*, the giant roundworm of humans, infects more than one billion people. *Enterobius vermicularis* is the pinworm, where anal irritation causes anal-oral transmission by contaminated fingers. *Necator* species are hookworms which enter skin directly from infected soil. *Trichuris* (whipworm) also is transmitted by ingestion of eggs from feces-contaminated soil.

372. The answer is b. *(Brooks, pp 682-683. Levinson, pp 365-366, 518. Murray-2009, pp 841-844. Ryan, pp 722-727.)* One of the leading causes of death among AIDS patients is central nervous system toxoplasmosis. It is thought that *Toxoplasma* infection is a result of reactivation of old or preexisting toxoplasmosis. Occasionally, the infection may be acquired by needle sharing. Because the disease is a reactivation of old or preexisting toxoplasmosis, routine quantitative tests for IgM antibody are usually negative, and IgG titers are low (≤1:256, IFA). More sophisticated methods, such as IgM capture or IgG avidity, may reveal an acute response.

373. The answer is b. *(Brooks, pp 663-666. Levinson, pp 366-368. Murray-2009, pp 850-852. Ryan, pp 695, 757-760.)* American trypanosomiasis (Chagas disease) is produced by *T cruzi*, which is transmitted to humans by the bite of an infected reduviid bug. They are introduced when infected bug feces are rubbed into the conjuctiva, the bug bite, or a break in the skin. Infants are often infected and demonstrate a unilateral swelling of the eyelids (Romana sign). After multiplication, the tissues most likely to be affected in the chronic stage of the disease are the cardiac muscle fibers and the digestive tract. A diffuse interstitial fibrosis of the myocardium results and may lead to heart failure and death. The inflammatory lesions in the digestive tract that are seen in the esophagus and colon produce considerable dilatation. Chagas disease has not been an important disease in the United States; most cases have been imported, although there are a few reports of endogenous disease in the southern United States. The other organs may be affected, but not at the rate the heart and digestive tract are invaded.

374. The answer is a. *(Brooks, pp 674-679. Levinson, pp 361-365. Murray-2009, pp 835-839. Ryan, p 712.)* The febrile paroxysms of *Plasmodium malariae* malaria occur at 72-hour intervals; those of *P falciparum* and *P vivax* malaria occur every 48 hours. The paroxysms usually last 8 to 12 hours with *P vivax* malaria but can last 16 to 36 hours with *P falciparum* disease. In *P vivax*, *P ovale*, and *P malariae* infections, all stages of development of the organisms can be seen in the peripheral blood; in malignant tertian (*P falciparum*) infections, only early ring stages and game-tocytes are usually found. *Schistosoma*, *Trypanosoma*, and *Wucheria* infections do not present with periodic symptoms in their disease progressions.

375. The answer is a. *(Brooks, pp 692-693. Levinson, p 382. Murray-2009, pp 874-875. Ryan, pp 807-808.)* The Chinese liver fluke, *C sinensis*, is a parasite of humans that is found in Japan, China, Korea, Taiwan, and Indochina. It has recently been renamed *Opisthorchis sinensis;* either name may appear in texts or the literature. Humans usually are infected by eating uncooked fish. The worms invade bile ducts and produce destruction of liver parenchyma. Anemia, jaundice, weakness, weight loss, and tachycardia may follow. Treatment is likely to be ineffectual in heavy infections, but chloroquine can destroy some of the worms. *Diphyllobothrium latum,* the fish tapeworm, travels from copepod to frog to water snail or rodent to a carnivore. *Diphyllobothrium latum* absorbs vitamin B_{12}, causing a host vitamin deficiency. *Plasmodium* species are transmitted via a mosquito vector. *Taenia* species are transmitted by ingestion of undercooked, larvae-containing beef or pork.

376. The answer is d. *(Brooks, pp 692-693. Levinson, p 382. Murray-2009, pp 874-875. Ryan, pp 807-808.)* The life cycle of *C sinensis (O sinensis)* is similar to that of other trematodes. A mollusk is characteristically the first intermediate host of trematodes. For *C sinensis,* snails perform this role. Cows and pigs are intermediate hosts for *Taenia* species. Mosquitoes serve as intermediate hosts for *Plasmodium* species. Ticks are not intermediate hosts for *Clonorchis* species.

377. The answer is b. *(Brooks, pp 674-679. Levinson, pp 361-365. Murray-2009, pp 838-839. Ryan, pp 711-722.)* The case history presented in the question is characteristic of infection with *P falciparum,* the causative agent of malignant tertian malaria. The long duration of the febrile stage rules out other forms of malaria. The presence of ringlike young trophozoites and crescent-like mature gametocytes—as represented in the illustration below—as well as the absence of schizonts is diagnostic of *P falciparum* malaria. Answer option A represents only RBCs and C represents trypanosomes and RBCs. Choice D represents a microfilarium and RBCs while E exhibits crenellated RBCs (round RBCs into shrunken, starry forms).

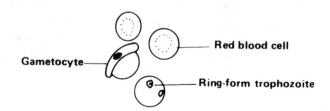

378. The answer is b. *(Brooks, pp 648-649. Levinson, pp 82, 366. Murray-2009, pp 638, 772-773. Ryan, pp 685-689.)* Both methenamine-silver and toluidine blue stain pneumocysts nonspecifically. These preparations are difficult to read because background material may nonspecifically stain black or blue. *Pneumocystis jiroveci* cannot be routinely cultured from human specimens. Both IFA and DFA tests are FDA-approved and available for detection of *P jiroveci*. The advantage of DFA is that it is quicker (45-60 minutes vs 3 hours), and there is less nonspecific fluorescence observed in the preparation. Recent evidence suggests that *Pneumocystis* is a fungus. Polymerase chain reaction (PCR), in sputum especially, increases sensitivity but reduces specificity. *Pneumocystis* cannot be cultured, either in cell culture preparations or by using artificial media that will allow other fungi to grow.

379. The answer is e. *(Brooks, pp 661-662. Levinson, pp 356-360. Murray-2009, pp 826-827. Ryan, pp 742-745.)* *Trichmonas vaginalis* is the only protozoan listed where the trophozoite is the diagnostic and infective stage that feeds on the mucosal surface of the vagina (bacteria and leukocytes). The trophozoite possesses a short, undulating membrane (one-half of the body) and four anterior flagella. No cyst stage exists. A persistent vaginitis with a frothy and foul-smelling discharge with burning, itching, and increased frequency of urination is common. Three to six million women in the United States are infected annually, while males are usually asymptomatic. Wet mounts examined in the laboratory reveal trophozoites with rapid, jerky, and nondirectional motion. *Balantidium coli* is a fish tapeworm. *Entamoeba histolytica* is an intestional amoeba. *Giardia lamblia* is a flagellated protozoan found in the duodenum and jejunum of humans. *Toxoplasma gondii* is a coccidian protozoan especially important in congenital infections when the pregnant woman becomes infected during pregnancy.

380. The answer is a. *(Brooks, pp 686t, 694. Levinson, pp 378-382. Murray-2009, pp 886-887. Ryan, pp 799-801.)* *Echinococcus granulosus* causes hydatid disease. The definitive hosts are dogs. Sheep, cattle, and humans are intermediate hosts. The adult tapeworm does not occur in humans. In the herbivores (infected by grazing where eggs have been deposited by carnivore feces) the eggs hatch and release hexacanths. These penetrate the gut and pass to other tissues (liver, viscera, muscle, and brain). Humans are only infected from dog feces and develop hydatid cysts, as described for herbivores. Diarrhea, therefore, does not occur with *E granulosis* human infections, whereas the other four choices can routinely present with diarrhea.

381. The answer is e. (*Brooks, pp 648-649. Levinson, pp 82, 366. Murray-2009, pp 638, 772-773. Ryan, pp 685-689.*) One of the multiple criteria for classification of AIDS is the development of PCP. *Pneumocystis* is a fungus formerly thought to be a parasite that was classified with the sporozoa. PCP may also be seen in patients with congenital or other acquired cellular immune dysfunction. Most patients with AIDS are given prophylactic aerosolized pentamidine or TMP-SMX for PCP. PCP is easily diagnosed in respiratory secretions by a DFA test. Both the microsporidia and *Cryptosporidium* are intestinal parasites that also infect patients with AIDS, but these microorganisms cause protracted diarrhea. Both *Blastocystis* and *Blastomyces* are yeasts and should not be confused with *Pneumocystis* or each other.

382. The answer is c. (*Brooks, pp 695. Levinson, pp 376-377. Murray-2009, pp 884-886. Ryan, pp 797-798.*) Consumption of raw fish causes endemic diphyllobothriasis in Scandinavia and the Baltic countries. While most people do not become ill, a small percentage (2%) develops vitamin B_{12} deficiency anemia. The adult fish tapeworm has an affinity for vitamin B_{12} and may induce a serious megaloblastic anemia. Parvovirus B19 causes acute hemolytic anemia primarily in immunosuppressed patients. *Yersinia* infection is common in Scandinavia but is not fish-borne and does not cause anemia. The larval stage of *T solium* is called *cysticercus*. Humans usually acquire cysticercosis by ingestion of food and water contaminated by infected human feces. Excessive consumption of ice-cold vodka may lead to headaches and memory loss, but otherwise has nothing to do with parasitemia.

383. The answer is e. (*Brooks, pp 688-691. Levinson, pp 387, 390. Murray-2009, pp 860-862. Ryan, pp 763, 774-777. Toy p 314.*) Strongyloidiasis may be observed in three phases: cutaneous, pulmonary, and intestinal. The pulmonary presentation of *Strongyloides* in patients with AIDS is the most common. Often, all body fluids will contain larvae. Prognosis is poor. *Necator* must be distinguished from *Strongyloides* by microscopy. Gross appearances are similar. *Ascaris* is a common roundworm which can be found in the small intestine and lungs, but not in all body fluids. *Hymenolepis* species are tapeworms, found only in the small intestine. Loiasis is an infection transmitted by the bite of deer flies found in equatorial Africa. They invade subcutaneous tissue and are migratory. Microfilariae are also found in the blood.

384. The answer is d. *(Brooks, pp 669-672. Levinson, pp 354-357, 517. Murray-2009, pp 822-824. Toy, p 314.)* *Entamoeba histolytica* is a pathogenic species that is capable of causing disease, such as colitis or liver abscess, in humans. *Entamoeba dispar* is indistinguishable from *E histolytica* by usual laboratory tests but only exists in humans as an asymptomatic carrier state and does not cause colitis. Infection with *E histolytica* is prevalent in Central and South America, southern and western Africa, the Far East, and India. Poor sanitation and lower socioeconomic conditions favor the spread of the disease. In the United States, those who travel to endemic areas, homosexual males, and institutionalized persons are at increased risk of infection. *Acanthamoeba* species are free-living amebas in soil and water and usually cause infections of skin, encephalitis, and kerititis. *Ascaris* is a nematode and is transmitted by ingestion. They hatch in the small intestine, and larvae migrate to the pulmonary alveoli. From here, they induce a cough and are swallowed by the host, maturing in the small intestine. *Balantidium coli* is a ciliate, infecting the lining of the large intestine, cecum, and terminal ilium. *Taenia* species (beef and pork) are ingested in undercooked meat. Only *T solium* (pork) may occasionally involve liver if cystericercosis occurs.

385. The answer is c. *(Brooks, pp 674-680. Levinson, pp 361-365. Murray-2009, pp 835-838. Ryan, pp 711-722.)* Prophylaxis for malaria should be considered whenever a person is traveling in a malaria-endemic area. Drugs consist of mefloquine or chloroquine and Fansidar. Other control measures such as draining swamps, protective clothing (although white clothing is not more protective than any other color, long sleeves and long trousers are beneficial) and netting, and insect repellents are also effective. There is no currently available vaccine for malaria. There are various drugs that can be used to treat active malaria (chloroquine [Aralen], see above). Antibiotics may be useful against bacteria but have no effect on the *Plasmodium* species. Tick repellents would not be useful since only mosquitoes are malarial vectors.

386. The answer is d. *(Brooks, pp 663-668. Levinson, pp 366-369. Murray-2009, pp 848-852. Ryan, p 902.)* African trypanosomiasis (sleeping sickness) is caused by *T brucei gambiense* and *T brucei rhodensiense* and transmitted by tsetse flies. From the fly's salivary glands, the trypomastigotes enter the host's blood and lymph and eventually the CNS. The trypomastigotes reproduce by binary fission and are infective for biting tsetse flies. During the course of trypanosome infection, the number of parasites in the blood and lymph tissues fluctuates according to the host's immune response. An increase in parasite number is related to the proliferation of parasite sub-populations that express an antigenically new or variant glycoprotein coat. Each parasite carries genes encoding multiple, variant surface glycoproteins (VSG) with only one VSG being expressed at any one time. These changes lead to evasion of the immune system and produce challenges for vaccine development. The other parasites listed do not exhibit this ability to change surface glycoproteins.

387. The answer is d. (*Brooks, pp 669-671. Levinson, pp 354-357, 517. Murray-2009, pp 822-824. Ryan, pp 733-738.*) Of the intestinal amebas, *E hartmanni, E coli, E polecki,* and *E nana* are considered nonpathogenic. *Entamoeba histolytica* is distinctively characterized by its pathogenic potential for humans, although infection with this protozoan is commonly asymptomatic (causing "healthy carriers"). Symptomatic amebiasis and dysentery occur when the trophozoites invade the intestinal wall and produce ulceration and diarrhea. Peritonitis can occur, with the liver the most common site of extraintestinal disease. The life cycle of the *ameba* is simple by comparison. There is encystment of the troph, followed by excystation in the ileocecal region. The trophs multiply and become established in the cecum, where encystation takes place and results in abundant amebas, cysts, and trophozoites. Infection is spread by the cysts, which can remain for weeks or months in appropriately moist surroundings.

388. The answer is e. (*Brooks, pp 665, 688. Levinson, pp 379-382. Murray-2009, pp 876-879. Ryan, pp 803, 808-813.*) Although the chronic stage of proliferation within tissues is distinctive in the different forms of schistosomiasis, a granulomatous reaction to the eggs and chemical products of the schistosome occurs in all forms of the disease. *Schistosoma haematobium* commonly involves the distal bowel and the bladder, as well as the prostate gland and seminal vesicles. Bladder calcification and cancer may ensue. *Shaematobium haematobium* infection has the flukes located in the vesicular plexis, and granulomatous formations occur in the bladder and ureters.

Hematuria is a common complaint. With prolonged infection, fibrosis, ureteral obstruction, and chronic renal failure may occur. *Schistosoma mansoni* affects the large bowel and the liver; presinusoidal portal hypertension, splenomegaly, and esophageal varices may be complications. Pulmonary hypertension, often fatal, may be seen with *S mansoni* and *S japonicum* disease. Eggs may be found in an unstained specimen of rectal mucosa or in stool. Urine microscopy and liver biopsy, when warranted, often prove positive. Schistosomiasis is best prevented by the elimination of the parasite in snails before human infection occurs.

389. The answer is d. (*Brooks, pp 337-339. Levinson, pp 176-177. Murray-2009, pp 411-414. Ryan, pp 434-437.*) In the United States, *B burgdorferi*, the causative agent of Lyme disease, has two principal vectors: *I scapularis* in the eastern and midwestern United States and *I pacificus* in the western United States. The ticks are tiny and can easily be missed. Fortunately, relatively few people who are bitten by ticks develop Lyme disease. Lyme disease, usually with joint involvement, is also seen in veterinary patients such as dogs, cats, and horses. White-tailed deer and small rodents are an important reservoir for these ticks. *Borrelia burgdorferi* has been isolated from mosquitoes and *Dermacentor* and *Amblyomma* ticks, as well as from several *Ixodes* species. However, the isolation of the bacterium from these ticks is not sufficient evidence to indicate that they transmit the disease to humans.

390. The answer is b. (*Brooks, pp 687, 692. Levinson, pp 392-393. Murray-2009, pp 863-865. Ryan, pp 695-779, 784-785.*) *Wuchereria bancrofti* is the cause of bancroftian filariasis or filarial elephantiasis. Control of the mosquito vectors (culex, anopheles, and Aedes) is the most significant mechanism to control human infections. A disease of the tropics and subtropics, adults live in the lymphatics of a host and cause lymph blockage of the feet, arms, genitals, and breasts. Enlargement of the affected body part (elephantiasis) can then occur. Babesiosis is caused by tick-borne *Babesia microti*. Leishmaniasis is spread by a sandfly (Phlebotomus) vector. Guinea worms (*Dracunculus medinensis*) has an aquatic life cycle involving copepods (water fleas). Dog tapeworms would routinely be transmitted by fecal contamination.

391 to 394. The answers are 391-e, 392-a, 393-d, 394-c. (*Brooks, pp 685, 688, 693. Levinson, pp 379-382. Murray-2009, pp 871-880. Ryan,* *pp 803, 809-813.)* The life cycle of the medically important trematodes (or flukes) involves a sexual cycle in humans and an asexual cycle in snails. The schistosomes can penetrate the skin, whereas *Clonorchis* and *Paragonimus* are ingested, usually in fish or seafood. These flukes can be easily differentiated morphologically by the appearance of the egg. Schistosome eggs have an identifiable spine, and both *Clonorchis* and *Paragonimus* eggs are operculated; that is, they have what appears to be a cover that opens. Serological tests are not useful. Many patients with schistosomiasis are asymptomatic, but disease may become chronic, resulting in malaise, diarrhea, and hepatosplenomegaly (an enlarged liver and spleen). *Clonorchis* infection usually causes upper abdominal pain but can also cause biliary tract fibrosis. Paragonimiasis is characterized by a cough, often with bloody sputum, and pneumonia. Praziquantel is the treatment of choice for these flukes.

395 to 398. The answers are 395-c, 396-e, 397-a, 398-b. *(Brooks, pp 660-662, 669-674. Levinson, pp 357-358, 390. Murray-2009, pp 821-826, 853-855, 860-862. Ryan, pp 695-696, 733-738, 745-748, 769-771, 774-777. Toy, p 332.)* It is not uncommon that repeated stool specimens do not reveal the suspected parasite. Also, microscopic analysis of stool may not reveal parasite load when such data are necessary. For these reasons, other techniques are available to identify parasites as well as to quantitate them.

The diagnosis of giardiasis is usually made by detecting trophozoites and cysts of *G lamblia* in consecutive fecal specimens. Alternatively, a gelatin capsule on a string (enterotest) can be swallowed, passed to the duodenum, and then retrieved after 4 hours. The string is then examined for *Giardia*. A recent innovation is the introduction of an EIA for *G lamblia*. The EIA is more sensitive than microscopy, can be performed on a single stool specimen, and does not depend on the presence of entire trophozoites and cysts.

During sigmoidoscopy, a curette or suction device may be used to scrape or aspirate material from the mucosal surface. Cotton swabs should not be used. A direct mount of this material should immediately be examined for *E histolytica* trophozoites, and then a permanent stain made for subsequent examination.

The Baermann technique may be helpful in recovering *Strongyloides* larvae. Essentially, fecal material is placed on damp gauze on the top of a glass funnel that is three-quarters filled with water. The larvae migrate through the damp gauze and into the water. The water may then be centrifuged to concentrate the *Strongyloides*.

Worm burdens may be estimated by a number of microscopic methods. While not often done, such procedures may provide data on the extent of infection or the efficacy of treatment of hookworms, *Ascaris,* or *Trichuris.* Thirty thousand *Trichuris* eggs per gram, 2000 to 5000 hookworm eggs per gram, and one *Ascaris* egg are clinically significant and suggest a heavy worm burden.

A cellophane tape swab is used to trap pinworms crawling out of the anus during the night. The tape is then examined microscopically for *Enterobius.*

399. The answer is c. (*Brooks, pp 682-684. Levinson, pp 365-366. Murray-2009, pp 841-844. Ryan, pp 695-696, 723-727, 746-748, 779-784, 809-813.*) Toxoplasmosis is generally a mild, self-limiting disease; however, severe fetal disease is possible if pregnant women ingest *Toxoplasma* oocysts. Consumption of uncooked meat may result in either an acute toxoplasmosis or a chronic toxoplasmosis that is associated with serious eye disease. Most adults have antibody titers to *Toxoplasma*, and thus would have a positive Sabin-Feldman dye test. The Sabin-Feldman dye test measures antibodies that render the membrane of living *T gondii* impermeable to methylene blue (no staining occurs). It is being replaced by IFA and ELISA tests. While we usually think of in utero infections of a developing fetus and the subsequent medical difficulties of the newborn infant, an equally important source of human exposure is raw or undercooked meat in which infective tissue cysts are frequently found. When a tissue cyst ruptures, numerous bradyzoites are released and grow, causing chorioretinitis, myocarditis, and polymyositis. Treatment is with pyrimethamine and sulfadiazine. Schistosomiasis is caused by blood flukes whose cercariae (larvae) penetrate skin in snail-infested water. Trichinosis is caused by the trichina worm whose larvae are found in uncooked pork. Larva migrans consists of subcutaneous migrating larvae of hookworms.

400 to 403. The answers are 400-d, 401-a, 402-b, 403-e. (*Brooks, pp 660, 685, 687t, 691. Levinson, pp 357-358, 379-382, 390-391. Murray-2009, pp 824-826, 855-856, 862-863, 876-879. Ryan, pp 695-696, 723-727, 746-748, 779-784, 809-813.*) All the diseases listed in the question have significant epidemiologic and clinical features. Trichinosis most often is caused by ingestion of contaminated pork products. However, eating undercooked bear, walrus, raccoon, or possum meat also may cause this disease. Symptoms of trichinosis include muscle soreness and swollen eyes. The described symptoms of the fur trapper would not fit the clinical presentations of giardiasis, schistosomiasis, toxoplasmosis, or visceral larva migrans.

Although giardiasis has been classically associated with travel in Russia, especially St Petersburg (Leningrad), many cases of giardiasis caused by contaminated water have been reported in the United States as well. Diagnosis is made by detecting cysts in the stool. In some cases, diagnosis may be very difficult because of the relatively small number of cysts present. Alternatively, an EIA may be used to detect *Giardia* antigen in fecal samples. The symptoms that were experienced by the correspondent would not fit the clinical presentation of schistosomiasis, toxoplasmosis, trichinosa, or visceral larva migrans.

Schistosomiasis is a worldwide public health problem. Control of this disease entails the elimination of the intermediate host snail and removal of streamside vegetation. Abdominal pain is a symptom of schistosomiasis. The symptoms that were experienced by the colonel would not fit the clinical presentation of giardiasis, toxoplasmosis, trichinosa, or visceral larva migrans.

Visceral larva migrans is an occupational disease of people who are in close contact with dogs and cats. The disease is caused by the nematodes *Toxocara canis* (dogs) and *Toxocara cati* (cats) and has been recognized in young children who have close contact with pets or who eat dirt. Symptoms include skin rash, eosinophilia, and hepatosplenomegaly. The symptoms that were experienced by the teenager would not fit the clinical presentation of giardiasis, toxoplasmosis, trichinosa or schistosomiasis.

404 to 408. The answers are 404-e, 405-a, 406-d, 407-c, 408-b. (*Brooks, pp 660, 661-662, 680, 690, 693. Levinson, pp 357-360, 382-383, 390-391. Murray-2009, pp 824-827, 862-863, 875-876. Ryan, pp 695-696, 741-748, 779, 781-784, 803, 805-807.*) *Trichmonas vaginalis*, an odd-looking protozoan, moves with a jerky, almost darting motion. Trichomoniasis, a bothersome vaginal infection, can be diagnosed by observing this organism in a wet mount of vaginal secretions. It may be washed out in the urine as well. *Trichmonas vaginalis* can be grown in special media, and there are now several products available for direct detection of the organism.

Trichinella spiralis causes trichinosis, a parasitic disease that is usually mild and results in muscle pain and a mild febrile illness. However, fulminant fatal cases have been described. Humans, who are accidental hosts, become infected by ingesting cysts that are in the muscle of animals. Most infections still come from pork, although regulations on pig feeding have markedly reduced the incidence. Laboratory diagnosis is by serology or demonstration of the larvae in the muscle tissue.

Paragonimus westermani is a lung fluke. This trematode infects lung tissue and is seen not only in sputum but also in feces because infected patients swallow respiratory secretions. Paragonimiasis is contracted by ingesting the metacercariae that are encysted in crabs or crayfish.

Giardia infection may be difficult to diagnose by stool examination, as patients may shed the cysts intermittently. When symptoms persist and the stool examination is negative, then duodenal contents may be sampled directly with the enterotest. The patient swallows a gelatin capsule that contains a coiled string. The other end is attached to the patient's face. The gelatin capsule dissolves, and Giardia organisms, if present, adhere to the string within a 4-hour period. The string is retrieved and examined microscopically. Alternatively, an enzymatic immunoassay can detect Giardia antigen directly in a single specimen of feces.

Babesia is a sporozoan parasite transmitted by the bite of I scapularis, the same tick that carries B burgdorferi. Reproduction of this parasite occurs in erythrocytes and may resemble Plasmodium species when blood smears are examined. Babesia is endemic in the northeastern United States, particularly in the islands of Massachusetts. Laboratory diagnosis is made by examining blood smears for this parasite, or by detection of specific antibody. Babesiosis clinically resembles malaria.

409. The answer is b. (Brooks, p 680. Levinson, pp 371-372. Murray-2009, pp 830-832.) Coccidian-like bodies have been identified in stools of some patients with diarrhea. These organisms appear to be similar to blue-green algae and were referred to as Cyanobacterium-like until they were recently reclassified as Cyclospora. They are larger than the microsporidia and resemble neither Giardia nor Prototheca nor other algae-like organisms. Unlike Cryptosporidium, these organisms fluoresce under ultraviolet light. The diarrhea can be prolonged and relapsing, and the treatment is usually trimethoprim-sulfamethoxazole. See the figure for an illustration of G lamblia.

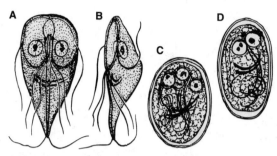

Giardia lamblia. A: "face" and B: "profile" of vegetative forms; C and D: cysts (binucleate [D] and quadrinucleate stages). 2000×
(Reproduced, with permission, from Brooks GF et al. Jawetz's Medical Microbiology. 24th ed. New York, NY: McGraw-Hill; 2007:660.)

410. The answer is c. *(Brooks, p 694. Levinson, p 377. Murray-2009, pp 886-889. Ryan, pp 799-801.)* *Echinococcus* is a small, three-segmented tapeworm found only in the intestines of dogs and other carnivores. Eggs leave these hosts and infect grazing animals. In the herbivore gut, the eggs hatch and the released forms penetrate the gut. Various organs (especially the liver) develop huge, fluid-filled cysts in which future scoleces form (hydatid sand). Dogs become infected when they feed on viscera of diseased sheep or cows. Hydatid disease in humans occurs only through ingestion of dog feces. Humans are only an intermediate host of this organism and never the final host. None of the other answer options are cestodes, or tapeworms.

Immunology

Questions

Questions 411 to 414

Hypersensitivity reactions are exaggerated or inappropriate immune responses that can sometimes result in damage to the host instead of providing protection. The four main types are represented below. Use these reactions to answer the following questions.

$C^* = $ complement

411. A 13-year-old male with cystic fibrosis develops repeated episodes of pneumonia resulting in multiple hospitalizations. Previous antibiotic treatment resulted in severe rash, fever, and systemic anaphylaxis almost immediately. A penicilloyl polylysine skin test yields positive results. Which of the following best illustrates the type of hypersensitivity reaction associated with this clinical scenario?

a. 1
b. 2
c. 3
d. 4

412. After playing in the bushes during a camping trip, a 7-year-old girl complains of intense itching and blistering of the hands, arms, and legs. Which of the following are the most likely medical condition and the correct hypersensitivity diagram from those presented above?

a. Contact dermatitis and 2
b. Contact dermatitis and 3
c. Contact dermatitis and 4
d. Arthus reaction and 1
e. Arthus reaction and 2
f. Arthus reaction and 3

413. Skin testing is useful in the diagnosis of which of the following?

a. 1 and 2
b. 1 and 3
c. 1 and 4
d. 2, 3, and 4

414. Rh disease and Goodpasture syndrome are best represented by which of the following?

a. 1 and 2
b. 2 and 3
c. 2 and 4
d. 2 only
e. 3 only

Questions 415 and 416

415. A 7-month-old male infant presents to the emergency department with severe middle ear and upper respiratory tract infections, which respond promptly to antibiotics. Two months later he is again admitted, this time with *Streptococcus pneumoniae* pneumonia. After several more episodes of bacterial infections, genetic testing is done and the presence of a defective B-cell tyrosine kinase gene (*btk* gene or *X-LA* gene) is revealed. In addition, physical examination detects very small tonsils. Which of the following is the most likely diagnosis?

a. Ataxia-telangiectasia
b. Bruton agammaglobulinemia
c. Chronic granulomatous disease
d. Late (C5, C6, C7, C8, C9) complement deficiency
e. Thymic aplasia (DiGeorge syndrome)

416. Which of the following pathogens presents the most serious threat to this child?

a. *Chlamydia trachomatis*
b. Measles virus
c. *Mycobacterium tuberculosis*
d. Varicella-zoster virus (VZV)

Questions 417 and 418

Flow cytometry of blood from an HIV-positive patient yielded a CD4:CD8 ratio less than 1.

417. This ratio best represents a major decline in which of the following cell types and its associated cell surface proteins?

a. B lymphocytes; MHC class I, IgM, B7, CD19, CD20
b. Cytotoxic T lymphocytes; MHC class I, TCR, CD3
c. Cytotoxic T lymphocytes; MHC class I, TCR, CD3, CD28
d. Helper T lymphocytes; MHC class I, TCR, CD3
e. Helper T lymphocytes; MHC class I, TCR, CD3, CD28
f. Macrophages; MHC class I, MHC class II, CD14

418. Which of the following best represents the "costimulatory signal" pair that occurs between cellular surface proteins associated with the reduced cell type represented in the CD4:CD8 ratio less than 1?

a. B7 (B cell) and CD28 (T cell)
b. B7 (B cell) and CD4 (T cell)
c. CD40L (B cell) and CD40 (T cell)
d. MHC class I (B cell) and CD4 (T cell)
e. MHC class II (B cell) and CD8 (T cell)

419. A young girl has had repeated infections with *Candida albicans* and respiratory viruses since she was 3 months old. As part of the clinical evaluation of her immune status, her responses to routine immunization procedures should be tested. In this evaluation, the use of which of the following vaccines is contraindicated?

a. Bacillus Calmette-Guerin (BCG)
b. Bordetella pertussis vaccine
c. Diphtheria toxoid
d. Inactivated polio
e. Tetanus toxoid

420. A 7-year-old male developed normally until 7 years of age, after which he suddenly starts suffering from progressive personality and intellect deterioration leading to dementia, and finally death within 1 year of symptoms. His history reveals a severe measles attack at the age of 1. Laboratory tests indicate elevated measles antibody levels in both the serum and cerebrospinal fluid (CSF) with no antibody to the M protein. A latent measles-like viral infection and, presumably, a defect in cellular immunity are associated with which of the following diseases?

a. Creutzfeldt-Jakob disease (CJD)
b. Epstein-Barr virus (EBV) infection
c. Multiple sclerosis (MS)
d. Progressive multifocal leukoencephalopathy (PML)
e. Subacute sclerosing panencephalitis (SSPE)

421. A 31-year-old patient suffering from recurrent episodic intestinal hemorrhages attributed to a severe form of Crohn disease decides to undergo surgery to resect his terminal ileum. The surgeon orders two units of blood to be preserved for possible use during the surgery. The patient decides to store one unit of his own blood and one unit of his 35-year-old brother's blood with the blood bank. This type of donation is most likely which of the following transplantation terminology (patient's blood:brother's blood)?

a. Allograft:allograft
b. Allograft:autograft
c. Autograft:allograft
d. Autograft:autograft
e. Autograft:isograft (syngeneic graft)

422. While learning to ride his tricycle, a young boy falls and scrapes his knee. About 3 weeks later he falls again, reinoculating the same wound with the same antigen. The following graph shows the sequential alteration in the type and amount of antibody produced after an immunization. (Inoculation of antigen occurs at two different times, as indicated by the arrows.) Curve A and curve B each represent a distinct type of antibody. The class of immunoglobulin represented by curve B has which of the following unique characteristics?

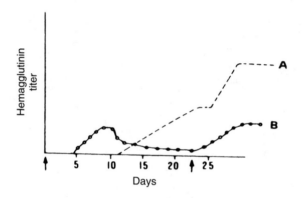

a. A composition of four peptide chains connected by disulfide links
b. A dimeric structure
c. An appearance in neonates at approximately the third month of life
d. An estimated molecular weight of 150,000
e. The human ABO isoagglutinin

423. A 27-year-old female presents to the emergency room with a temperature of 103°F, severe fatigue, weight loss, and joint pain. During the history and physical examination, the patient reports that she stopped taking her aspirin and corticosteroids to control her condition. A butterfly-type rash over her cheeks, sensitivity to light, and a heart murmur are apparent. The patient also reports a history of a progressively developing arthritis and glomerulonephritis. Laboratory tests further indicate anemia, leukopenia, and thrombocytopenia. This condition is best diagnosed by the presence of which of the following?

a. Anticentromere antibodies
b. Anti-dsDNA antibodies
c. Antimitochondrial antibodies
d. Antineutrophil antibodies
e. Anti-TSH receptor antibodies

424. A 29-year-old highly promiscuous male with a fever, rash, weight loss, general malaise, and a purulent urethral discharge presents to an STD clinic for the first time. Suspecting a gonococcal infection, the physician obtains a specimen and sends it to the laboratory for an initial enzyme-linked immunosorbent assay (ELISA) test, a widely used method for detecting antigen. The figure below demonstrates an ELISA for detection of antigen. One of the problems with ELISA is nonspecific reactivity due to nonspecific antibody present in the reaction. Of the four steps depicted, A, B, C, and D, which one may be the major cause of nonspecificity?

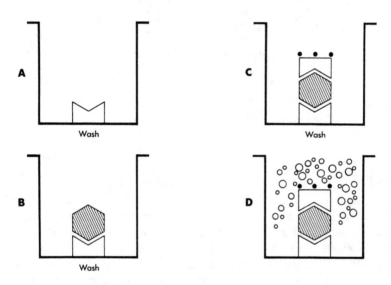

a. A
b. B
c. C
d. D

425. An Ouchterlony gel diffusion plate shows the reaction of a polyspecific serum against several antigen preparations. The center well in Figure 1 contains polyspecific antiserum, first bleed; the center well in Figure 2 contains polyspecific antiserum, second bleed; NS is normal saline. In this situation, cross-reaction can be recognized between antigen X and which of the following antigens?

Figure 1   Figure 2

a. A
b. B
c. C
d. D
e. E

426. A 1-year-old male patient presents with marked susceptibility to opportunistic infections with bacteria such as *Escherichia coli* and *Staphylococcus aureus* and fungal *Aspergillus*. Examination findings reveal granulomatous abscesses in the lungs, ataxia, nystagmus, and photophobia. Biochemical analysis reveals the deficiency of the central enzyme in the respiratory burst pathway via an inability to reduce nitroblue tetrazolium (NBT) dye. The deficient enzyme and reaction are represented by which of the following?

a. $NADPH + 2O_2 \xrightarrow{\text{NADPH oxidase}} NADP^+ + 2O_2^- + H^+$

b. $2O_2^- + 2H^+ \xrightarrow{\text{Superoxide dismutase}} H_2O_2 + O_2$

c. $H_2O_2 + Cl^- \xrightarrow{\text{Myeloperoxidase}} H_2O + OCl^-$

d. $\frac{1}{2}O_2 + \text{arginine} \xrightarrow{\text{NO synthase}} NO + \text{citrulline}$

e. $2H^+ + 2e^- + \frac{1}{2}O_2 \xrightarrow{\text{Oxidase}} H_2O$

f. $2H_2O_2 \xrightarrow{\text{Catalase}} 2H_2O + O_2$

427. Chromosomal analysis of a patient suffering from a lymphoma reveals the following result:

(Reproduced, with permission, from Parslow TG, et al. Medical Immunology. 10th ed. New York, NY: McGraw-Hill; 2001:113.)

According to the above figure, the patient has which of the following?

a. Anaplastic large cell lymphoma
b. Burkitt lymphoma
c. Follicular lymphoma
d. Mantle cell lymphoma

428. Which of the following statements best applies to the following diagram?

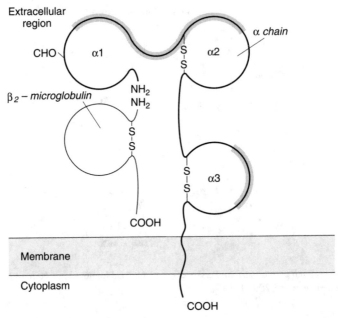

(Modified, with permission, from Parslow TG, et al. Medical Immunology. *10th ed. New York, NY: McGraw-Hill; 2001:85.)*

a. Depicts the cell-membrane MHC product associated with narcolepsy
b. Essential for the transplacental passage of antibody
c. Found on memory T and B lymphocytes
d. Present on macrophages but not neutrophils
e. Represents the secretory component associated with IgA
f. Required for recognition of processed antigen by TH1 and TH2 lymphocytes

429. A 19-year-old college student develops a rash. She works part-time in a pediatric AIDS clinic. Her blood is drawn and tested for specific antibody to the chicken pox virus (varicella-zoster). Which of the following antibody classes would you expect to find if she is immune to chicken pox?

a. IgG
b. IgA
c. IgM
d. IgD
e. IgE

Questions 430 to 432

430. A 34-year-old male patient visits a physician with complaints of fatigue, weight loss, night sweats, and "swollen glands." The physician observes that he has an oral yeast infection. Which of the following tests would most likely reveal the cause of the patient's problems?

a. A human T-lymphotropic virus type I (HTLV-I) test
b. A test for *C albicans*
c. A test for CD8 lymphocytes
d. A test for infectious mononucleosis
e. An HIV ELISA test

431. The figure below demonstrates a Western blot for HIV. Based on these results, and assuming a repeatedly reactive ELISA HIV screening test, which of the following is the best course of action?

gp 160
gp 120
p 66
p 51
gp 41
p 24
p 17

a. Consider anti-HIV therapy.
b. Inform the patient that the test is falsely positive.
c. Order an HIV RNA test.
d. Repeat the test immediately.
e. Wait for 6 weeks and repeat the test.

432. A 30-year-old male patient requests a routine HIV test. The HIV ELISA is weakly positive and is repeated with the same results. The Western blot result is as shown in the preceding figure. The patient denies any risk factors for HIV. Which of the following is the most likely cause of a falsely positive HIV test?

a. A recent flu shot
b. A yeast infection
c. Naturally occurring HIV antibody
d. Test cross-reactivity with Epstein-Barr virus
e. Test cross-reactivity with HTLV

433. Patients with C5 through C9 complement deficiencies are most likely to be susceptible to which of the following infections?

a. AIDS
b. Giardiasis
c. Histoplasmosis
d. Neisserial infection
e. Pneumococcal infection

434. As part of the management of a 28-year-old male with acute onset of Crohn disease of the small bowel, you decide to treat him with a new cocktail of mouse-human chimeric antibodies to reduce his intestinal inflammation and cachexia. To which of the following sets of proteins are these antibodies directed?

a. IL-1, IL-2, IL-3
b. IL-2, IL-12, TNF-α
c. IL-2, TGF-β, TNF-α
d. IL-1, IL-6, TNF-α
e. IL-2, IL-3, IL-12

435. A mother and newborn are exposed to a pathogen while at the hospital for a routine checkup and breastfeeding clinic. This same pathogen had infected the mother about a year previously, and she had successfully recovered from the subsequent illness. Immunity may be innate or acquired. Which of the following best describes acquired immunity with respect to the newborn?

a. Complement cascade
b. Increase in C-reactive protein (CRP)
c. Inflammatory response
d. Maternal transfer of antibody
e. Presence of natural killer (NK) cells

436. A 35-year-old male patient presents with numerous subcutaneous hemorrhages. History and physical examination reveals that he has been taking sedormid (a sedative) for the past week. Laboratory tests indicate normal hemoglobin and white blood cell levels with significant thrombocytopenia (very low platelet count). You suspect that he has developed a drug-induced type II hypersensitivity reaction. This reaction may occur if the drug does which of the following?

a. Activates T cytotoxic cells
b. Acts as a hapten
c. Induces mast cell degranulation, releasing mediators such as histamine, leukotrienes, and prostaglandins
d. Induces oxygen radical production through the respiratory burst pathway
e. Persists in macrophages

437. After learning of a family history of humoral immunity deficiency during an office visit from a patient 6 months pregnant, a radial immunodiffusion assay is ordered on fetal serum. The test reveals no humoral immunity problems and normal results in all respects. According to this test, the normal level of which fetally made immunoglobulin is the highest in the fetus?

a. IgA
b. IgD
c. IgE
d. IgG
e. IgM

438. Antibodies (immunoglobulins) are extremely important proteins involved in the adaptive immune response whose functions involve the neutralization of toxins and viruses, the opsonization of microbes, and the activation of complement. Which of the following best characterizes immunoglobulins?

a. Digestion of an IgG antibody molecule with papain yields two F(ab) arms, which are unable to agglutinate or precipitate antigen, by cleaving the antibody unit on the C terminus side of the sulfhydryl bridge binding the heavy chain.
b. In humans, there are approximately twice as many Ig molecules with κ than λ light chains.
c. In the three-dimensional structure of Ig, there is little if any flexibility in the hinge region between the Fc and two F(ab) portions.
d. Normally, IgG makes up 20% of the antibody concentration and migrates in the gamma globulin fraction of serum protein separation.
e. Pepsin digestion of an IgG molecule cleaves the antibody unit on the N terminus side of the sulfhydryl bridge binding the heavy chains.
f. The two arms of an antibody molecule are different in that they recognize different epitopes.

439. A 31-year-old male patient complains of fatigue, yeast infection in his mouth, and enlarged lymph nodes under his arms. He says that he was involved in "high-risk" behavior 6 years ago while on a trip to eastern and southern Africa. He also indicates that his "HIV test" was negative. Which of the following options is most appropriate?

a. Initiate treatment for HIV disease.
b. Order a test for human T-cell leukemia virus (HTLV).
c. Order an HIV-1 RNA PCR.
d. Order an HIV test that would include antibodies to HIV-1 and HIV-2.
e. Repeat the test for HIV-1.

440. A laboratory analysis report of a specific fraction of a patient's lymphocytes indicates the following:

HLA, B, and C+, PHA+, CD3−, CD16+, CD11a/CD18+, CD56+, and in vitro blastogenesis with IL-12

What are the lymphocytes this set describes?

a. B lymphocytes
b. Cytotoxic T lymphocytes
c. Natural killer cells
d. T helper 1 (TH1) subset
e. T helper 2 (TH2) subset

441. The complement system plays a key role in the host defense process. Which of the following components of this system is the most important in chemotaxis?

a. C1q
b. C3a
c. C3b
d. C4a
e. C5a

442. A 7-year-old child presents to your clinic during flu season with a severe headache, sinus congestion, fever, sore throat, and cough. Respiratory secretions reveal detectable levels of the cytokine interferon. Which of the following is the mechanism of action of this cytokine?

a. Binds extracellular virus particles and prevents cellular adherence.
b. Up regulates the synthesis of secretory proteins that bind and inhibit the virus particles.
c. Disrupts viral and cellular protein synthesis, leading to cellular apoptosis.
d. Inhibits viral protein synthesis by degrading viral mRNA.
e. Down regulates cellular protein synthesis, leading to decreased levels of viral receptors on the cytoplasmic membrane.

443. Soon after birth, a newborn undergoes heart transplantation surgery at a local medical center. Transplantation of tissue and organs is a common procedure whose success depends largely on the "self" versus "nonself" interactions. Survival of allografts is increased by choosing donors with few major histocompatibility complex (MHC) mismatches compared to recipients and by use of immunosuppression in recipients. Which of the following procedures is the most useful measure of immunosuppression?

a. Administration of corticosteroids to recipient
b. Administration of immunoglobulin to recipient
c. Destruction of donor B cells
d. Destruction of donor T cells
e. Lymphoid irradiation of donor

444. Relative to the primary immunological response, secondary and later booster responses to a given hapten-protein complex can be associated with which one of the following?

a. Antibodies that are less efficient in preventing specific disease
b. Decreased antibody avidity for the original hapten-protein complex
c. Increased antibody affinity for hapten
d. Lower titers of antibody
e. Maintenance of the same subclass, or idiotype, of antibody produced

445. You are managing a 3-year-old female patient with a fever of unknown origin. Her serum is tested for antibodies against *Haemophilus influenzae*. A precipitation test conducted by the clinical laboratory yields the following results:

Serum (antibody) dilutions

Undiluted serum	1:2	1:4	1:8	1:16	1:32	1:64	1:128	1:256
±	+	+	+	+	+	+	−	−

From this data, which of the following can be concluded?

a. Postzone occurs at undiluted 1:2; zone of equivalence occurs at 1:2 to 1:64; and prozone occurs at 1:128.

b. The negative reactions at 1:128 and 1:126 are false negatives.

c. The patient has antibodies against *H influenzae*, the titer is 64, and the dilution 1:64.

d. The patient has antibodies against *H influenzae*, the dilution is 64, and the titer 1:64.

e. The patient does not have antibodies against *H influenzae* since the reaction is negative with undiluted serum.

f. The patient should be immunized against *H influenzae*.

g. The test needs to be repeated because the results cannot be interpreted.

446. Of the five immunoglobulin classes, IgA is the main immunoglobulin of secretions from the genital, respiratory, and intestinal tracts. As a result, IgA antibody is the first line of defense against infections at the mucous membrane. It is usually an early specific antibody. Which of the following statements most accurately describes IgA?

a. Complement fixation tests for IgA antibody will be positive if specific IgA antibody is present.

b. IgA can be destroyed by bacterial proteases.

c. IgA is absent in colostrum.

d. IgA is not found in saliva; therefore, an IgA diagnostic test on saliva would have no value.

e. IgA is a small molecule with a molecular weight of 30,000 kDa.

447. A 60-year-old male presents with severe jaundice to the local walk-in clinic. History and physical examination reveals a 30-year history of alcohol consumption and drug abuse. Blood tests reveal elevated AST and ALT levels and the presence of hepatitis B and, as a result, reduced complement levels. Complement is a series of important host proteins that provide protection from invasion by foreign microorganisms. Which of the following best describes complement?

a. Complement inhibits phagocytosis.
b. Complement is activated by IgE antibody classes.
c. Complement plays a minor role in the inflammatory response.
d. Complement protects the host from pneumococcal infection through C1, C2, and C4.
e. Microorganisms agglutinate in the presence of complement but do not lyse.

448. Radial immunodiffusion and immunoelectrophoresis is performed on a young patient to evaluate the function of his humoral immune system. Which of the following immunoglobulins has no known function, is found in the serum in low concentrations, and is present on the surface of B lymphocytes (may function as an antigen receptor)?

a. IgG
b. IgA
c. IgM
d. IgD
e. IgE

449. A young patient with severe recurrent pyogenic bacterial infections, but with normal T-cell and B-cell numbers, arrives at the hospital. Testing reveals that this patient's CD4 T-helper cells have a defect in CD40 ligand. As a result, humoral immunity evaluation reveals a significant elevation in the levels of which immunoglobulin that is present as a monomer on B-cell surfaces, as a pentamer in serum, and is initially seen in the primary immune response?

a. IgG
b. IgA
c. IgM
d. IgD
e. IgE

450. A patient with a long history of consuming poorly cooked pork meat presents with generalized myalgia and a low-grade fever. Striated muscle biopsy reveals multiple cysts. Eosinophilia is also present with elevated levels of which of the following immunoglobulins most likely involved in parasitic infections?

a. IgG
b. IgA
c. IgM
d. IgD
e. IgE

451. A patient with cerebellar problems and spider angiomas is diagnosed with a combined T-cell and B-cell deficiency known as ataxia-telangiectasia. In addition to a defect in this patient's DNA repair enzymes, which immunoglobulin is the primary antibody in saliva, tears, and intestinal and genital secretions, and is also deficient in this illness?

a. IgG
b. IgA
c. IgM
d. IgD
e. IgE

452. With four subclasses, which immunoglobulin is the predominant antibody in the secondary immune response and has the greatest concentration of the five immunoglobulin classes in the fetus?

a. IgG
b. IgA
c. IgM
d. IgD
e. IgE

453. A 15-year-old boy is bitten by an *Ixodes* tick while camping with his parents and presents 1 week later with fatigue, fever, headache, and a reddish rash over his trunk and extremities. Positive IgM antibody (1:200) to *Borrelia burgdorferi* is associated with which of the following?

a. Acute Lyme disease
b. Fifth disease
c. Possible hepatitis B infection
d. Possible subacute sclerosing panencephalitis (SSPE)
e. Susceptibility to chicken pox

454. A small child presents with a low-grade fever, coryza, sore throat, a bright red rash on his cheeks, and a less intense erythematous rash on his body. Elevated IgG and IgM antibody titers to parvovirus suggest a diagnosis of which of the following?

a. Acute Lyme disease
b. Fifth disease
c. Possible hepatitis B infection
d. Possible subacute sclerosing panencephalitis (SSPE)
e. Susceptibility to chicken pox

455. Blood from a woman at a local pregnancy clinic is analyzed for antibody titers to known pathogens. A negative varicella antibody titer in this young woman signifies which of the following?

a. Acute Lyme disease
b. Fifth disease
c. Possible hepatitis B infection
d. Possible subacute sclerosing panencephalitis (SSPE)
e. Susceptibility to chicken pox

456. A patient with severe jaundice and liver failure has an increased antibody titer to delta agent. You should suspect which of the following?

a. Acute Lyme disease
b. Fifth disease
c. Possible hepatitis B infection
d. Possible subacute sclerosing panencephalitis (SSPE)
e. Susceptibility to chicken pox

457. A pediatric patient with progressively developing degenerative neurologic disease/disorder has an elevated cerebrospinal fluid (CSF) antibody titer to measles virus. You should suspect which of the following?

a. Acute Lyme disease
b. Fifth disease
c. Possible hepatitis B infection
d. Possible subacute sclerosing panencephalitis (SSPE)
e. Susceptibility to chicken pox

458. A 2-year-old patient presents to the pediatrician for a routine visit. History and physical examination reveals recurrent infections, and enlarged small blood vessels of the skin and conjunctivas. In addition, the physician notices irregular movements most akin to staggering. Suspecting an immune dysfunction, molecular testing reveals a defect in DNA repair enzymes. This autosomal recessive immune deficiency disorder usually is associated with which of the following?

	Humoral	**Cellular**
a.	Normal	Normal
b.	Normal	Deficient
c.	Deficient	Normal
d.	Deficient	Deficient
e.	Elevated	Elevated

459. A 10-month-old male infant with recurrent *H influenzae* infections presents to the emergency room with otitis media, sinusitis, and in severe respiratory distress. Immunological and genetic testing reveals the absence of B cells and a destructive mutation in the tyrosine kinase gene. This X-linked recessive immune disorder is usually associated with which of the following?

	Humoral	**Cellular**
a.	Normal	Normal
b.	Normal	Deficient
c.	Deficient	Normal
d.	Deficient	Deficient
e.	Elevated	Elevated

460. Amniocentesis conducted during genetic counseling of a pregnant woman reveals a fetal adenosine deaminase deficiency. This autosomal recessive immunodeficiency is usually associated with which of the following?

Humoral	Cellular
a. Normal	Normal
b. Normal	Deficient
c. Deficient	Normal
d. Deficient	Deficient
e. Elevated	Elevated

461. A young child with spastic paralysis presents to the emergency room. Blood tests reveal hypocalcemia. This immune disorder is usually associated with which of the following?

Humoral	Cellular
a. Normal	Normal
b. Normal	Deficient
c. Deficient	Normal
d. Deficient	Deficient
e. Elevated	Elevated

462. A 10-month-old patient with recurrent pyogenic infections, eczema, and severe bleeding (thrombocytopenia) is diagnosed with Wiskott-Aldrich syndrome. This immune disorder is usually associated with which of the following?

Humoral	Cellular
a. Normal	Normal
b. Normal	Deficient
c. Deficient	Normal
d. Deficient	Deficient
e. Elevated	Elevated

463. An autograft of a burn victim is best described by which one of the following?

a. Transplant from one region of a person to another region
b. Transplant from one person to a genetically identical person
c. Transplant from one species to the same species
d. Transplant from one species to another species

464. Transplantation involving tissue from two brothers possessing identical HLA genes is best described by which one of the following?

a. Allograft: transplant from one species to the same species
b. Autograft: transplant from one region of a person to another region
c. Isograft: transplant from one person to a genetically identical person
d. Xenograft: transplant from one species to another species

465. A 21-year-old patient in severe kidney failure receives a kidney from his 30-year-old brother. This type of transplantation is best described by which of the following?

a. Allograft: transplant from one species to the same species
b. Autograft: transplant from one region of a person to another region
c. Isograft: transplant from one person to a genetically identical person
d. Xenograft: transplant from one species to another species

466. During the infancy days of cardiac transplantation, nonhuman primate hearts were transplanted into humans to save lives. This type of transplantation is best described by which one of the following?

a. Allograft: transplant from one species to the same species
b. Autograft: transplant from one region of a person to another region
c. Isograft: transplant from one person to a genetically identical person
d. Xenograft: transplant from one species to another species

467. Humoral immunity evaluation mainly consists of measuring the amount of IgG, IgM, and IgA in the patient's serum. These three immunoglobulins represent three distinct isotypes. An isotype is characterized by which of the following?

a. Determinant exposed after papain cleavage to an F(ab) fragment
b. Determinant from one clone of cells and probably located close to the antigen-binding site of the immunoglobulin
c. Determinant inherited in a Mendelian fashion and recognized by cross-immunization of individuals in a species
d. Heavy-chain determinant recognized by heterologous antisera
e. Species-specific carbohydrate determinant on the heavy chain

468. An allotype is characterized by which of the following?

a. Determinant exposed after papain cleavage to an F(ab) fragment
b. Determinant from one clone of cells and probably located close to the antigen-binding site of the immunoglobulin
c. Determinant inherited in a Mendelian fashion and recognized by cross-immunization of individuals in a species
d. Heavy-chain determinant recognized by heterologous antisera
e. Species-specific carbohydrate determinant on the heavy chain

469. Antibodies produced from hybridomas are extremely useful clinically for their monoclonal properties. These antibodies have the same idiotype. An idiotype is characterized by which of the following?

a. Determinant exposed after papain cleavage to an F(ab')2 fragment
b. Determinant from one clone of cells and probably located close to the antigen-binding site of the immunoglobulin
c. Determinant inherited in a Mendelian fashion and recognized by cross-immunization of individuals in a species
d. Heavy-chain determinant recognized by heterologous antisera
e. Species-specific carbohydrate determinant on the heavy chain

470. A 30-year-old male presents to the emergency room with difficulty in breathing and abdominal pain. Upon physical examination, you notice diffuse areas of nondependent, nonpitting swelling without pruritus, with predilection for the face, especially the perioral and periorbital areas. You also notice swelling in the mouth, pharynx, and larynx. Laboratory analysis of blood drawn from this patient indicates a complement problem. Which of the following is most likely?

a. High C4, C2, and C3
b. High C1 and normal level of C1 esterase inhibitor
c. High C1 esterase inhibitor and high C4
d. High C1 esterase inhibitor and low C4
e. Low C1 esterase inhibitor and high C4
f. Low C1 esterase inhibitor and low C4
g. Low C4 and high C2

471. A 45-year-old businesswoman arrives in your office with vague abdominal complaints. She has noticed melenic stool. Upon performing a sigmoidoscopy, you find a 4-cm mass in the upper colon. You should immediately order a blood test for which of the following tumor markers?

a. α-Fetoprotein
b. Antitumor antibody
c. Antitumor light chains
d. Carcinoembryonic antigen
e. Human chorionic gonadotropin
f. Prostate-specific antigen

Questions 472 and 473

472. An 18-year-old male heroin addict, who practices the sharing of needles at a "shooting gallery," is positive in the screening test for AIDS. This patient is most likely to be immunodeficient because of which one of the following?

a. A genetic defect in chromosome 14
b. A low T-helper lymphocyte count
c. An atrophied thymus
d. NADPH enzyme deficiency
e. Insufficient B-cell maturation

473. Since a false positive result is possible in the screening test in the previous vignette, the physician orders a confirmatory test. Which of the following best describes the standard confirmatory test, and what this test checks for, respectively?

a. Complement fixation test; antibodies against the virus
b. Enzyme-linked immunosorbent assay; antigens of the virus
c. Radioimmunoassay; specific antibodies against the virus
d. Western blot; antigens of the virus
e. Western blot; specific antibodies against the virus

474. A pregnant 21-year-old Rh-negative female is about to deliver. The baby's father is determined to be Rh-positive. To reduce the chance for the development of hemolytic disease of the newborn, which of the following procedures should you order?

a. Administration of anti-Rh antibodies to the fetus postdelivery
b. Administration of anti-Rh antibodies to the mother postdelivery
c. Immediate blood transfusion of the suspected father
d. Immediate blood transfusion of the mother with Rh-positive blood
e. Infusion of immune serum globulin into the fetus
f. Intravenous infusion of the Rh antigen into the mother

Questions 475 and 476

475. An 8-month-old male infant with a history of chronic diarrhea, otitis media, and several episodes of pneumonia presents to your clinic with gingivostomatitis (due to herpes simplex virus) and oral candidiasis (thrush). You immediately order an x-ray and a blood workup. X-ray and laboratory blood analysis reveal the absence of a thymic shadow and absence of B lymphocytes, respectively. History taken from the infant's mother reveals a rash evident at birth. Which of the following diseases is most likely present in this infant?

a. Ataxia-telangiectasia
b. Bruton agammaglobulinemia
c. Chediak-Higashi syndrome
d. Chronic granulomatous disease
e. Chronic mucocutaneous candidiasis
f. Hereditary angioedema
g. Severe combined immunodeficiency syndrome (SCID)
h. Thymic aplasia (DiGeorge syndrome)
i. Wiskott-Aldrich syndrome

476. Which of the following is the best therapy for the infant in the previous vignette?

a. Antifungal agents
b. Blood transfusion
c. Bone marrow transplant
d. IgG from pooled random donors
e. Immunization with attenuated vaccines

477. A 5-year-old child arrives at the emergency department minutes after being bitten by a black widow spider. You immediately inject gamma globulin in the form of an antivenom. This type of immunization is referred to as which of the following?

a. Artificial active immunization
b. Artificial passive immunization
c. Natural active immunization
d. Natural passive immunization
e. Adoptive immunization

478. A patient with an increased susceptibility to viral, fungal, and protozoa infection would be expected to have a deficiency in which of the following cell types?

a. B lymphocytes
b. Macrophages
c. Natural killer cells
d. Neutrophils
e. T lymphocytes

Questions 479 and 480

An 18-year-old female visits her local medical clinic presenting with a now chronic productive cough, general malaise, and fever. Previous visits for this same problem resulted in prescriptions for penicillin and cephalosporins, which proved ineffective. Suspecting *Mycoplasma pneumoniae*, caused by an organism that lacks a cell wall, complement fixation tests are ordered. Complement fixation (CF) testing is an important serological tool. One has to understand the conditions under which complement is bound, and RBCs are lysed.

479. Anti-*Mycoplasma* antibody + complement + hemolysin-sensitized red blood cells (RBCs) + anti-RBC antibody results in which of the following?

a. Complement is bound; RBCs are lysed
b. Complement is bound; RBCs are not lysed
c. Complement is not bound; RBCs are lysed
d. Complement is not bound; RBCs are not lysed
e. Complement is not bound; RBCs are agglutinated

480. Anti-*Mycoplasma* antibody + *Mycoplasma* antigen + complement + hemolysin-sensitized RBCs + anti-RBC antibody results in which one of the following?

a. Complement is bound; RBCs are lysed.
b. Complement is bound; RBCs are not lysed.
c. Complement is not bound; RBCs are lysed.
d. Complement is not bound; RBCs are not lysed.
e. Complement is not bound; RBCs are agglutinated.

481. While walking through a field, a 28-year-old woman is stung by a bee. Within 10 minutes, she has asthmatic-like symptoms. This type of hypersensitivity reaction can be correctly characterized by which of the following sequence of steps?

a. Allergen, chemical mediators, sensitization, allergen, IgE, symptoms
b. Allergen, IgE, sensitization, allergen, chemical mediators, symptoms
c. Allergen, sensitization, IgE, allergen, chemical mediators, symptoms
d. Sensitization, allergen, chemical mediators, allergen, IgE, symptoms
e. Sensitization, IgE, allergen, symptoms, allergen, chemical mediators

482. Findings of IgG antibodies to core antigen, antibodies to e antigen, and antibodies to surface antigen in a hepatitis B patient reflects which of the following?

a. Acute infection (incubation period)
b. Acute infection (acute phase)
c. Postinfection (acute phase)
d. Immunization
e. HBV carrier state

483. Findings of HBsAg positive and HBeAg positive test results in a hepatitis B patient reflects which of the following?

a. Acute infection (incubation period)
b. Acute infection (acute phase)
c. Postinfection (acute phase)
d. Immunization
e. HBV carrier state

484. Findings of HBsAg positive, HBeAg positive, and IgM core antibody positive in a hepatitis B patient reflects which of the following?

a. Acute infection (incubation period)
b. Acute infection (acute phase)
c. Postinfection (acute phase)
d. Immunization
e. HBV carrier state

485. Findings of HBsAg positive, no antibodies to HBsAg, and other tests variable in a hepatitis B patient reflects which of the following?

a. Acute infection (incubation period)
b. Acute infection (acute phase)
c. Postinfection (acute phase)
d. Immunization
e. HBV carrier state

486. Findings of antibodies to HBsAg in a hepatitis B patient reflects which of the following?

a. Acute infection (incubation period)
b. Acute infection (acute phase)
c. Postinfection (acute phase)
d. Immunization
e. HBV carrier state

487. A 15-year-old male is rushed to the emergency room with a temperature of 103°F, severe headache, and stiff neck. Upon physical examination, a petechial rash is observed all over his body. Suspecting meningitis, the physician orders a lumbar puncture, revealing gram-negative diplococci (*Neisseria meningitidis*) on Gram stain. The physician wishes to use a more sensitive test to confirm this as the causative agent. Which of the following tests combines features of gel diffusion and immunoelectrophoresis and is applicable only to negatively charged antigens?

a. Coagglutination (COA)
b. Counterimmunoelectrophoresis (CIE)
c. Enzyme-linked immunosorbent assay (ELISA)
d. Latex agglutination (LA)
e. Radioimmunoassay (RIA)

488. A 21-year-old female presents to the emergency room with a high fever, hypotension, and a diffuse, macular, sunburn-like rash that is desquamating. She is also vomiting, has profuse diarrhea, leukocytosis, thrombocytopenia, and elevated BUN and creatinine levels. History from her roommate reveals that these symptoms started soon after the patient began packing her nose to stop chronic nose bleeds. Suspecting *S aureus*, a nasal swab specimen is obtained and sent to the laboratory. Which of the following rapid tests will be ordered and depends on the presence of protein A on certain strains of *S aureus*?

a. Coagglutination (COA)
b. Counterimmunoelectrophoresis (CIE)
c. Enzyme-linked immunosorbent assay (ELISA)
d. Latex agglutination (LA)
e. Radioimmunoassay (RIA)

489. A 50-year-old building contractor arrives in your office complaining of abdominal pain that has increased in severity over the last 3 months. He has noticed melenic stool. Ordering a sigmoidoscopy, a 10-cm mass is visualized in the transverse colon. Surgery is immediately done and the tumor excised. As part of the patient's postsurgical follow through of this resected carcinoma of the colon, blood is obtained and sent to the laboratory to monitor levels of the tumor marker known as carcinoembryonic antigen (CEA). Which of the following tests involves the measurement of very small quantities of CEA through competition of radiolabeled and unlabeled antigen for the same limited amount of antibody?

a. Coagglutination (COA)
b. Counterimmunoelectrophoresis (CIE)
c. Enzyme-linked immunosorbent assay (ELISA)
d. Latex agglutination (LA)
e. Radioimmunoassay (RIA)

490. A 13-year-old male arrives at his doctor's office with a severe sore throat and very high fever. On physical examination, the physician observes his pharynx to be inflamed with a significant exudate along with tender cervical lymph nodes. Laboratory tests reveal a leukocytosis. Suspecting Group A β-hemolytic *Streptococcus pyogenes*, a throat swab and culture are obtained. Using a rapid diagnostic kit recently obtained, the physician decides to test the specimens himself. This test involves inert particles that are sensitized with either antigen or antibody. Which of the following tests is used extensively to detect microbial antigens rapidly (5 minutes or less)?

a. Coagglutination (COA)
b. Counterimmunoelectrophoresis (CIE)
c. Enzyme-linked immunosorbent assay (ELISA)
d. Latex agglutination (LA)
e. Radioimmunoassay (RIA)

491. A 7-month-old baby who is failing to thrive is brought into a neighborhood clinic. History reveals that the baby's mother died of AIDS 2 months ago. Blood is obtained and sent to the laboratory to check for HIV infection. The physician orders a test whose detection system is based on enzymatic activity. Which of the following tests is a heterogeneous immunoassay?

a. Coagglutination (COA)
b. Counterimmunoelectrophoresis (CIE)
c. Enzyme-linked immunosorbent assay (ELISA)
d. Latex agglutination (LA)
e. Radioimmunoassay (RIA)

Questions 492 to 496

A 29-year-old pregnant female gives birth to a stillborn child. History reveals that the woman continued to have close contact with her five cats, by emptying litter boxes and feeding them raw meat, during pregnancy, against her physician's advice. An autopsy is conducted, and multiple cysts are found in the fetal brain, lungs, liver, and eyes. As a confirmatory test, the pathologist orders an enzyme immunoassay to detect the presence of *Toxoplasma gondii*. The diagram below presents the various steps (labeled A-F) of the enzyme immunoassay.

492. Failure of or improper methods for which step in the process is the primary cause of high background color?

a. A
b. B
c. C
d. D
e. E
f. F

493. Where is unlabeled antibody attached if this enzyme immunoassay is intended for detection of antigen?

a. A
b. B
c. C
d. D
e. E
f. F

494. What is the location of the "solid phase"?

a. A
b. B
c. C
d. D
e. E
f. F

495. Addition of reagent at which step will cause color in the positive control well and reactive patient specimens?

a. A
b. B
c. C
d. D
e. E
f. F

496. What is the location of the patient's specimen in the diagram?

a. A
b. B
c. C
d. D
e. E
f. F

497. An 18-year-old male patient with acute lymphocytic leukemia fails all standard chemotherapies. Cells from an HLA-nonidentical donor are used to perform a bone marrow transplant. Prior to transplantation, the patient is given broad-spectrum antibiotics and an immunosuppressive regimen. Within 2 to 4 weeks, lymphocyte and granulocyte numbers begin to rise, confirming bone marrow cell engraftment. However, 1 month later, the patient develops diarrhea, jaundice, and a severe maculopapular rash. Physical examination reveals hepatosplenomegaly. Which of the following is most likely occurring?

a. Acute rejection
b. Chronic rejection
c. Cyclosporine A toxicity
d. Graft versus host disease (GVHD)
e. Hyperacute rejection

498. A 27-year-old male patient (blood group O) arrives at the emergency room with a massive intestinal bleed (hematochezia). Within hours he has lost half of his blood volume, and you decide to transfuse. Due to human error, you transfuse blood group AB into him and within minutes he develops a fever, chills, dyspnea, and a dramatic drop in blood pressure. This reaction is most likely due to which of the following?

a. A cell-mediated response against AB antigens.
b. IgG production by the recipient in response to AB antigens.
c. Preformed anti-A and anti-B antibodies in the recipient.
d. Preformed anti-A and anti-B antibodies of the blood donor.
e. Preformed isohemagglutinins of the IgG isotype.

499. During a clinic office visit, a 35-year-old male stockbroker shows signs of excessive nervousness and irritability and complains that the office is too hot. History and physical examination reveals the presence of a goiter and exophthalmia. Laboratory analysis of his blood reveals high antibody titers against the thyroid-stimulating hormone (TSH) receptor. Which of the following is the most likely diagnosis?

a. Goodpasture syndrome
b. Graves disease
c. Hashimoto disease
d. Juvenile onset diabetes mellitus
e. Myasthenia gravis
f. Pernicious anemia
g. Rheumatoid arthritis
h. Systemic lupus erythematosus (SLE)

500. A 9-year-old female with a recent history of weight loss and vision problems arrives at the hospital. Soon after, it is determined that she has low blood glucose, and autoantibodies against β cells are detected in her serum. Which of the following is the most likely diagnosis?

a. Goodpasture syndrome
b. Graves disease
c. Hashimoto disease
d. Juvenile onset diabetes mellitus
e. Myasthenia gravis
f. Pernicious anemia
g. Rheumatoid arthritis
h. Systemic lupus erythematosus (SLE)

501. A 35-year-old woman with fever, weight loss, fatigue, and painful joints and muscles presents to her physician's office. The physician notes that she has marked photosensitivity and a rash on the cheeks and over the bridge of her nose. Laboratory tests reveal anemic conditions and the presence of anti-DNA antibodies. Which of the following is the most likely diagnosis?

a. Goodpasture syndrome
b. Graves disease
c. Hashimoto disease
d. Juvenile onset diabetes mellitus
e. Myasthenia gravis
f. Pernicious anemia
g. Rheumatoid arthritis
h. Systemic lupus erythematosus (SLE)

Immunology

Answers

411 to 414. The answers are 411-a, 412-c, 413-c, 414-d. *(Kindt, pp 372-396. Levinson, pp 460-467.)* Reactions to small amounts of drugs can occur, as illustrated in the skin test using penicilloyl polylysine to reveal a penicillin allergy or type I hypersensitivity reaction. In Question 412, the girl was likely exposed to poison ivy or poison oak (contact dermatitis) which is attributed to a type IV hypersensitivity reaction. The Arthus reaction is a localized type of reaction mediated by aggregates of antibody and antigen and is characteristic of type III hypersensitivity reactions. In Question 413, only hypersensitivity reactions type I and IV are associated with skin tests. Type I is commonly referred to as a challenge in which a specific antigen is injected intradermally into a sensitized individual, creating a "wheal and flare" (erythema and edema) reaction. Type IV hypersensitivity is commonly associated with tuberculin injections to recognize the presence of delayed type hypersensitivity. In Question 414, Rh disease and Goodpasture syndrome are the result of antibodies that have formed against normally present host antigens on red blood cells and the kidney's glomerular basement membrane, respectively. Thus, these two diseases are associated with type II reactions. The diagrams in 1, 2, 3, and 4 represent types I, II, III, and IV hypersensitivity, respectively. The table below describes these reactions in detail.

Mediator	HYPERSENSITIVITY REACTIONS Type	Reaction
Antibody (IgE)	I (immediate, anaphylactic)	IgE antibody is induced by allergen and binds to mast cells and basophils. When exposed to the allergen again, the allergen cross-links the bound IgE, which induces degranulation and release of mediators, eg, histamine.
Antibody (IgG)	II (cytotoxic)	Antigens on a cell surface combine with antibody; this leads to complement-mediated lysis, eg, transfusion or Rh reactions, or autoimmune hemolytic anemia.
Antibody (IgG)	III (immune complex)	Antigen-antibody immune complexes are deposited in tissues, complement is activated, and polymorphonuclear cells are attracted to the site. They release lysosomal enzymes, causing tissue damage.
Cell	IV (delayed)	Helper T lymphocytes sensitized by an antigen release lymphokines upon second contact with the same antigen. The lymphokines induce inflammation and activate macrophages, which, in turn, release various mediators.

(Reprinted, with permission, from Levinson W, Jawetz E. Medical Microbiology. 7th ed. New York, NY: McGraw-Hill; 2002: 415.)

415 and 416. The answers are 415-b, 416-a. (Kindt, pp 284, 498. Levinson, pp 463-465, 478, 479t.) Bruton agammaglobulinemia is a congenital defect that becomes apparent at approximately 6 months of age, when maternal IgG is diminished. It occurs in males and is characterized by a defective *btk* gene, very small tonsils, low levels of all five classes of immunoglobulins, and no mature B cells. Thus, the child is unable to produce immunoglobulins and develops a series of bacterial infections characterized by recurrences and progression to more serious infections such as septicemia. The most common organisms responsible for infection are *H influenzae* and *S pneumoniae*. Treatment consists of pooled IgG. Cell-mediated immunity is not affected, and the child is able to respond normally to diseases that require this immune response for resolution, such as the measles virus, varicella-zoster virus, and *M tuberculosis*. The other diagnoses do not describe the specific clinical scenario outlined in this case. Also, it is important to note that since the main defect in this child's immunity is in the B-cell line, in that, the child is unable to produce immunoglobulins. The organism that would be most dangerous to the child is *C trachomatis* because the B-cell line (antibodies) is typically responsible for its elimination from the host.

Note: Immunodeficiency is characterized by unusual and recurrent infections:

- B-cell (antibody) deficiency—bacterial infections

- T-cell deficiency—viral, fungal, and protozoal infections

- Phagocytic cell deficiency—pyogenic infections (bacterial), skin infections, systemic bacterial opportunistic infections

- Complement deficiencies—pyogenic infections (bacterial)

417 and 418. The answers are 417-e, 418-a. *(Kindt, pp 30-40. Levinson, pp 406-415.)* Cells can be differentiated based on unique cell surface markers (antigens). In this case, a CD4:CD8 ratio of less than 1 indicates a significant reduction in the helper T-lymphocyte population. The surface proteins that best represent this pool are MHC I, TCR, CD3, and CD28. CD4 is also associated with helper T lymphocytes. B lymphocytes have MHC I, IgM, B7 CD19, and CD20. Cytotoxic T lymphocytes have MHC I, TCR, CD3, and CD8, while macrophages have MHC I, MHC II, and CD14. An important fact to remember is that all healthy cells other than mature red cells have class I MHC. The B7 surface protein on the antigen-presenting cell (B cell) is the costimulatory molecule and must interact with the CD28 on the helper T cell for full activation to occur. (See the figures.)

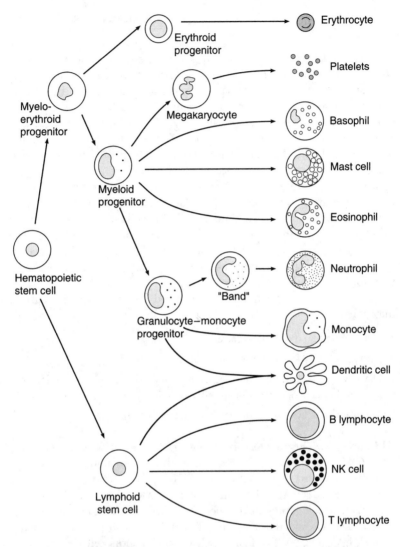

Schematic overview of hematopoiesis, emphasizing the erythroid, myeloid, and lymphoid pathways. This highly simplified depiction omits many recognized intermediate cell types in each pathway. All of the cells shown here develop to maturity in the bone marrow, except T lymphocytes, which develop from marrow-derived progenitors that migrate to the thymus. A common lymphoid stem cell serves as the progenitor of T and B lymphocytes and of natural killer (NK) cells. Dendritic cells arise from both the myeloid and lymphoid lineages. (Reproduced, with permission, from Parslow TG, et al. Medical Immunology. 10th ed. New York, NY: McGraw-Hill; 2001:3.)

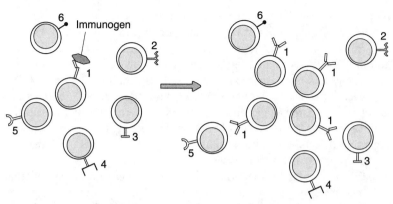

Clonal selection of lymphocytes by a specific immunogen. **Left:** The unimmunized lymphocyte population is composed of cells from many different clones, each with its own antigen specificity, indicated here by the distinctive shapes of the surface antigen receptors. **Right:** Contact with an immunogen leads to selective proliferation (positive selection) of any clone or clones that can recognize that specific immunogen. *(Reproduced, with permission, from Parslow TG, et al. Medical Immunology. 10th ed. New York, NY: McGraw-Hill; 2001:62.)*

419. The answer is a. *(Kindt, pp 2-3, 475-490. Levinson, pp 94-96, 244-247.)* Recurrent severe infection is an indication for clinical evaluation of immune status. Live vaccines, including BCG attenuated from *M tuberculosis,* should not be used in the evaluation of a patient's immune competence because patients with severe immunodeficiencies may develop an overwhelming infection (disseminated disease) from the vaccine. For the same reason, oral (Sabin) polio vaccine is not advisable for use in such persons. The other vaccines listed are acellular and should be safe to use in this clinical scenario described.

420. The answer is e. *(Kindt, pp 475-484. Levinson, pp 244-247, 273-274.)* Measles-like virus has been isolated from the brain cells of patients with SSPE. The role of the host immune response in the causation of SSPE has been supported by several findings including the following: (1) progression of disease despite high levels of humoral antibody; (2) presence of a factor that blocks lymphocyte-mediated immunity to SSPE-measles virus in SSPE-cerebrospinal fluid (CSF); (3) lysis of brain cells from SSPE patients by SSPE serum or CSF in the presence of complement (a similar mechanism could cause in vivo tissue injury). SSPE is particularly common in those who acquired measles before 2 years of age and is very rare after measles vaccination.

Higher-than-normal levels of serum antibodies (Ab) to measles virus and local synthesis of measles Ab in CSF, as evidenced by the oligoclonal IgG, imply a connection between the virus and multiple sclerosis (MS). However, the other studies have implicated the other viruses. Several studies of cell-mediated hypersensitivity to measles and other viruses in MS have been done, but the results have been conflicting. Definite conclusions regarding defects in cellular immunity in this disease cannot be reached until further research is completed.

CJD is caused by the prion which is an altered host protein that becomes infectious in nature. It is characterized by myoclonic jerking along with characteristic EEG changes. PML is associated with the JC virus (JCV), while this clinical scenario is not characteristic of EBV infection.

421. The answer is c. (*Kindt, pp 426-440. Levinson, pp 470-475.*) Transplantation terminology is being tested in this question. An autograft is a transfer of an individual's own tissue to another site in the body. An isograft (syngeneic graft) is the transfer of tissue between genetically identical individuals, such as monozygotic twins. An allograft is the transfer of tissue between genetically different members of the same species (ie, brother to sister, dizygotic twins, etc), while a xenograft is the transfer of tissue between different species (eg, pig valve to human heart). In this case, one unit is the patient's own blood (an autologous donation) while the second unit is his older brother's blood (most like an allograft donation). If his brother had been an identical twin, then (e) would be the correct answer.

422. The answer is e. (*Kindt, pp 16-18, 481-482. Levinson, pp 436-437.*) The graph presented in the question exhibits hemagglutinating antibody responses to primary and secondary immunization with any standard antigen. Curve B represents the early response to primary immunization, which is chiefly an IgM response. Rechallenge elicits an accelerated response that mainly involves IgG and occurs 2 to 5 days after reimmunization. IgM has a molecular weight of 900,000 and is a pentamer that the fetus can produce quite early in gestation. IgM (and IgG) have the ability to activate complement, appear along with sIgD as the B-cell receptor on B lymphocytes, and like IgA require J chains to join the Fc chains of each monomer together. The letter (a) is a feature of all antibody molecules and is not *unique* to IgM. IgA is associated with the J chain that helps to form its dimeric structure. The fetus does not begin to produce its own IgG until about the third month of life when maternal IgG is catabolized (IgG half-life is approximately 23 days). In addition, (d) describes the estimated molecular weight of the IgG molecule.

423. The answer is b. (*Kindt, pp 403, 410-412. Levinson, pp 466, 473-474.*) This clinical case represents a patient suffering with systemic lupus erythematosus (SLE). The diagnosis of SLE is best supported by detecting the presence of anti-dsDNA and anti-Smith (anti-Sm) antibodies. The presence of anti-dsDNA antibodies are very specific for SLE and represent a poor prognosis for disease. Antinuclear antibodies (ANA) can also be detected using fluorescent antibody tests. The other antibodies listed are related to other autoimmune diseases as follows: anticentromere antibodies in CREST syndrome and occasionally in systemic scleroderma, antimitochondrial antibodies in primary biliary cirrhosis, antineutrophil antibodies in antineutrophil cytoplasmic antibodies (ANCA)-associated vasculitis (systemic vasculitis), and anti-TSH receptor antibodies in Graves disease (hyperthyroidism).

424. The answer is a. (*Kindt, pp 155-158. Levinson, pp 67, 234, 452-453.*) ELISA (enzyme-linked immunosorbent assay) methods can be used to detect either antigens or antibodies. If antigen is to be detected, then specific antibody is initially bound to the plate (see A in the diagram presented with the question). If antibody is to be detected, then antigen is bound to the solid phase. The bound antigen and antibody then "captures" the analyte to be detected. One of the major causes for high background in ELISA tests is the failure to wash off unbound antigen or antibody (see B in the diagram presented with the question). ELISA is routinely used to screen patient sera for different antibodies (including anti-HIV-1 antibodies). In this case, the well is initially coated with HIV-1 antigen, and the patient sera is tested for anti-HIV-1 antibodies.

425. The answer is a. (*Kindt, pp 151-152. Levinson, pp 451, 453.*) In the Ouchterlony agar-gel diffusion test, an antigen and a series of antibodies (or an antibody and a series of antigens) are allowed to diffuse toward each other. At the zone of optimal proportions of the reactants, a precipitin line occurs. Cross-reactions between antigens or antibodies tested can be detected by: (1) a shortening of the major precipitin band contiguous to the cross-reacting substance, or (2) the identity of precipitin reaction between the two cross-dressing substances. The figures presented in the question illustrate both types of cross-reactions. In the first bleed pattern shown in the question, cross-reaction between antigen X and antigen A is recognizable only by a shortening of the precipitin band between the center well and X on the A well side (relative to the band going directly into the normal saline well). In the second bleed pattern, full cross-reaction of X and A is apparent. No other cross-reactions are seen.

426. The answer is a. (*Kindt, pp 66, 495t, 501-503. Levinson, pp 57t, 479-481.*) The patient in this case has chronic granulomatous disease (CGD), an X-linked (65%) or autosomal recessive (35%) inherited disease. Patients with CGD are not able to generate a respiratory burst after granulocyte and monocyte stimulation. Thus, they are unable to kill microorganisms. Answers a, b, and c are all involved in the respiratory burst; however, the central enzyme is the NADPH oxidase (answer a). Without this enzyme, hydrogen peroxide (answer b), superoxide (answer c), and other microbial reactive oxygen species would not be generated. Answer d depicts the synthetic pathway for nitric oxide, a potent vasodilator. Answers e and f are reactions involving common metabolic enzymes in various bacteria.

427. The answer is b. (*Kindt, pp 527-531, 535. Levinson, pp 426-434.*) Immunoglobulin gene rearrangement errors can contribute to the development of many types of leukemia and lymphoma. Some genetic alterations are characteristic of particular histologic entities: t(8;14) in Burkitt lymphoma, t(14;18) in follicular lymphoma, t(11;14) in mantle cell lymphoma, and t(2;5) in anaplastic large cell lymphoma.

428. The answer is c. (*Kindt, pp 193-195. Levinson, pp 440-441.*) The figure shown in the question is a schematic representation of the MHC class I molecule, which has a CD8 binding site (α3) and a peptide-binding site (α1 and α2). MHC class I is active on all nucleated cells.

429. The answer is a. (*Kindt, pp 85-89. Levinson, pp 428-434.*) The initial response to a new infection is with an IgM class antibody. IgM develops quickly and usually disappears within a few months. The secondary response is IgG and reflects the patient's immune status or, in the case of chicken pox, a vaccination given.

430 to 432. The answers are 430-e, 431-a, 432-a. (*Kindt, pp 155-158. Levinson, pp 328, 452-456.*) A male patient with the presentation as outlined in Question 429 (fatigue, weight loss, and lymphadenopathy) must be tested for antibodies to HIV. While other antibody tests may be relevant after the primary diagnosis, they must be considered after HIV is ruled out. Certainly, infectious mononucleosis is a possibility, but its occurrence in this age group is not as frequent as HIV. Patients are tested first by an ELISA screening test. ELISA is the most sensitive test available (99.7%-99.9%) and is usually positive 3 to 12 weeks postinfection. If this test is positive (X2), then a confirmatory Western blot is performed. A Western blot separates the immune response into antibody production for specific components of the virus, that is, envelope, gag, and so forth. The following table shows the various bands that could be seen on a widely used Western blot and their identification by specific antigen source. There are at least three schemes for interpreting Western blots. A Western blot is deemed positive when any two of the following bands are present: p24, gp41, gp120, and/or gp160. Assuming technical competence in the laboratory, one of the more common reasons for falsely positive ELISA and Western blots is an influenza vaccination within the past few months. A rare patient may have antibody to the cell line used to grow virus. Unlike Lyme disease, there is no reported cross-reactivity with Epstein-Barr virus (EBV) or HTLV. There appears to be no naturally occurring antibody to retroviruses.

Antigen	Source
gp 160	Env gene product
gp 120	Env fragment
gp 41	Transmembrane fragment
gp 31	
gp 51	Pol gene product
p 66	
p 24	Core protein (gag)

Abbreviations: gp, glycoprotein; p, protein; env, envelope; pol, polymerase.

433. The answer is d. (*Kindt, pp 168, 185-186, 502. Levinson, pp 448, 480-482.*) Patients with complement deficiencies such as C5 through C9, which form the membrane attack complex (MAC), are predisposed to disseminated meningococcal (neisserial) disease. These patients may also be susceptible to gonococcal (neisserial) infection. There appears to be no disposition to AIDS or to fungal, parasitic, or pneumococcal infections.

434. The answer is d. (*Kindt, pp 346-347. Levinson, pp 444t.*) The acute-phase response is a primitive, nonspecific defense reaction, mediated by the liver, which increases innate immunity and other protective functions in stressful times. It can be triggered by chronic autoimmune disorders such as rheumatoid arthritis and Crohn disease. This response occurs when hepatocytes are exposed to IL-6 and IL-1 or TNF-α. LPS is a potent inducer of these cytokines. They are responsible for fever, somnolence, loss of appetite, and, if the response is prolonged, anemia and cachexia (wasting). A traditional assay known as the *erythrocyte sedimentation rate* (ESR) may be used as an indicator of an acute-phase response. The ESR involves measuring the rate at which the red blood cells fall through plasma, which increases as fibrinogen concentration rises. Currently, Crohn disease may be treated with infusions of a drug known as inflix-imab, which is a mouse-human chimeric antibody against human TNF-α or adalimumab, a fully humanized monoclonal antibody against human TNF-α. The FDA has approved these monoclonal antibody drugs in the treatment of Crohn disease, rheumatoid and psoriatic arthritis, ankylosing spondylitis, moderate to severe chronic psoriasis, and juvenile idiopathic arthritis.

435. The answer is d. (*Kindt, pp 99-100. Levinson, pp 403, 405.*) Maternal transfer of antibody (secretory IgA in the colostrum of breast milk), however, is passive but still confers specific immunity. It is termed *passive acquired* immunity. Natural immunity is nonspecific. The natural immune functions described are not specific for a certain antigen. For example, certain proteins such as C-reactive protein (CRP) are acute-phase reactants. While elevated CRP is seen in infection, it is not disease specific.

436. The answer is b. (*Kindt, pp 77-78. Levinson, pp 403-404.*) Haptens (incomplete antigens) are not themselves antigenic, but when coupled to a cell or carrier protein become antigenic and induce antibodies that can bind the hapten alone (in the absence of the carrier protein). They are small molecules that are generally less than 1000 kDa. While haptens react with antibodies, they are not immunogenic because they do not activate T cells and cannot bind the MHC. Haptens are significant in disease; penicillin is a hapten and can cause severe life-threatening allergic reaction by destruction of erythrocytes. Catechols in the oils of poison ivy plants are haptens and cause a significant skin inflammatory response. Chloramphenicol is a hapten that can lead to the destruction of leukocytes and cause agranulocytosis. Sedormid is a hapten that can cause thrombocytopenia and purpura (bleeding) through the destruction of platelets.

437. The answer is e. (*Kindt, pp 87, 95-100. Levinson, pp 430-431, 436.*) The radial immunodiffusion and immunoelectrophoresis are two tests used to evaluate humoral immunity. Evaluating humoral immunity consists of measuring the levels of IgM, IgG, and IgA in the patient's serum. Whereas total IgG is greater than total IgM in the fetus due to the maternal transfer of IgG and not IgM across the placenta, it is important to remember that IgM is the antibody produced in the greatest amounts by the fetus. The fetus also produces IgG and IgA, but the fetus produces greater amounts of IgM than these other two important antibodies.

438. The answer is b. (*Kindt, pp 85-89, 115-116. Levinson, pp 427, 430f.*) The hinge region consists mostly of cysteine and proline residues, allowing for the formation of interchain disulphide bonds and flexibility, respectively. There appears to be considerable flexibility in the hinge region between the Fc and the two F(ab) portions of the molecule. This allows the molecule to assume either a T shape or a Y shape. The two arms of the antibody are identical and possess the same paratopes; hence, they will recognize identical epitopes. Each variable and constant heavy and light chain consists of the same amino acid sequences. IgG is the most abundant antibody in the serum. It migrates in the gamma globulin fraction during serum protein separation and composes 80% of the antibody concentration in the serum. Two enzymes, papain and pepsin, can digest an IgG antibody molecule by cleaving (hydrolysis) the antibody molecule on the N and C terminus sides, respectively, of the sulfhydryl bridge binding the heavy chains. Finally, antibodies protect the host by neutralizing (preventing adherence), opsonizing (promoting phagocytosis), and activating complement (lysis). (See the figure.)

Schematic model of an IgG1 (κ) human antibody molecule showing the basic four-chain structure and domains (V_H, C_H1, etc). Sites of enzymatic cleavage by pepsin and papain are shown. *(Reproduced, with permission, from Parslow TG, et al. Medical Immunology. 10th ed. New York, NY: McGraw-Hill; 2001:96.)*

439. The answer is d. *(Kindt, pp 508-509, 512. Levinson, pp 322-340.)* HIV-2 disease is very rare in the United States. However, HIV-2 is present in Africa, the Far East, and some parts of the Caribbean. Many of the screening tests for HIV-1 will not detect antibodies to HIV-2. Either a separate HIV-2 antibody test or a combination HIV-1/2 is necessary. While HTLV disease is also seen in the same geographic areas, the symptoms displayed by this patient are more akin to HIV disease. While an HIV-1 RNA PCR is a useful test for monitoring the results of HIV therapy, it is not approved for diagnosis, nor will it detect HIV-2 nucleic acid.

440. The answer is c. *(Kindt, pp 30, 35-36, 360-363. Levinson, pp 229, 421-422.)* NK cells do not express a cell surface TCR/CD3 complex and are CD4–. About half of human NK cells are CD8+. Also, most NK cells express an Fc IgG receptor, known as CD16, and CD56, a neural cell adhesion molecule variant. NK cells are generally CD16+, CD56+, and CD3–, which contrasts them with T cells which are CD3+, CD16–, and CD56–. Also, B cells are associated with CD19 and CD20.

441. The answer is e. *(Kindt, pp 175-176, 338-339. Levinson, pp 446-449.)* C3a and C5a are potent mediators of inflammation; that is, they have anaphylatoxin activity. This activity is characterized by smooth-muscle contraction and the degranulation of mast cells and basophils leading to the release of histamine and other vasoactive substances, causing increased vascular (capillary) permeability. C5a is the most potent of these anaphylatoxins; however, it also serves another role as a potent chemotactic agent, attracting polymorphonucleated neutrophils and macrophages to the site of inflammation.

442. The answer is d. *(Kindt, pp 9, 59, 322, 540. Levinson, pp 228-229, 241.)* Alpha and beta interferons are proteins that can induce an antiviral state in uninfected cells via the production of secondary protein factors that inhibit viral protein synthesis by degrading only viral mRNA (not host mRNA). Also, they can increase the expression of MHC class I proteins, which enable an infected cell to present viral antigens and facilitate killing by cytotoxic T lymphocytes (CTLs), and they can stimulate the production of gamma interferon. In addition, gamma interferon increases MHC class II expression and antigen presentation in all cells and activates NK cells to kill virus-infected cells. Interferons have no direct effect on extracellular virus particles.

443. The answer is a. *(Kindt, pp 33, 426-440. Levinson, pp 442-444.)* Allograft rejection is primarily a T-cell response to foreign tissue. Many immunosuppressive measures exist, including cyclosporine, tacrolimus, sirolimus, azathioprine, monoclonal antibodies, radiation, and corticosteroids. Commonly used, the corticosteroids reduce inflammatory response and are generally administered by cytotoxic drugs, such as cyclosporine. Corticosteroids function as immunosuppressive agents by inhibiting cytokine production, such as IL-1 and TNF, and also by lysing certain T-cell types. Lymphoid irradiation is usually done so that the bone marrow is shielded. This removes lymphocytes from lymph nodes and spleen while allowing the patient to have the capacity to regenerate new T and B cells. Likewise, antilymphocyte globulin will destroy the recipient's lymphocytes, especially T cells. Destruction of donor B cells and T cells would not play a role in the immunosuppression of the graft recipient. In graft crises, monoclonal antibody to CD3 is sometimes given. This targets mature T lymphocytes for destruction.

444. The answer is c. *(Kindt, pp 77-78. Levinson, pp 403-404.)* With repeated immunization, higher titers of all antibodies are observed, and, as priming is repeated, the immune response recruits B cells of progressively greater affinity. The affinity of antibody for a hapten-protein complex rises, cross-reactivity also rises, and the response becomes wider in specificity. As the number of antigenic sites detected per reacting particle increases, the avidity increases. In addition to shifts in the class of immunoglobulin synthesized in response to an antigen (IgM-IgG), shifts also may occur in the idiotype of antibody.

445. The answer is c. *(Kindt, pp 151-153. Levinson, pp 450-452.)* In precipitation reactions, both the antigen and the antibody are soluble. The antibody cross-links antigen molecules, creating an increasing lattice that eventually forms an insoluble precipitate. The antigen must be divalent, and the antigen/antibody proportion is critical in order for detectable precipitate to form. The prozone is the zone of antibody excess. The postzone is the zone of antigen excess. The zone of equivalence is the zone where the proportion of antibody and antigen is optimal for precipitate formation. Titer is the reciprocal of the highest dilution (ratio) of antibody (or antigen) at which there is still a detectable reaction. (See figure below.)

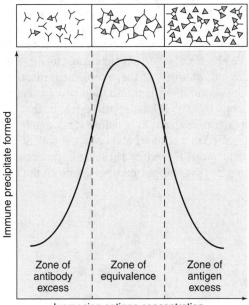

(Modified and reproduced, with permission, from Stites D, Terr A, Parslow T (eds). Basic and Clinical Immunology. 9th ed. Originally published by Appleton & Lange. Copyright© 1997 by The McGraw-Hill Companies.)

446. The answer is b. *(Kindt, pp 96t, 99-100. Levinson, pp 426-427, 429.)* Each secretory IgA molecule has a molecular weight of 400,000 and consists of two H2L2 units and one molecule each of J chain and secretory component. Some IgA exists in serum as a monomer H2L2 with a molecular weight of 160,000. Some bacteria, such as *Neisseria*, can destroy IgA-1 by producing protease. It is the major immunoglobulin in milk, saliva, tears, mucus, sweat, gastric fluid, and colostrum. IgA does not fix complement, so one would anticipate that a complement fixation test would not be useful for IgA antibody. It is important to remember that of the five classes of immunoglobulins, only IgG and IgM are complement-fixing/activating antibodies.

447. The answer is d. (*Kindt, pp 9, 55, 168-187. Levinson, pp 446-449.*) Both IgG and IgM activate complement by the classic pathway, while IgA activates it by the alternative pathway. IgA, IgD, and IgE cannot activate complement. Complement is a system of several proteins that is activated by either an immune or a nonimmune pathway. Both of these pathways result in the production of many biologically active components that cause cell lysis and death. Thus, it plays a significant role in the inflammatory process. In addition, products of the complement cascade are associated with enhancing opsonization, neutralization of invading pathogens, and clearance of debris by the CR1 on erythrocytes. In this clinical case, the patient is suffering from severe liver failure. This significant reduction in liver function has led to a reduced ability by the patient to produce sufficient complement proteins, and as a result the patient is predisposed to infections caused by pyogenic bacteria. See figure on the following page.

The classic and alternative pathways of the complement system indicate that proteolytic cleavage of the molecule at the tip of the arrow has occurred; a line over a complex indicates that it is enzymatically active. Note that the nomenclature of the cleavage products of C2 is undecided. Some call the large fragment C2a and others call it C2b. The C3 convertase is depicted here as C4b,2b. Note that proteases associated with the mannose-binding lectin cleave C4 as well as C2. *(Reprinted, with permission, from Levinson W, Jawetz E. Medical Microbiology and Immunology. 7th ed. NewYork, NY: McGraw-Hill; 2002:401.)*

448 to 452. The answers are 448-d, 449-c, 450-e, 451-b, 452-a.
(*Kindt, pp 95-100, 170-173. Levinson, pp 426-437.*) IgG antibody provides an
"immune history." That is, IgG antibody persists in most people and indicates
the antigens to which they have been exposed. IgG is not formed early in
infection but is a secondary response arising weeks to months after antigenic
challenge. IgG also has a built-in memory. Even people with very low levels
of specific IgG will respond to an antigen challenge with an IgG response.

IgM antibody, in contrast, arises early in infection and then disappears
within a couple of months. IgM is intravascular and does not cross the placental barrier. For this reason, infants with specific IgG responses to disease must
be tested for IgM to determine whether their immune systems have produced
antibody or whether the test was positive because of passively transferred IgG
from mother to child. The clinical case described in Question 448 is of a young
patient with hyper-IgM syndrome. This immune deficiency presents early in
life with severe pyogenic infections, resembling those seen in X-linked
hypogammaglobulinemia; however, unlike X-linked hypogammaglobulinemia (very low levels of all immunoglobulins, virtual absence of B cells, found
in young boys with female carriers being immunologically normal), hyper-IgM
syndrome patients have a high IgM concentration, low IgG, IgA, and IgE concentrations, and normal T- and B-cell numbers. The problem exists in a muta-
tional defect in the CD40 ligand in CD4-positive helper T cells, leading to
failure of normal interaction between this ligand on T cells and CD40 on B-cell
surfaces. This failure leads to an inability of the B cells to class switch from IgM
production to other antibodies. Treatment includes pooled gamma globulin.

IgA antibody is involved in local immunity at the level of the mucous
membrane. It also arises early in disease, is short lived, and will disappear
similarly as IgM.

IgE antibody is characteristically seen in parasitic infections, particularly worm (helminth) infections because of the attraction of eosinophils to
the site of the infestation. Certain allergies are due to excessive production
of IgE. The patient in this case has irichinosis as a result of consuming
undercooked pork and ingesting the parasite *Trichinella spiralis*. IgE specific
for worm proteins binds to receptors on eosinophils, promoting the release
of worm-destroying enzymes involved in the antibody-dependent cellular
cytotoxicity (ADCC) response.

IgD antibody consists of two light chains and two heavy chains. Its role
is not known, but it can be found on the surface of lymphocytes, where it
may act as a surface receptor.

IgG is susceptible to proteolytic enzymes, which may explain why it is present in such low levels in serum. In addition, the fetus has more total IgG, than IgM, as a result of maternal placental IgG transfer, even though IgM is produced in greater amounts by the fetus.

453 to 457. The answers are 453-a, 454-b, 455-e, 456-c, 457-d. *(Kindt, pp 455-460, 448-454. Levinson, pp 176-177, 246, 257, 266, 273-274, 294-298.)* Borrelia burgdorferi, the causative agent of Lyme disease, elicits an acute antibody response. IgM appears within days to a few weeks following tick bite, and IgG appears a few weeks later. IgG persists; IgM does not. Cross-reactions occur with other treponemes.

Fifth disease is a viral exanthem commonly seen in children 8- to 12-years-old. Children are ill for a few days but recover without incident, usually within about 1 week. Unfortunately, if a pregnant female acquires the disease in the first trimester of pregnancy, the fetus is at risk. The causative agent is thought to be a parvovirus (Parvovirus B19). Fifth disease is also known as erythema infectiosum or slapped cheek syndrome. The four other maculopapular or macular rash diseases of childhood are measles, roseola, rubella, and scarlet fever.

Adults with no titer to varicella (VZV) are at risk for acquisition of chicken pox. If they are health care workers, there is additional risk of transmitting VZV to immunodeficient children. Antibodies to VZV are readily detected by both enzyme immunoassay (EIA) and fluorescent antibody (FA) techniques.

Delta agent is a recently discovered antigen associated with HBsAg. Its presence usually correlates with HBsAg chronic carriers who have chronic active hepatitis. EIA and radioimmunoassay (RIA) tests are available to detect antibodies to delta agent.

SSPE is thought to be caused by a measles-related virus present in the central nervous system. Most SSPE patients show elevated measles virus antibodies in serum and CSF. In patients with multiple sclerosis (MS), lower CSF antibody titers have been observed, suggesting a possible etiologic role for measles virus in MS.

458 to 462. The answers are 458-d, 459-c, 460-d, 461-b, 462-d. *(Kindt, pp 185-186, 493-504. Levinson, pp 30, 476-482.)* Immunodeficiency disorders can be categorized according to whether the defect primarily involves humoral immunity (bone marrow derived, or B lymphocytes) or cellular immunity (thymus derived, or T lymphocytes) or both. Swiss-type hypogammaglobulinemia, ataxia-telangiectasia, the Wiskott-Aldrich syndrome, and severe combined immunodeficiency disorders all involve defective B-cell and T-cell function. Infantile X-linked agammaglobulinemia is caused chiefly by deficient B-cell activity, whereas thymic hypoplasia is mainly a T-cell immunodeficiency disorder.

In Question 458, this 2-year-old patient has ataxia (staggering)-telangiectasia (spider angiomas), an autosomal recessive immune disorder associated with both a lymphopenia (cellular) and IgA deficiency (humoral). Question 459 describes a patient with X-linked hypogammaglobulinemia or Bruton agammaglobulinemia, which only occurs in boys and is characterized by low levels of all immunoglobulin classes and the absence of almost all B cells. Pre-B cells are present; however, they fail to differentiate into B cells. Cell-mediated immunity is relatively normal. Recurrent bacterial infections occur after about 6 months of age when protective maternal IgG antibody declines. The fetus represented in Question 460 has severe combined immunodeficiency disease (SCID) characterized by defects in early stem cell differentiation. As a result, B cells and T cells are both defective, immunoglobulins are very low, and tonsils and lymph nodes are absent. Thymic aplasia or DiGeorge syndrome marks the young child in Question 461. Failed development of the thymus and the parathyroids lead to hypoparathyroidism, hypocalcemia, and ultimately a spastic paralysis (strong muscle contractions or tetany). Finally, Wiskott-Aldrich syndrome (Question 462), an X-linked defect, is associated with reduced IgM levels and variable cellular-mediated immunity.

463 to 466. The answers are 463-a, 464-c, 465-a, 466-d. (*Kindt, pp 33, 426-440, 443-444. Levinson, pp 442, 444.*) Transplantation from one region of a person to another region of that same person is an *autograft* and has the best chance of succeeding. When a transplant is done between monozygotic twins, it is an *isograft* and has a complete MHC compatibility and a good chance of success. *Allografts* are between members of the same species, and *xenografts* are between members of different species. Both of these transplants have a high rate of rejection unless immunosuppression accompanies the transplant.

467 to 469. The answers are 467-d, 468-c, 469-b. (*Kindt, pp 101-102. Levinson, pp 426, 431.*) Isotypes are determined by antigens of the immunoglobulin classes found in all individuals of one species. In addition to heavy-chain isotypes of IgA, IgD, IgE, IgG, and IgM, two light-chain isotypes exist for κ and λ chains.

Allotypes are differentiated by antigenic determinants that vary among individuals within a species and are recognized by cross-immunization of individuals in a species. Allotypes include the Gm marker of IgG and the Inv marker of light chains.

Idiotypes are antigenic determinants that appear only on the F(ab) fragments of antibodies and appear to be localized at the ligand-binding site; thus, anti-idiotype antisera may block reactions with the appropriate hapten. The carbohydrate side chains of immunoglobulins are relatively nonimmunogenic. New determinants may be exposed after papain cleavage of immunoglobulins, but these determinants are not included in the classification of the native molecule.

470. The answer is f. *(Kindt, pp 186. Levinson, pp 448, 461, 479-480.)* This patient has a classic case of hereditary angioedema. This disease is characterized by a deficiency of complement control proteins such as C1 esterase inhibitor, leading to overactive complement (reduced C4 levels). Uncontrolled generation of vasoactive peptides (C3a and C5a) causes increased blood vessel permeability, causing hereditary angioedema. Edema, especially of the larynx, obstructs the airways. Abdominal pain may indicate that the patient has angioedema of the gut.

471. The answer is d. *(Fauci, pp 483, 577-578. Kindt, pp 536-537. Levinson, p 476.)* The best-characterized human tumor-associated antigens are the oncofetal antigens. Carcinoembryonic antigen (CEA) is a glycoprotein and member of the immunoglobulin gene superfamily and is elevated in colorectal cancer. α-Fetoprotein (AFP) is analogous to albumin and elevated in hepatocellular carcinoma. Prostate-specific antigen (PSA) is elevated in prostatic cancer. CEA, AFP, and PSA are all glycoproteins. Melena refers to altered (black) blood per rectum, indicative of an upper gastrointestinal bleed. A patient's tumor markers are best used clinically in the monitoring of the efficiency of the anti-tumor therapy and remission periods posttreatment.

472 and 473. The answers are 472-b, 473-e. *(Kindt, pp 493-495, 500-502. Levinson, pp 322-330, 456.)* HIV infection affects mainly the immune system and the brain. The main immunologic feature of HIV infection is progressive depletion of the CD4 subset of T lymphocytes (T-helper cells), causing a reversal in the normal CD4:CD8 ratio, leading to immunodeficiency. Currently, ELISA is the basic screening test to detect anti-HIV antibodies. Repeated reactive ELISA tests should be confirmed using either Western blot or immunofluorescence. The Western blot detects specific antibodies against the various HIV proteins (antigens). As stated previously, Western blot is positive when two or more of the p14, gp41, gp120, or gp160 bands are present in the gel.

474. The answer is b. *(Kindt, pp 389-391. Levinson, pp 455-459.)* Anti-Rh antibodies (IgG are reactive at 98.6°F [37°C]) are the leading cause of hemolytic disease of the newborn (HDN). Currently, Rh immunization can be suppressed in antepartum or postpartum Rh– women if high-titer anti-Rh immunoglobulin (RhIg) is administered within 72 hours after the potentially sensitizing dose of Rh+ cells (ie, the birth of the child). The other choices will do nothing to prevent the development of HDN in future pregnancies.

475 and 476. The answers are 475-g, 476-c. *(Kindt, pp 29-30, 440-442, 494-498. Levinson, pp 443, 479-480.)* Immune deficiency disorders occur as a result of impaired function in one or more of the major immune system components such as B lymphocytes, T lymphocytes, B and T lymphocytes, phagocytic cells, and complement. Unusual and recurrent infections are the hallmark of immunodeficiency. SCID occurs as a result of an early defect in stem cell differentiation and may be caused as a result of defective IL-2 receptors, adenosine deaminase deficiency, or failure to make MHC class II antigens. This condition is characterized by B- and T-cell deficiency and presents with recurrent infections. The other disorders listed do not have both B- and T-cell deficiency with an absence of a thymus gland. Definitive treatment of SCID consists of stem cell transplantation, with the ideal donor being a sibling with identical human leukocyte antigens (HLA).

477. The answer is b. *(Kindt, pp 95-98, 477-480. Levinson, pp 58-59, 402-403.)* There are three forms of immunity: active, passive, and adoptive. Active immunity involves an individual making his or her own antibodies, either naturally, by infection, or artificially by immunizations. Passive immunity refers to the transfer of preformed antibodies from one individual to another either naturally (transplacental or enteromammary antibodies from mother to fetus) or artificially through gamma globulin injections such as antitoxins, anti-Rh, and antivenoms (black widow spider bites and the like, etc).

Finally, adoptive immunity refers to the transfer of lymphoid cells from an actively immunized donor and does not involve antibody transfer.

478. The answer is e. *(Fauci, pp 2054-2058. Kindt, pp 495-500. Levinson, pp 478-480.)* Patients with T-cell defects are generally susceptible to viral, fungal, and protozoan infections. This can be especially visible in patients with primary immunodeficiency diseases such as SCID. For further explanation of immunodeficiencies, please refer to the answer explanations for Questions 414 and 415, 457 to 461, 474 and 475.

479 and 480. The answers are 479-c, 480-b. *(Kindt, pp 168-175. Levinson, pp 453-455.)* The complement fixation (CF) test is a two-stage test. The first stage involves the union of antigen with its specific antibody, followed by the fixation of complement to the antigen-antibody structure. In order to determine whether complement has been "fixed," an indicator system must be employed to determine the presence of free complement. Free complement binds to the complexes formed when red blood cells (RBCs) are mixed with anti-RBC antibody; this binding causes lysis of the cells. Complement that has been fixed before addition of RBCs and anti-RBC antibody cannot cause lysis.

481. The answer is b. *(Kindt, pp 372-388. Levinson, pp 460-463.)* This is an example of a type I hypersensitivity reaction. Type I hypersensitivity is also referred to as anaphylaxis or immediate-type hypersensitivity. Major components include IgE, mast cells/basophils, and pharmacologically active mediators. Exposure to antigen causes IgE production, followed by sensitization of mast cells and basophils. Subsequent encounter with the same allergen (antigen) leads to chemical mediator release (histamine and the like, etc) and also leads to clinical symptoms associated with asthma, allergic rhinitis, and so on. This reaction can occur within minutes and can be extremely severe and life-threatening.

482 to 486. The answers are 482-c, 483-a, 484-b, 485-e, 486-d. *(Kindt, pp 477-479. Levinson, pp 292-301.)* The following table presents the patterns of hepatitis B virus (HBV) serologic markers observed in various stages of infection with HBV. The diagnosis of HBV infection is usually based on three tests: hepatitis B surface antigen (HBsAg), antibodies to surface antigen (HBsAg), and antibodies to core antigen (HBcAg). Tests are available, however, for e antigen and antibodies to e antigen. Variety of testing methods are available and include enzyme immunoassay, radioimmunoassay, hemagglutination, latex agglutination, and immune adherence. The delta agent has recently been described. The delta agent exacerbates infection with HBV, apparently in a synergistic manner. Commercial tests are now available for the delta agent.

Interpretation	Serologic Markers					
	HBsAg	Anti-HBeAg	IgM Anti-HBc	Total Anti-HBc	Anti-HBe	HBs
Acute infection						
Incubation period	+[a]	+[a]	–	–	–	–
Acute phase	+	+	+	+	–	–
Early convalescent phase	+	–	+	+	+	–
Convalescent phase	–	–	+	+	+	–
Late convalescent phase	–	–	–[b]	+	+	+
Long past infection	–	–	–	+[c]	+ or –	+[c]
Chronic infection						
Chronic active hepatitis	+[d]	+ or –	+ or –	+[d]	+ or –	–[d]
Chronic persistent hepatitis	+[e]	+ or –	+ or –	+	+ or –	–
Chronic HBV carrier state	+[e]	+ or –	+ or –	+	+ or –	–
HBsAg immunization	–	–	–	–	–	+

[a]HBsAg and HBeAg are occasionally undetectable in acute HBV infection.
[b]IgM anti-HBc may persist for over a year after acute infection when very sensitive assays are employed.
[c]Total anti-HBc and anti-HBs may be detected together or separately long after acute infection.
[d]HBsAg-negative chronic active hepatitis may occur where total anti-HBc and anti-HBs may be detected together, separately, or not at all.
[e]HBsAg-negative chronic persistent hepatitis and chronic HBV carriers have been observed.

487 to 491. The answers are 487-b, 488-a, 489-e, 490-d, 491-c. (Kindt, pp 145-164. Levinson, pp 65-67, 234, 450-459.) Of the many methods available for antigen and antibody detection, LA, ELISA, RIA, CIE, and COA are the most widely used. Latex agglutination (LA) employs latex polystyrene particles sensitized by either antibody or antigen. LA is more sensitive than CIE and COA, but slightly less sensitive than either RIA or EIA. LA has been used to detect *H influenzae, N meningitidis,* and *S pneumoniae* antigens in cerebrospinal fluid. LA has also been used for detection of cryptococcal antigen. Most recently, LA has been widely used for rapid detection of group A streptococcal antigen directly from the pharynx. The test is rapid (5 minutes), sensitive (approximately 90%), and specific (99%).

Coagglutination (COA), also an agglutination test, is slightly less sensitive than LA but is less susceptible to changes in environment (eg, temperature). Most strains of coagulase-positive staphylococci have protein A in their cell wall. Protein A binds the Fc fragment of microbial antigens in body fluids. COA has also been used to rapidly type or group bacterial isolates.

Enzyme immunoassays (EIAs) can be either homogeneous (EMIT) or heterogeneous (ELISA). EMIT has been used primarily for assays of low-molecular-weight drugs. Its primary use in microbiology has been for assays of aminoglycoside antibiotics. EIAs vary as to the solid support used. A variety of supports can be used, such as polystyrene microdilution plates, paddles, plastic beads, and tubes. The number of layers in the antibody-antigen sandwich varies; usually as additional layers are added, detection sensitivity is increased. The two most common enzymes are horseradish peroxidase (HRP) and alkaline phosphatase (AP). β-Galactosidase has also been employed. *O*-phenylenediamine is the most common substrate for HRP and p-nitrophenyl phosphate for AP. Because EIAs are usually read in the visible color range, the tests can be read qualitatively by eye or quantitatively by machine.

Counterimmunoelectrophoresis (CIE) was originally used for "Australia antigen" (HBsAg) but was soon replaced by RIA. For a decade, CIE was used to detect antigens in body fluids. CIE is not an easy technique. Its success depends on the control of many variables, including solid support, voltage, current, buffer, affinity and avidity of antibodies, charge on the antigen, and time of electrophoresing.

Radioimmunoassay involves the radiolabeling of either antibody or antigen (Ag) using ^{131}Iodine (^{131}I) or ^{125}I (radioisotopes). It measures very small quantities and can be used to detect hormones, carcinoembryonic antigen (CEA), hepatitis B Ag, steroids, prostaglandins, and morphine-related drugs in patient sera.

492 to 496. The answers are 492-c, 493-a, 494-f, 495-e, 496-b. *(Kindt, pp 155-158. Levinson, pp 450-454.)* The enzyme immunoassay (EIA, ELISA) has become a common method for the detection of either antibody or antigen in a patient specimen. The technique is based on building a "sandwich." For example, the following sandwich is made on what is called the *solid phase*. The solid phase is usually a plastic microtiter plate but can be a plastic paddle or even a nitrocellulose membrane. First, whole *Toxoplasma* organisms or purified antigenic components of *Toxoplasma* are added to the plate and the plate is washed off. Failure of one or more of the washing steps or inadequate washing usually causes high background color in the developed plate.

The *Toxoplasma* antigen-antibody complex must be detected by the addition of a second antibody to which is linked an enzyme such as horseradish peroxidase or alkaline phosphatase. The nature of this second antibody is dependent on whether one wishes to measure IgG or IgM. If the test is for IgG, then the second antibody is antihuman IgG conjugated to an enzyme. Following another wash cycle, the enzyme substrate is added to the plate and color develops in those wells where the sandwich is complete. If the patient's serum does not contain specific antibody, then the sandwich is not completed and there is no development of color. If the EIA is for detection of antigen, then the layers of the sandwich are as follows:

Specific antibody
Patient specimen (contain antigen)
Enzyme-labeled antibody specific for the antigen
Enzyme substrates

There are many variations of the test using a variety of antibodies, indicators such as fluorescence, and magnetic beads as solid phases. EIA is more sensitive than agglutination methods or complement fixation and slightly less sensitive than radioimmunoassay.

497. The answer is d. *(Kindt, pp 19, 33, 367-368, 441-442. Levinson, pp 442-444.)* GVHD occurs due to attack by the graft against the recipient. There are three requirements for GVHD rejection: (1) histocompatibility differences between the graft (donor) and host (recipient), (2) immunocompetent graft cells, and (3) immunodeficient host cell. Immunocompetent graft cells may be "passenger" lymphocytes or major cells transplanted, and must be present in the graft. Prevention of GVHD is essential, as there is no adequate treatment once it is established.

498. The answer is c. (*Kindt, pp 398-391. Levinson, pp 456-458, 464.*) All blood for transfusion should be carefully matched to avoid transfusion reaction. As shown in the tables below, persons with group O blood have no A or B antigens on their erythrocytes and are thus considered to be universal donors. In contrast, persons with group AB blood have neither A nor B antibody and thus are universal recipients.

ABO BLOOD GROUPS		
Group	**Antigen on Red Cell**	**Antibody in Plasma**
A	A	Anti-B
B	B	Anti-A
AB	A and B	No anti-A or anti-B
O	No A or B	Anti-A and anti-B

COMPATIBILITY OF BLOOD TRANSFUSIONS BETWEEN ABO BLOOD GROUPS[a]				
	Recipient			
Donor	**O**	**A**	**B**	**AB**
O	Yes	Yes	Yes	Yes
A (AA or AO)	No	Yes	No	Yes
B (BB or BO)	No	No	Yes	Yes
AB	No	No	No	Yes

[a]"Yes" indicates that a blood transfusion from a donor with that blood group to a recipient with that blood group is compatible, that is, no hemolysis will occur. "No" indicates that the transfusion is incompatible and that hemolysis of the donor's cells will occur.
(*Reprinted, with permission, from Levinson W, Jawetz E. Medical Microbiology and Immunology. 7th ed. New York, NY: McGraw-Hill; 2002:412.*)

499 to 501. The answers are 499-b, 500-d, 501-h. (*Fauci, pp 1960-1967, 2037-2040, 2071-2073. Kindt, pp 403, 408-411, 442-443. Levinson, pp 470-474.*) Loss of tolerance by the immune system to certain self-components can lead to the formation of antibodies, causing tissue and organ damage. Such diseases are referred to as *autoimmune diseases*. There are a host of autoimmune diseases characterized by the autoantibodies. The presence of a "butterfly" rash is a classic cutaneous sign of SLE and is characterized by a rash over the bridge of the nose and on the cheeks.

Bibliography

Brooks GF, Carroll KC, Butel JS, et al, eds. *Jawetz's Medical Microbiology.* 24th ed. New York, NY: McGraw-Hill; 2007.

Engleberg NC, DiRita V, Dermody TS, eds. *Schaechter's Mechanism of Microbial Disease.* 4th ed. Philadelphia, PA: Lippincott, Williams & Wilkins; 2007.

Fauci, AS, Braunwald E, Kasper DL, et al, eds. *Harrison's Principles of Internal Medicine.* 17th ed. New York, NY: McGraw-Hill; 2008.

Kindt TJ, Goldsby RA, Osborne BA, et al, eds. *Kuby Immunology.* 6th ed. New York, NY: WH Freeman and Co; 2007.

Levinson W. *Medical Microbiology and Immunology.* 10th ed. New York, NY: McGraw-Hill; 2008.

Li X, Brown N, Chau AS, et al. Changes in susceptibility to posaconazole in clinical isolates of *Candida albicans. J Antimicrob Chemother. 2004*; 53:74-80.

Mokrousov I, Narvskaya O, Otten T, Limeschenko E, Steklova L, Vyshnevskiy B. High prevalence of KatG Ser315Thr substitution among isoniazid-resistant Mycobacterium tuberculosis clinical isolates from northwestern Russia, 1996 to 2001. *Antimicrob Agents Chemother.* 2002 May; 46(5):1417-1424.

Murray PR, Baron EJ, Pfaller MA, et al, eds. *Manual of Clinical Microbiology.* 8th ed. Washington, DC: ASM Press; 2003.

Murray PR, Baron EJ, Jorgensen JH, et al. *Medical Microbiology.* 6th ed. St. Louis, MO: Mosby; 2009.

Ryan KJ, Ray CG, eds. *Sherris Medical Microbiology.* 4th ed. New York, NY: McGraw-Hill; 2004.

Toy EC. *Case Files: Microbiology.* 2nd ed. New York, NY: McGraw-Hill; 2008.

Index